Breast Imaging

Guest Editor

ROBYN L. BIRDWELL, MD, FACR

RADIOLOGIC CLINICS OF NORTH AMERICA

www.radiologic.theclinics.com

Consulting Editor
FRANK H. MILLER, MD

September 2010 • Volume 48 • Number 5

SAUNDERS an imprint of ELSEVIER, Inc.

W.B. SAUNDERS COMPANY
A Division of Elsevier Inc.

1600 John F. Kennedy Boulevard • Suite 1800 • Philadelphia, Pennsylvania 19103-2899

http://www.theclinics.com

RADIOLOGIC CLINICS OF NORTH AMERICA Volume 48, Number 5
September 2010 ISSN 0033-8389, ISBN 13: 978-1-4377-2595-7

Editor: Barton Dudlick
Developmental Editor: Donald Mumford

Radiologic Clinics of North America (ISSN 0033-8389) is published bimonthly by Elsevier Inc., 360 Park Avenue South, New York, NY 10010-1710. Months of issue are January, March, May, July, September, and November. Periodicals postage paid at New York, NY and additional mailing offices. Subscription prices are USD 361 per year for US individuals, USD 545 per year for US institutions, USD 176 per year for US students and residents, USD 421 per year for Canadian individuals, USD 684 per year for Canadian institutions, USD 520 per year for international individuals, USD 684 per year for international institutions, and USD 253 per year for Canadian and foreign students/residents. To receive student and resident rate, orders must be accompanied by name of affiliated institution, date of term and the signature of program/residency coordinatior on institution letterhead. Orders will be billed at individual rate until proof of status is received. Foreign air speed delivery is included in all *Clinics* subscription prices. All prices are subject to change without notice. **POSTMASTER:** Send address changes to *Radiologic Clinics of North America*, Elsevier Health Sciences Division, Subscription Customer Service, 3251 Riverport Lane, Maryland Heights, MO63043. **Customer Service: Telephone: 1-800-654-2452** (U.S. and Canada); **1-314-447-8871** (outside U.S. and Canada). **Fax: 1-314-447-8029. E-mail: journalscustomerservice-usa@ elsevier.com** (for print support); **journalsonlinesupport-usa@elsevier.com** (for online support).

Reprints. For copies of 100 or more of articles in this publication, please contact the Commercial Reprints Department, Elsevier Inc., 360 Park Avenue South, New York, New York 10010-1710. Tel.: (+1) 212-633-3812; Fax: (+1) 212-462-1935; E-mail: reprints@elsevier.com.

Radiologic Clinics of North America also published in Greek Paschalidis Medical Publications, Athens, Greece.

Radiologic Clinics of North America is covered in *MEDLINE/PubMed (Index Medicus), EMBASE/Excerpta Medica, Current Contents/Life Sciences, Current Contents/Clinical Medicine, RSNA Index to Imaging Literature, BIOSIS, Science Citation Index,* and *ISI/BIOMED.*

Printed in the United States of America.

Contributors

CONSULTING EDITOR

FRANK H. MILLER, MD
Professor of Radiology; Chief, Body Imaging
Section and Fellowship Program and GI
Radiology; and Medical Director MRI, Department
of Radiology, Northwestern University Feinberg
School of Medicine, Chicago, Illinois

GUEST EDITOR

ROBYN L. BIRDWELL, MD, FACR
Associate Professor of Radiology, Harvard
Medical School; Section Head, Division of Breast
Imaging, Brigham and Women's Hospital, Boston,
Massachusetts

AUTHORS

LAWRENCE W. BASSETT, MD, FACR
Iris Cantor Professor of Breast Imaging,
Department of Radiological Sciences, David
Geffen School of Medicine at University of
California Los Angeles, Los Angeles, California

WENDIE A. BERG, MD, PhD, FACR
American Radiology Services, Inc, Johns Hopkins
Green Spring, Lutherville, Maryland

ROBYN L. BIRDWELL, MD, FACR
Associate Professor of Radiology, Harvard
Medical School; Section Head, Division of
Breast Imaging, Brigham and Women's Hospital,
Boston, Massachusetts

JOHN M. BOONE, PhD
Professor and Vice Chair (Research) of Radiology;
Professor of Biomedical Engineering, Department
of Radiology, University of California, Davis School
of Medicine, Sacramento, California

RACHEL F. BREM, MD
Professor and Vice Chair, Department of
Radiology; Director, Breast Imaging and
Interventional Center, The George Washington
University, Washington, DC

CARL J. D'ORSI, MD
Professor of Radiology and Hematology/
Oncology; Emeritus Director Breast Imaging;
Director Breast Imaging Research, Section of
Breast Imaging, Winship Cancer Institute, Emory
University, Atlanta, Georgia

STEPHEN FEIG, MD
Professor, Department of Radiological Sciences;
Director of Breast Imaging, University of California
Irvine Medical Center, Orange, California

DIANNE GEORGIAN-SMITH, MD
Associate Professor of Radiology, Division of
Breast Imaging, Department of Radiology,
Brigham and Women's Hospital, Harvard Medical
School, Boston, Massachusetts

MARK A. HELVIE, MD
Department of Radiology, University of Michigan
Health System, Ann Arbor, Michigan

ANNE C. HOYT, MD
Associate Professor, Department of Radiological
Sciences, David Geffen School of Medicine at
University of California Los Angeles,
Los Angeles, California

J. DIRK IGLEHART, MD
Department of Surgery, Brigham and Women's
Hospital; Department of Cancer Biology,
Dana-Farber Cancer Institute, Boston,
Massachusetts

DANIEL B. KOPANS, MD, FACR
Professor, Department of Radiology, Harvard
Medical School; Senior Radiologist, Breast
Imaging Division, Massachusetts General
Hospital, Boston, Massachusetts

THOMAS J. LAWTON, MD
Director, Seattle Breast Pathology Consultants,
Seattle, Washington; Consultant Pathologist,
Clarient Inc, Aliso Viejo, California

KAREN K. LINDFORS, MD, MPH
Professor of Radiology and Chief of Breast
Imaging, Department of Radiology, University
of California, Davis School of Medicine,
Sacramento, California

MARTHA B. MAINIERO, MD
Associate Professor, Department of Diagnostic
Imaging, Rhode Island Hospital, The Warren Alpert
Medical School of Brown University,
Providence, Rhode Island

HELGA MARQUES, MS
Center for Statistical Sciences, Brown University,
Providence, Rhode Island

CAROLYN E. MOUNTFORD, DPhil
Center for Clinical Spectroscopy, Department
of Radiology, Brigham and Women's Hospital and
Harvard Medical School, Boston, Massachusetts

MARY S. NEWELL, MD
Assistant Professor of Radiology; Assistant
Director, Section of Breast Imaging; Director,
Breast MRI; Associate Director, Breast Cancer
Center; Winship Cancer Institute, Emory
University, Atlanta, Georgia

THOMAS OSHIRO, PhD
Assistant Professor, Medical Physicist,
Department of Radiological Sciences, David
Geffen School of Medicine at University
of California Los Angeles, Los Angeles,
California

LAUREN R. RECHTMAN, MA
Department of Radiology Breast Imaging and
Interventional Center, The George Washington
University, Washington, DC

MARK ROSEN, MD, PhD
Associate Professor, Division of Body MRI,
Department of Radiology, University of
Pennsylvania School of Medicine,
Philadelphia, Pennsylvania

ALAN G. SECHTIN, MD
American Radiology Services, Inc, Johns Hopkins
Green Spring, Lutherville, Maryland

EDWARD A. SICKLES, MD
Professor Emeritus of Radiology, University
of California San Francisco (UCSF) Medical
Center, San Francisco, California

SUSAN WEINSTEIN, MD
Associate Professor, Division of Breast Imaging,
Department of Radiology, University
of Pennsylvania School of Medicine
Philadelphia, Pennsylvania

ZHENG ZHANG, PhD
Center for Statistical Sciences, Brown University,
Providence, Rhode Island

MARGARITA L. ZULEY, MD
Associate Professor, Department of Radiology;
Medical Director, Breast Imaging Magee-Womens
Hospital of University of Pittsburgh Medical
Center, Pittsburgh, Pennsylvania

Contents

Mammography screening is one of the major medical accomplishments of the past 40 years. In light of the downstream consequences of any screening test, it was critical that mammography screening be challenged. There have been many legitimate challenges, as well as many challenges that are not scientifically based but have gained credibility because of repetition. The latter have led to a great deal of confusion among women and their physicians. The aim of this review is to dispel many of the misunderstandings that have developed in the past 4 decades and, hopefully, reduce the confusion that has occurred. Mammography screening does not find all breast cancers and does not find all cancers early enough to result in a cure, but it is a major advance, and women should not be denied access to its benefits.

Although there currently is no evidence of reduced breast cancer mortality for screening women at high risk with mammography, magnetic resonance (MR) imaging, or ultrasonography (US), the presumptive evidence of early cancer detection provided by numerous observational studies has led to the publication of guidelines and recommendations for the selective use of these imaging modalities. In general, annual screening mammography is recommended for women of appropriately high risk beginning at age 30 years, supplemental screening with MR imaging is recommended for a subset of women at very high risk, and screening US is suggested for women for whom MR imaging is appropriate but unavailable, impractical, or poorly tolerated. The use of screening US remains controversial among women who have no substantial risk factors other than dense breasts.

Screening mammography performed annually on all women beginning at age 40 years has reduced breast cancer deaths by 30% to 50%. The cost per year of life saved is well within the range for other commonly accepted medical interventions. Various studies have estimated that reduction in treatment costs through early screening detection may be 30% to 100% or more of the cost of screening. Magnetic resonance imaging (MRI) screening is also cost-effective for very high-risk women, such as BRCA carriers, and others at 20% or greater lifetime risk. Further studies are needed to determine whether MRI is cost-effective for those at moderately high (15%–20%) lifetime risk. Future technical advances could make MRI more cost-effective than it is today. Automated whole-breast ultrasonography will probably prove cost-effective as a supplement to mammography for women with dense breasts.

Current day digital mammography acquisition units have already been shown to be equal or better than screen film systems for the detection and classification of breast lesions. The optimal multimodality breast imaging diagnostic workstations and connectivity to existing picture and archiving communication systems and information systems is still a work in progress, but with more and more facilities transitioning to digital imaging it is only a matter of time until these hurdles are overcome.

This article addresses the essential components of the clinical image evaluation process for mammography examinations. The American College of Radiology Mammography Accreditation Program has specified 8 categories of image evaluation that are addressed in this article. While focused on the 2-view screening examination, the same general principles should apply to diagnostic mammograms. This article specifically focuses on the clinical image evaluation process as it applies to digital mammography.

This article discusses recent developments in advanced derivative technologies associated with digital mammography. Digital breast tomosynthesis, its principles, development, and early clinical trials, are reviewed. Contrast-enhanced digital mammography and combined imaging systems with digital mammography and ultrasound are also discussed. Although all these methods are currently research programs, they hold promise for improving cancer detection and characterization if early results are confirmed by clinical trials.

Masses due to cystic lesions of the breast are extremely common findings on mammography, ultrasonography, and magnetic resonance imaging. Although many of these lesions can be dismissed as benign simple cysts, requiring intervention only for symptomatic relief, complex cystic and solid masses require biopsy. Perhaps, the most challenging are complicated cysts, that is, cysts with internal debris. When the debris is mobile or a fluid-debris level is seen, complicated cysts can be dismissed as benign findings. As an isolated finding, homogeneous complicated cysts can be classified as probably benign, with intervention only considered with interval development or enlargement, abscess is suspected, or if suspicious features develop. When multiple and bilateral complicated and simple cysts are present (ie, at least three, with at least one in each breast), a benign, BI-RADS 2, assessment is usually appropriate. Clustered microcysts are common benign findings in pre- and perimenopausal women, though short-interval surveillance may be appropriate for many such lesions in post-menopausal women, particularly if the lesion is new or rather small or deep (ie, diagnostic uncertainty).

The status of axillary lymph nodes is a key prognostic indicator in patients with breast cancer and helps guide patient management. Sentinel lymph node biopsy is increasingly being used as a less morbid alternative to axillary lymph node dissection. However, when sentinel lymph node biopsy is positive, axillary dissection is typically performed for complete staging and local control. Axillary ultrasound and ultrasound-guided fine needle aspiration (USFNA) are useful for detecting axillary nodal metastasis preoperatively and can spare patients sentinel node biopsy, because those with positive cytology on USFNA can proceed directly to axillary dissection or neoadjuvant chemotherapy. Internal mammary nodes are not routinely evaluated, but when the appearance of these nodes is abnormal on imaging, further treatment or metastatic evaluation may be necessary.

Readers may feel less than satisfied when they discover that there is no consensus on the appropriate recommendations for follow-up of risk lesions following percutaneous core biopsy. The significance of this article is in the details of the methodologies and results, and much less in the numbers. The overall goal is to emphasize the flaws in current studies.

Breast cancer is the most common solid tumor diagnosed in women. In the past decades, great strides have been made in breast cancer screening. While multiple screening trials have shown the benefits of screening mammography, there are limitations to x-ray mammography. Given these inherent limitations, efforts have been made to develop adjunctive imaging techniques, including screening ultrasonography, gamma-specific breast imaging, breast tomosynthesis, dedicated breast computed tomography, and breast magnetic resonance (MR) imaging. This article addresses the current indications and advanced imaging applications of breast MR imaging.

Dedicated breast computed tomography (DBCT) is a burgeoning technology that has many advantages over current breast-imaging systems. Three-dimensional visualization of the breast mitigates the limiting effects of superimposition noted with mammography. Postprocessing capabilities will allow application of advanced technologies, such as creation of maximum-intensity projection and subtraction images, and the use of both computer-aided detection and possible computer-aided diagnosis algorithms. Excellent morphologic detail and soft tissue contrast can be achieved, due in part to the isotropic image data that DBCT produces. The expected cost should be more reasonable than magnetic resonance imaging. At present, because the breast is not compressed, patients find it more comfortable than mammography. Physiologic information can be obtained when intravenous contrast material is used and/or when DBCT is combined with single photon emission-computed tomography or positron emission tomography. DBCT provides an excellent platform for multimodality systems including integration with interventional and therapeutic procedures. With a slightly altered design, the DBCT platform may also be useful for external-beam radiation with image guidance.

Nuclear medicine imaging of the breast is a US Food and Drug Administration-approved imaging modality that is being integrated into clinical practice to increase the armamentarium of tools available to diagnose breast cancer. The authors' practice, and others that have integrated nuclear medicine imaging of the breast into their clinical protocols, has found it to be a critical tool in optimally evaluating women for breast cancer. This physiologic/metabolic approach of nuclear medicine breast imaging studies, and their utility in clinical situations make them an important part of the entire spectrum of modalities for optimal breast cancer diagnosis.

Contrast-enhanced magnetic resonance imaging (MRI), MR spectroscopy, and nuclear medicine sestamibi imaging using technetium-99 m methoxyisobutyl isonitrile or positron emission tomography (PET) techniques provide information beyond that of structural imaging by displaying tumor neoangiogenesis, tumor metabolites, increased numbers of tumor cellular mitochondria, and hypermetabolic tumor cells. Much needs to be learned at the molecular level of normal cellular pathways either suppressed or enhanced by tumor-specific molecular changes. These discoveries will allow realization of true individualized patient tumor detection, treatment, and surveillance.

GOAL STATEMENT

The goal of the *Radiologic Clinics of North America* is to keep practicing radiologists and radiology residents up to date with current clinical practice in radiology by providing timely articles reviewing the state of the art in patient care.

ACCREDITATION

The *Radiologic Clinics of North America* is planned and implemented in accordance with the Essential Areas and Policies of the Accreditation Council for Continuing Medical Education (ACCME) through the joint sponsorship of the University of Virginia School of Medicine and Elsevier. The University of Virginia School of Medicine is accredited by the ACCME to provide continuing medical education for physicians.

The University of Virginia School of Medicine designates this educational activity for a maximum of 15 *AMA PRA Category 1 Credits*™ for each issue, 90 credits per year. Physicians should only claim credit commensurate with the extent of their participation in the activity.

The American Medical Association has determined that physicians not licensed in the US who participate in this CME activity are eligible for a maximum of 15 *AMA PRA Category 1 Credits*™ for each issue, 90 credits per year.

Credit can be earned by reading the text material, taking the CME examination online at http://www.theclinics.com/home/cme, and completing the evaluation. After taking the test, you will be required to review any and all incorrect answers. Following completion of the test and evaluation, your credit will be awarded and you may print your certificate.

FACULTY DISCLOSURE/CONFLICT OF INTEREST

The University of Virginia School of Medicine, as an ACCME accredited provider, endorses and strives to comply with the Accreditation Council for Continuing Medical Education (ACCME) Standards of Commercial Support, Commonwealth of Virginia statutes, University of Virginia policies and procedures, and associated federal and private regulations and guidelines on the need for disclosure and monitoring of proprietary and financial interests that may affect the scientific integrity and balance of content delivered in continuing medical education activities under our auspices.

The University of Virginia School of Medicine requires that all CME activities accredited through this institution be developed independently and be scientifically rigorous, balanced and objective in the presentation/discussion of its content, theories and practices.

All authors/editors participating in an accredited CME activity are expected to disclose to the readers relevant financial relationships with commercial entities occurring within the past 12 months (such as grants or research support, employee, consultant, stock holder, member of speakers bureau, etc.). The University of Virginia School of Medicine will employ appropriate mechanisms to resolve potential conflicts of interest to maintain the standards of fair and balanced education to the reader. Questions about specific strategies can be directed to the Office of Continuing Medical Education, University of Virginia School of Medicine, Charlottesville, Virginia.

The faculty and staff of the University of Virginia Office of Continuing Medical Education have no financial affiliations to disclose.

THE AUTHORS/EDITORS LISTED BELOW HAVE IDENTIFIED NO FINANCIAL OR PROFESSIONAL RELATIONSHIPS FOR THEMSELVES OR THEIR SPOUSE/PARTNER

Lawrence W. Bassett, MD, Robyn L. Birdwell, MD (Guest Editor); Carl J. D'Orsi, MD; Barton Dudlick, (Acquisitions Editor); Stephen Feig, MD; Dianne Georgian-Smith, MD; Anne C. Hoyt, MD; J. Dirk Iglehart, MD; Theodore E. Keats, MD (Test Author); Karen K. Lindfors, MD, MPH; Martha B. Mainiero, MD; Helga Marques, MS; Frank H. Miller, MD (Consulting Editor); Carolyn E. Mountford, DPhil; Mary S. Newell, MD; Thomas Oshiro, PhD; Lauren R. Rechtman, MA; Mark Rosen, MD, PhD; Alan G. Sechtin, MD; Edward A. Sickles, MD; Susan Weinstein, MD; and Zheng Zhang, PhD.

The authors/editors listed below have identified the following financial or professional relationships for themselves or their spouse/partner:

Wendie A. Berg, MD, PhD is a consultant for Naviscan, Inc., SuperSonic, and Imagine; is an industry funded research/investigator for Naviscan, Inc; and has a complimentary license for E-Film from Merge Healthcare.

John M. Boone, PhD is an industry funded research/investigator for Fuji Medical Systems, Hologic Corporation, and Creativ Microtech, and owns stock in Artemis.

Rachel F. Brem, MD is a consultant for U-Systems and Philips, and is on the Advisory Committee/Board for and owns stock in Dilon and iCAD.

Mark A. Helvie, MD is an industry funded research/investigator for General Electric.

Daniel B. Kopans, MD receives research support from General Electric, and receives invention royalties without patent from Cook, Inc.

Thomas J. Lawton, MD is a consultant for Clarient, Inc.

Margarita L. Zuley, MD has received a grant from Hologic, Inc.

Disclosure of Discussion of Non-FDA Approved Uses for Pharmaceutical Products and/or Medical Devices.

The University of Virginia School of Medicine, as an ACCME provider, requires that all faculty presenters identify and disclose any off-label uses for pharmaceutical and medical device products. The University of Virginia School of Medicine recommends that each physician fully review all the available data on new products or procedures prior to clinical use.

TO ENROLL

To enroll in the Radiologic Clinics of North America Continuing Medical Education program, call customer service at 1-800-654-2452 or sign up online at http://www.theclinics.com/home/cme. The CME program is available to subscribers for an additional annual fee USD 245.

Radiologic Clinics of North America

THE CLINICS ARE NOW AVAILABLE ONLINE!

Access your subscription at:
www.theclinics.com

Preface
Breast Imaging

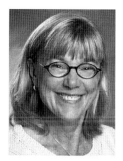

Robyn L. Birdwell, MD
Guest Editor

It has been decades since the presence of a doctor sitting in a dark room peering at low-resolution film mammograms was representative of all that was available for imaging of the breast. "Mammography" alone no longer encompasses the work performed by those radiologists and technologists who dedicate all or some of their careers to the field of breast care. "Breast Imaging" is a more appropriate subspecialty title and, perhaps, adding "and Intervention" would even better describe all that women may expect when they make an appointment for imaging evaluation of the breast.

The presentations included in this issue of *Radiologic Clinics of North America* were chosen in an attempt to include both updated information on topics familiar to the imager as well as data related to emerging technologies. Included are treatises on the efficacy and costs of screening for breast cancer; the basics, practical issues, and advances in digital mammography; the ultrasound depiction of cystic breast masses and the ACRIN 6666 experience; an in-depth assessment of the mixed literature regarding management of risk lesions found at core biopsy; the increasing role played by ultrasound in both imaging and interventional procedures directed toward lymph node assessment; both current and advanced imaging with breast MRI; some early experience with breast CT; and molecular imaging as it applies to the breast.

It is hoped that the reader will be both educated and inspired by the magnitude of interest, energy, resources, and imagination that play such important roles in furthering the understanding of breast disease and providing both diagnostic and therapeutic intervention.

It has been an honor and an educational experience for me to serve as the Guest Editor for this, the eighth *Radiologic Clinics of North America* issue dedicated to breast imaging. The exceptional group of authors who gave of their valuable time and extraordinary expertise has created a body of information that should serve to enhance the breast imaging literature for the novice as well as the expert.

Robyn L. Birdwell, MD
Department of Radiology
Brigham and Women's Hospital
75 Francis Street
Boston, MA 02115, USA

E-mail address:
rbirdwell@partners.org

Radiol Clin N Am 48 (2010) xi
doi:10.1016/j.rcl.2010.08.003

The 2009 US Preventive Services Task Force (USPSTF) Guidelines are not Supported by Science: The Scientific Support for Mammography Screening

Daniel B. Kopans, MD[a,b,*]

KEYWORDS

- USPSTF guidelines • Mammography screening
- Scientific support • Breast cancer screening

Mammography screening is one of the major medical accomplishments of the past 40 years. In the United States, before 1990, the death rate from breast cancer had been unchanged for the preceding 40 years. In the middle of the 1980s there was a sudden increase in the incidence of breast cancer that was initially believed to represent an epidemic until it was realized that this was caused by the start of mammography screening[1] in sufficient numbers to affect national statistics. There was no new epidemic of breast cancer. Mammography screening was simply detecting cancers that had been building up in the population (prevalence cancers) that had not yet been clinically detected, and it was also detecting cancers from the future (early detection) that had not reached clinical detection thresholds. This sudden increase in incidence was a marker for the onset of screening on a national scale. Periodic screening is unlikely to detect rapidly growing cancers that are soon to be lethal because of the well-known phenomenon of length bias sampling. It is more likely to interrupt moderate and slower growing cancers. These are no less lethal (see later discussion), but have sufficiently slow growth characteristics that they can be interrupted before metastatic spread, and future death can be prevented. Thus, it is not surprising that 5 to 7 years after the onset of mammography screening, the death rate from breast cancer in the United States suddenly began to decrease.[2] According to data from the Surveillance Epidemiology and End Results (SEER) program of the National Cancer Institute, the death rate as of 2005 (national statistics lag behind) from breast cancer is now down by almost 30% since 1990 (**Fig. 1**).

This decline in deaths is predominantly a result of mammography screening. In 2005, Berry and colleagues[3] published a summary of 7 computer models that had been queried to determine whether the decrease in breast cancer deaths was a result of mammography screening or

[a] Department of Radiology, Harvard Medical School, Shattuck Street, Boston, MA, USA
[b] Breast Imaging Division, Massachusetts General Hospital, 15 Parkman Street, Mailstop: Level 2, Suite 219, Boston, MA 02114, USA
* Breast Imaging Division, Massachusetts General Hospital, 15 Parkman Street, Mailstop: Level 2, Suite 219, Boston, MA 02114.
E-mail address: dkopans@partners.org

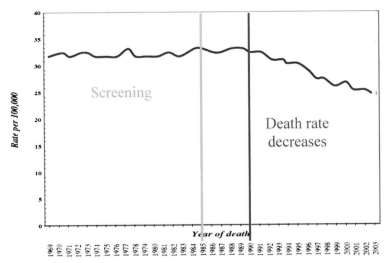

Fig. 1. The breast cancer death rate has decreased in relationship to mammography screening. The death rate was unchanged for decades until mammography screening began in the mid-1980s. Soon after the death rate began to decrease and it has continued to decrease as more and more women participate in screening. By 2005 it was down by 30%. (*Adapted from* Surveillance, Epidemiology, and End Results [SEER] Program [www. seer.cancer.gov] SEER∗Stat Database: Mortality - All COD, Public-Use With State, Total U.S. [1969–2003], National Cancer Institute, DCCPS, Surveillance Research Program, Cancer Statistics Branch, released April 2006. Underlying mortality data provided by NCHS [www.cdc.gov/nchs].)

improvements in breast cancer therapy. The computers provided an estimate of the portion of the benefit that was caused by mammography that ranged from 28% to 65% (median 46%). These, however, were computer models and not direct measures. They did, however, show that the contribution of mammography screening in these models was as high as 65%. It is unclear why anyone would rely on computer models when direct measurements are available to determine what happens when screening is introduced for the general public. There have been 4 studies that have directly measured the effect of mammography screening in real populations. In 2001 Tabar and colleagues[4] published their study of the 2 counties in Sweden that had been involved in the Two County Mammography Screening Trial in the 1980s. The investigators looked at the death rate from breast cancer in the prescreening era from 1968 to 1977 during which there was no mammography screening. They compared this with the death rate from 1977 to 1987 during which the Two County Trial was screening part of the population aged 40 to 74 years, and both periods were compared with the period 1988 to 1996 when all women aged 40 to 69 years were invited to participate in mammography screening. The death rate from breast cancer in these 3 periods is similar to a dose-response curve. As more women participated in screening, the death rate from breast cancer declined. When the women who actually participated in screening during the final period

(general population) were evaluated, the death rate (a measure that is independent of cancer detection rates and overdiagnosis/pseudodisease bias) decreased relative to the initial prescreening period by 63%. This is not computer modeling, but an actual measure in a real population. When all women who were offered screening (some women refused) were evaluated, the death rate was still decreased by 50%.

The investigators found a slight decrease in the number of deaths in the same period among women aged 20 to 39 years, who were never invited for screening and therefore had no mammograms, and they also found only a slight decrease in deaths among women in the screening ages who had refused to be screened. These latter 2 groups had access to all of the new therapeutic approaches in the same period of time, with no major decline in deaths. This suggests that mammography screening was the primary reason that the number of deaths had decreased in the 29 years encompassed by the review.

In 2002, Duffy and colleagues[5] published a similar study that included women in 7 counties, which amounted to 30% of the women in Sweden. Their results were similar to the Two County review. There was a major decline in breast cancer deaths among the women who participated in screening with only a small decline among women who refused screening in the same period, but had access to new therapies.

In 2003, Otto and colleagues[6] published an analysis of the effects of mammography screening and the use of adjuvant therapy on the death rate from breast cancer in the Netherlands. In the Netherlands, care is based on municipal health systems. Breast cancer mortality had been increasing at approximately 0.3% each year despite the introduction of modern adjuvant therapies. It was not until mammography screening was introduced into each municipality that the death rate began to decline by 1.7% each year. This was direct evidence that the decline in breast cancer mortality is the result of screening with little effect from improvements in therapy.

These direct measures of death rate in these general populations before and after the introduction of mammography screening are not conclusive proof that mammography screening is the main reason that the death rates have declined. As noted later, comparisons of populations at differing points in time (historical controls) are subject to many biases that could confound the interpretation. However, mammography has been shown to decrease deaths in randomized controlled trials (RCT; the most rigorous of scientific studies), and these service screening studies show that mammography screening has fulfilled the expectation that the death rate should decline when it is introduced into the general population. Were all women aged 40 year and older to participate in screening, the studies and estimates of potential benefit suggest that the death rate from breast cancer could be decreased by 50%.[7] No one has ever suggested that mammography screening is the ultimate solution to breast cancer, but there is clear evidence that mammography screening can and is saving tens of thousands of lives each year.

OPPOSITION TO SCREENING

Despite these clear benefits, the past decades have witnessed numerous issues that have been raised concerning the efficacy of mammographic screening that have clouded physician's and the public's understanding of the test. The most recent effort to reduce access to screening came in November 2009 when the United States Preventive Services Task Force (USPSTF) dropped support for screening women aged 40–49 years and supported biennial instead of annual screening for women aged 50–74 years. This latest effort to prevent access for women to mammography screening is scientifically unsupportable

(see later discussion). However, some of the issues raised are important.

Screening is very different from caring for individuals who are ill. Screening involves healthy individuals, most of whom do not have breast cancer. There are negative consequences that accompany screening. Some of these are economic and psychological. Women must take time away from home, family, and work to have the study. There is anxiety associated with having a test to look for cancer. As with any test, there are false-positive mammography screening examinations. False-positive studies can cause harms among women that they would not have faced had they not undergone the test in the first place. Although most of these can be resolved with a few additional mammographic projections or ultrasound, some lesions detected at screening require a biopsy to determine whether they are benign or malignant, adding physical trauma to the list of incurred harms. As discussed later, there are clearly some indolent cancers that may not be lethal that are nonetheless treated as if they could be lethal because it is not yet possible to determine which lesions, diagnosed as cancer, do not need to be treated. None of these unnecessary interventions would have occurred were it not for screening. These harms need to be considered because they involve women who may never develop breast cancer. The benefit is that some women will not die from breast cancer because it is found at screening and interrupted before successful metastatic spread. The bottom line is that mammography screening saves lives, but it is not without negative consequences. Women should understand that screening is not a guarantee that they will not die from breast cancer, but that screening can prevent many breast cancer deaths. In a recent study from Harvard, almost 75% of the women who died of breast cancer were among the 25% who were not being screened with mammography.[8]

In light of the downstream consequences of any screening test, it was critical that mammography screening be challenged. There have been many legitimate challenges, as well as many challenges that are not scientifically based but have gained credibility because of repetition. The latter have led to a great deal of confusion among women and their physicians. The aim of this review is to dispel many of the misunderstandings that have developed in the past 5 decades and, hopefully, reduce the confusion that has occurred. Mammography screening does not find all breast cancers and does not find all cancers early enough to result in a cure, but it is a major advance, and women should not be denied access to its benefits.

THE ISSUES

Mammography screening has undergone greater scrutiny than any other screening test. It has been shown to be able to detect cancers at a smaller size and earlier stage than waiting for a lump to develop.[9] It has been shown in RCTs to be able to reduce deaths from breast cancer,[10] and when mammography screening is provided in the general population, the death rate declines dramatically.[2,4–6] None of the issues raised in opposition to screening have negated the scientific evidence supporting its benefit.

How to Prove a Benefit from Screening

In the 1960s the fundamental question was raised: How do we know that screening will save lives? Comparing survival data between women screened and women who have not been screened is subject to too many possible biases to be scientifically acceptable. The only way to prove that screening saves lives is through the use of RCTs. A large population of women is divided randomly into 2 groups. If the allocation is truly random, the same number of women will be destined to die each year from breast cancer over time in both groups. If one group is screened, and if there are statistically significantly fewer deaths in the screened group, over time, and because this is the only difference between the 2 groups, then this mortality reduction is proof that screening reduces deaths. RCTs are the only way to eliminate such biases as leadtime, length bias sampling, selection bias, and so forth.[11]

RCT Underestimate Benefit

The first RCT of breast cancer screening, the Health Insurance Plan of New York (HIP), showed a 23% decrease in breast cancer deaths for 32,000 women aged 40 to 64 years invited to be screened.[12] What many do not realize is that the RCTs of mammography screening are actually trials of the invitation to be screened. Because no one can be coerced to participate in screening, some women who are invited decline to be screened. To avoid introducing selection bias into the trial, these women are still counted as having been screened. Even if they die of breast cancer they are still counted as deaths among the screened group even though they were never actually screened (noncompliance). Similarly, no one can stop women who are allocated to the unscreened control group from going out and getting a mammogram on their own outside of the trial (contamination). These women are still counted as having not been screened even if the mammogram outside the trial saved their lives. As a result of noncompliance and contamination, the RCT actually underestimates death reduction.

Population (Service) Screening

In the 1970s the question was raised: How can we possibly screen millions of women? This resulted in the Breast Cancer Detection Demonstration Project (BCDDP).[9] Approximately 275,000 women were screened every year for 4 years in several centers across the United States. The BCDDP showed that mammography can indeed find breast cancer at a smaller size and earlier stage than clinical examination. It also showed that large numbers of women could be screened efficiently, and at low cost. This has been confirmed by the experience of the past 20 years during which hundreds of millions of screening mammograms have been performed efficiently and effectively.

Radiation Risk

In 1976 concern was raised that the radiation from mammography would cause more cancers than would be cured.[13] This proved to be a marked overestimate of risk. Nevertheless, in the late 1970s and 1980s, there were major efforts to dramatically lower the doses used for mammography. The use of 1 rad or more per exposure in the HIP trial was reduced to less than 300 mrad per exposure as today's standard. Subsequent studies showed that radiation risk for the breast is highly age related. It is not surprising that the immature undifferentiated breast is more radiosensitive than the mature differentiated organ. This is clearly seen among women who were treated with mantle radiation for Hodgkin disease while in their teens. They have a 35% risk of developing breast cancer in the next 20 years.[14] However, women more than 30 years, who received the same treatment had no excess risk. By the time a woman is 40 years there is no direct evidence of any radiation risk to the breast from mammography and, even the theoretic risk is much less than the smallest benefit derived from detecting breast cancer earlier.[15] Although not conclusive proof, if mammograms were causing cancers, that there have been hundreds of millions of mammograms performed since the 1980s should lead to an increasing incidence of breast cancer. In fact, the incidence of breast cancer is decreasing.

Screening Using Clinical Breast Examination

It has been suggested that much of the benefit from screening may come from performing clinical breast examination (CBE), because the screening used in the HIP study included CBE, and it has been suggested that perhaps all that was needed was CBE to find cancers. There are no other RCT data for CBE since the HIP to support this concept. Earlier detection is a relative phenomenon. It is likely that finding breast cancers earlier than the usual situation will save some lives. Before the 1960s many women with breast problems kept them secret. Mastectomy was the only treatment option and a woman with a lump feared that she would go into hospital for surgery under general anesthesia, and would be put to sleep not knowing if, when she awoke, she would still have her breast. Women feared the diagnosis so much that they would often delay seeking care until the cancer was large and advanced. Any form of earlier detection, such as the CBE performed in the HIP trial, would likely result in reduced deaths. However, as breast cancer became highly visible as a major health concern, cancers began to be found by the individual women at a smaller size. It is unlikely that, at the present time, CBE adds much in terms of downstaging. There have been no RCTs since the HIP study that have included CBE that have shown any independent benefit for CBE. The RCTs of mammography screening in Sweden (5 trials) confirmed that deaths can be reduced by at least 20% by mammography screening alone.[16]

Confusing Guidelines in the Past

In the 1980s several organizations were issuing various guidelines for screening that were confusing to women and their physicians. In 1989 The American Cancer Society, the National Cancer Institute, the American College of Surgeons, the American College of Radiology, and other groups got together and developed the Consensus Guidelines that recommended screening women aged 40 to 49 years every 1 to 2 years and women aged 50 years and older every year. This consensus did not end the debates. There were still some who did not believe that screening benefited women aged 40 to 49 years, and there were no direct data that could accurately determine the appropriate interval between screens.

The Age of 50 Years Becomes a Scientifically Unsubstantiated Breast Cancer Threshold

Because breast cancer is fairly clearly related, at least in part, to hormones, investigators had wondered how menopause might affect the value of screening. None of the RCTs were designed to evaluate women with regard to their hormone (menopausal) status. Consequently, the age of 50 years was chosen as a surrogate for menopause. Although the trial was not designed to permit age stratification, the data in the HIP study were broken into 2 groups[17,18] and women aged 40 to 49 years were evaluated as a separate subgroup. In the early years of follow-up of these younger women, there was no evidence of any difference in deaths between the screened women and the control women. It was not until 5 to 7 years after the first screen that the curves began to diverge with fewer deaths among the screened women than the controls. Although there were questions raised as to which cancers and cancer deaths to include in the follow-up studies[19] and with regard to the timing of analysis after the screening began, it was argued that because the data did not show a statistically significant benefit for women aged 40 to 49 years, there was no benefit. This unplanned, retrospective subgroup analysis of data that lacked statistical power to permit such analysis is the basis for the fallacy that continues today that screening is less effective before the age of 50 years than for women aged 50 years and older. As discussed later, analysts who wanted it to appear as if something suddenly changed at the age of 50 years divided screening data into 2 groups: those younger than 50 years and those aged 50 years and older, making it seem as if the findings jumped suddenly at the age of 50 years when, in fact, there are no ungrouped data (analyzed by individual ages) that show that any of the parameters of screening change abruptly at the age of 50 years, or any other age.

The RCTs of Mammography Screening Demonstrate a Statistically Significant Decrease in Breast Cancer Deaths

In the 1980s a trial was undertaken in 2 counties in Sweden in which part of the population, randomly chosen, was offered mammography screening and the other part of the population was not invited for screening and acted as unscreened controls. In 1985, preliminary results were published showing a statistically significant 30% decrease in breast cancer deaths among women aged 40 to 74 years as a result of mammography screening.[20] There were also trials being conducted in Stockholm, Malmo, and Gothenburg in Sweden, and another screening trial in Edinburgh, Scotland. In 1994, Shapiro published an analysis of these trials which, when combined, showed a 25% mortality reduction for screening women aged 40 to 74 years.[21] The RCTs, when analyzed as they were designed, were showing a statistically significant benefit (mortality reduction) for screening women beginning at the age of 40 years and continuing up to the age of 74 years.

Major Flaws in the Canadian National Breast Screening Study

Based on the results of age stratification in the HIP trial that had raised questions about the benefit of mammography screening for women aged 40 to 49 years, an RCT was undertaken in Canada to try to answer the specific question as to whether or not mammography screening could reduce deaths from breast cancer among women aged 40 to 49 years. The preliminary results of this trial were published at the end of 1992.[22] Not only did the trial fail to show any early benefit, but, incongruously, there were more breast cancer deaths among women in the mammography arm of the trial.

The Canadian National Breast Screening Study (CNBSS) was given great credibility and was the primary reason that, at the end of 1993, the National Cancer Institute (NCI) decided to drop support for screening women aged 40 to 49 years. Despite hopes that it would resolve the question concerning women aged 40 to 49 years, a careful review of the design and execution of the CNBSS showed that it had major flaws. It was seriously underpowered. This meant that there were not enough women expected to participate in the trial to have enough women who would develop breast cancer, and enough women who would be expected to die from breast cancer to be able to show a statistically significant decrease in deaths among the screened women that was anything less than 40%. Without any contamination or noncompliance, the CNBSS1 did not even plan to recruit sufficient numbers of women to be able to show anything less than a 40% or higher decrease in deaths.[23] The HIP trial had suggested a 25% benefit was likely so that the CNBSS1, before it even began, lacked the power that was needed to prove a benefit. Furthermore, this was a trial of mammography screening yet, by the trial's own review, the quality of the mammography was poor.[24,25] Their own reference physicist stated that the quality of the mammography in the CNBSS, a trial of mammography screening, was far from state-of-the-art, but was even poorer than the quality of mammography being practiced in Canada at the same time.[26]

Although the poor quality of the mammography in the CNBSS was a major problem, it is overshadowed by the design and execution of the CNBSS. To produce 2 identical groups, RCTs require random allocation of the participants. It is well established that randomization must be blinded. Those performing the random assignment can have no information about the participants. This is critical to avoid any compromise of the randomization process and potentially biasing the trial. Almost in complete disregard for this fundamental requirement, the participants in the CNBSS were given a CBE before allocation, and the allocation into the screened group or the control group was then done on open lists. This meant that the nurses and clerks who were assigning women to be in the mammography screening group or the unscreened control group knew, before allocation, which women had clinically evident breast lumps as well as which women had palpable axillary lymph nodes signifying advanced incurable cancer. It is likely that the findings on the clinical examination biased the allocation and indeed there was an excess of advanced cancers allocated at the start of the trial to the mammography group.[27] A study by an analyst at the National Cancer Institute showed that there were statistically significantly more women with 4 or more positive axillary lymph nodes who were allocated to the mammography group.[28] Thus, it is not surprising that there were more deaths among women in the screened group. Given the importance of strict blinded allocation in RCTs, the major failures in the CNBSS raise significant doubt about its conclusions. It is unclear why the CNBSS, a truly compromised trial, continues to be described as a well-performed trial (see later discussion).

In 1993, the NCI, for the First Time in Its History, Ignored the Advice of the National Cancer Advisory Board and Dropped Support for Screening Women Aged 40 to 49 Years

Based on the preliminary data from the CNBSS1, the NCI, at the start of 1993, convened an International Workshop on Breast Cancer Screening. The stated aim was to review all the data with regard to breast cancer screening. One of the major issues was support for screening women aged 40 to 49 years. For unexplained reasons, I was the only expert invited to argue in support of screening these women. The NCI required that a mortality reduction from screening had to appear within 5 years of the start of a trial. This was an overly optimistic goal because it is well known that, because of length bias sampling, periodic screening tests are more likely to find moderate and slower growing cancers rather than fast-growing cancers. This meant that it would be unlikely for a benefit to appear so soon after the start of the screening trials. The HIP trial seemed to show an immediate benefit for women aged 50 to 64 years, so it was assumed that screening should be able to show an immediate benefit. Given length biased sampling, it was the immediate benefit seen for the older women that should have been questioned, rather than the delayed benefit that was found among the younger women. Furthermore, none of the RCTs were designed to permit legitimate subgroup analysis of women aged 40 to 49 years to guide medical recommendations because they had not been powered to support age stratification. Even the CNBSS1 was underpowered. In fact, in an analysis that I presented to the 1993 Workshop, we showed that the RCT cannot be legitimately used to analyze women aged 40 to 49 years as a subgroup and expect a statistically significant benefit within 5 years of the start of screening[29] as the NCI had required. The NCI had set a requirement that was mathematically impossible to achieve given the numbers of women at these ages in the RCT. The trials, when analyzed as they had been designed, showed a statistically significant benefit for screening women aged 40 to 74 years. There was in fact a decrease in breast cancer deaths that was evident among women aged 40 to 49 years even though the trials were not designed to analyze them separately, but because this benefit was not statistically significant it was discounted. The summary of the workshop did not support screening women in their 40s and gave only passing mention of the power problem[30] even though it showed that what the NCI required was scientifically unsupportable.

At the end of 1993, the National Cancer Advisory Board (NCAB), having been informed of the problems with the CNBSS1, and the inappropriate use of subgroup analyses to make medical recommendations, voted 13 to 1 and advised the NCI to not change their guidelines. For unexplained reasons, the NCI Director, for the first time in the history of the NCI, ignored the advice of the NCAB, and dropped support for screening women aged 40 to 49 years. When asked by a Congressional Panel as to why he had ignored the NCAB he stated that the vote (13 to 1) was "not unanimous."[31] I would speculate that because the NCI Director had been advising the Clinton administration[32] that their health care package, being formulated at the end of 1993, would not have to pay for women aged 40 to 49 years and could screen women aged 50 years and older every 2 years, had he not changed the guidelines, the Clinton Health package, unveiled the next month, would have been financially out of balance.

The Age of 50 Years was Established as a Threshold for Screening Even Though None of the Parameters of Screening Change Abruptly at the Age of 50 Years or Any Other Age

Following the NCI decision, numerous articles were published that supported the concept that the age of 50 years was a valid threshold for initiating screening.[33–39] However, there are actually no data to support this. The age of 50 years is nothing more than an arbitrary threshold, but it continues to be used as if there was scientific support for its use when there is none.[40] The age of 50 years was supported as a real threshold by grouping all women aged 49 years and younger as if they were a uniform group and comparing them with all women aged 50 years and older as if they were a uniform group. Such dichotomous analyses make variables that change gradually with increasing age, such as breast cancer detection rates, appear to change suddenly at the age of 50. The clear example of how this can be misleading is seen in an often-quoted paper from the University of California.[41] The actual data in the paper show that the breast cancer detection rate increases steadily with increasing age with no abrupt change at any age as would be expected. However, the investigators decided to group the data and analyze it dichotomously. Furthermore, they added the results for screening women in their 30s to the results for women in their 40s. This made it appear as if the cancer detection rate jumped suddenly from 2 cancers per 1000 for women aged 30 to 49 years to 10 cancers per 1000 women for women aged 50 to 74 years. No explanation is given for including women in their 30s because no one was suggesting that women in their 30s should be screened. However, their inclusion clearly pulls down the detection rate among women less than the age of 50 years just as grouping women aged 60 years and older with women aged 50 to 59 years makes it appear that there is a large jump in cancer detection at the age of 50 years when there was actually no evidence of this in the ungrouped data. Clearly, this analysis was misleading for many readers. Even a well-known commentator on public health issues was misled when he wrote in a review of this paper

The yield [of cancers] of the first mammogram was five times higher in women 50 years of age and older (10 cancers per 1000 studies compared with 2 cancers per 1000 studies)… Clearly mammography is much more efficient in detecting breast cancers in older women.[42]

There are other concepts that have been used to buttress the importance of age 50 years as having biologic significance such as the importance of breast density. This is actually a measure of the x-ray attenuation of the breast tissues on mammograms and has nothing to do with the firmness of the tissues on clinical examination. It is still suggested that, because young women (<50 years) are believed to have firm breasts, they must be dense breasts and dense tissue can hide a cancer. In fact, there is no relationship between breast density on mammography and firmness on clinical examination. There is no question that large numbers of young women have dense breast tissues, but the percentage of women with dense breasts decreases gradually with increasing age with no sudden change at the age of 50 years or any other age.[43] There are many women in their 50s, 60s, 70s, and 80s who still have dense breasts and there also many women less than the age of 50 years who have fatty (not dense) breasts. Once again, by grouping the data dichotomously, and analyzing all women as 2 groups, breast density (which actually changes gradually with increasing age) is made to appear to change abruptly at the age of 50 years. Furthermore, although breast tissue density does reduce the sensitivity of mammography, it does not eliminate it, and many early cancers are found among women with dense breasts, regardless of age.

Years of Life Lost to Breast Cancer and Relative Versus Absolute Numbers of Cancers

Other arguments have been made against screening women aged 40 to 49 years. It is argued that breast cancer is not an important problem for women in their 40s. In fact, at least 41% of the years of life lost as a result of breast cancer are from cancers diagnosed in women less than 50 years of age.[44] It is argued that because the incidence of breast cancer doubles at age 50 years, breast cancer is not an important problem before the age of 50 years. Approximately 1 woman in 1000 will be diagnosed with breast cancer each year during their 40s, 2/1000 among women in their 50s, 3/1000 among women in their 60s and 4/1000 among women in their 70s. I suspect that most women will not see a big difference between 1/1000 and 2/1000 even though the incidence doubles. What is never pointed out is that the incidence of breast cancer among women aged 70 to 80 years is twice the incidence among women in their 50s yet we do not disparage the importance of screening for women in their 50s.

Although the incidence of breast cancer increases with increasing age (with no abrupt change at the age of 50 years), the absolute number of women diagnosed with breast cancer at a given age is based on the number of women at that age (total number of women at a specific age with breast cancer = incidence at that age × number of women at that age). In 1995 there were actually more women aged 40 to 49 years who were diagnosed with breast cancer than there were women aged 50 to 59 years, but this was overlooked by comparing women in their 40s with all women aged 50 to 74 years. No decade of life accounts for more than 25% of all breast cancers each year but women in their 40s were (and continue to be) singled out as being unimportant.

Age Creep: A Lie that Persists

In 1995 de Koning and colleagues[45] wrote a paper suggesting that decreased deaths among women in their 40s in the RCTs was because the participants reached the age of 50 years during the trials, and screening began to work. This was subsequently termed age creep.[46,47] This concept was restated by de Koning at the 1997 Consensus Development Conference (see later discussion). However, when the Swedish trialists provided him with more complete data he announced to the Consensus Development Conference that he now realized that the benefit was actually primarily due to screening before age 50 years. Although he reaffirmed this to me in an e-mail,[48] he has yet to publish a retraction. Even though age creep actually did not exist in the RCTs, it is still used as an argument against screening women aged 40 to 49 years.

1997 CONSENSUS DEVELOPMENT CONFERENCE TO REVIEW THE NCI GUIDELINES THAT NO LONGER SUPPORTED SCREENING WOMEN AGED 40 TO 49 YEARS

In 1997 the NCI convened a Consensus Development Conference to review their policy concerning women aged 40 to 49 years. Although convened to review the latest follow-up data from the RCTs, the Panel summary, presented to the media on the final day of the conference, somehow failed to include any of the new Swedish data. Even though the RCTs were not designed to permit separate subgroup analysis of women aged 40 to 49 years, with longer follow-up the Malmo trial showed a 35% statistically significant benefit for screening women in their 40s, and Gothenburg showed a 44% statistically significant benefit. The 5 Swedish trials together showed a 29% statistically significant benefit for screening women in their 40s.[49] Ignoring these facts (they were not even mentioned to the media), the Panel suggested that any benefit from screening women aged 40 to 49 years was because of CBE. This was problematic in that none of the Swedish trials included CBE, yet they showed a statistically significant mortality reduction of 29%. The public was told that the Panel could find no reason to encourage women in their 40s to be screened. Having heard much of the testimony at the Consensus Development Conference himself, Dr Richard Klausner, the Director of the National Cancer Institute, was surprised at the Panel conclusion (I was seated next to him), and he asked a reporter to ask him his opinion. He then stated that he disagreed with the Panel conclusion and would have the NCAB review the new data. The NCAB undertook a review and several months later the NCI once again threw its support behind screening for women aged 40 to 49 years. Once again, the truth was corrupted. To this day, Dr Klausner's statement at the Consensus Development Conference has been forgotten, and writers and reporters continue to insist that the 1997 guideline change was not based on science but on congressional pressure.[50]

A Cochrane Review Raises Questions About Screening for Women at Any Age

In 2000 Gotzsche and Olsen[51] published an article suggesting that the RCT did not show a benefit from screening for women at any age. Because of the amount of criticism engendered by their review, the *Lancet*, allowed them to publish the same material again in 2001[52] asserting that they had re-reviewed the data and were correct in their first analysis. These analysts reached their conclusions by dropping the results from 4 of the Swedish Trials and claiming that the Malmo trial showed no benefit when it actually did show a screening benefit. Even though the Canadian NBSS1 was completely compromised by major trial violations (see earlier discussion) the investigators called it fairly well done and, because it showed no benefit, they concluded that there was no benefit from screening for women at any age. This stimulated multiple re-analyses of the data in multiple countries. These repeat analyses concluded that these Danish analysts were incorrect and that there was an approximately 30% reduction in breast cancer deaths as a result of screening.[53,54]

The American College of Physicians Advises Women in Their 40s to be Screened Based on Their Risk of Developing Breast Cancer

In 2007, The American College of Physicians (ACP) advised women in their 40s to consider their risk for developing breast cancer when deciding whether or not to be screened.[55] The committee that promulgated the guidelines never explained why women aged 40 to 49 years were being advised separately given that the age of 50 years has no biologic or screening significance (see earlier discussion). Furthermore, the RCT of mammography screening did not stratify by risk so there are no data that show that screening only high-risk women will actually saves lives. The third major fallacy in these guidelines is that, depending on what is considered increased risk, only 10% to at most 25% of women who develop breast cancer would fall into the ACP high-risk group.[56] If the ACP guidelines were followed, 75% to 90% of women who develop breast cancer would not be screened.[57]

Breast Cancers do not Melt Away

There has always been concern that mammography screening might lead to overdiagnosis; namely the detection of insignificant nonlethal cancers that, in the absence of screening, would have gone undetected and not bothered the individual during her lifetime. Most of the studies have suggested that this is a minor possibility[58] until 2008 and 2009 when it was suggested that mammography finds numerous cancers that, if left undiscovered, would melt away. Both papers made major methodological errors. In the first paper[59] the investigators compared the incidence of breast cancer in a cohort of women in the prescreening era (1992–1997) with the incidence of breast cancer among screened women in a totally different cohort at a later period of time (1996–2001). This use of historical controls can be dangerously misleading. The investigators compared the incidence of breast cancer as if it were a constant over time and that the higher incidence among the second cohort was to the result of mammography finding cancers that would have never bothered the women had they remained undiscovered and been left alone. Not only did they forget about the effect of prevalence cancers adding to the data (see later discussion) but they discounted that the incidence of breast cancer had been increasing in the past 50 years even before there was any screening so that a more recent cohort would be expected to have a higher incidence than one from earlier years.

The second paper[60] recognized that when screening begins, there are a large number of cancers diagnosed in the first year. This includes future cancers detected by the screening 1 or more years before they would have been detected in the absence of screening. It also includes a prevalence bump. These are cancers that have been building up in the population. Some of these are even palpable, but have gone undetected, or ignored by the patient and/or her doctor. Because cancers arise in the population at a fairly steady (although increasing) rate, once everyone is being screened, the annual rate of detection should return to the level before the start of screening and before the prevalence bump, but the incident cancers should be at a smaller size and earlier stage because the screening is detecting them at a new threshold. The investigators noted that once screening began, the incidence did not return to the prescreening baseline, but remained somewhat increased. They incorrectly attributed this to excess melt away cancers that were only found because of screening. In fact, the investigators made a fundamental mistake. In the countries whose data they evaluated, screening is offered to women aged 50 years and older. Every year a new cohort of women reaches the age of 50 years and begins screening. This means that every year there is a new prevalence bump that would add breast cancers to the annual incidence more than the number that would be seen if only the same women (cohort) were being screened without the new women. The suggestion that the failure to return to baseline is because of unimportant breast cancers detected by mammography is not supported by these analyses.

The only way to accurately evaluate overdiagnosis is in RCTs where the cohort of women is the same and they are studied over the same time period. In the RCTs the highest estimate of overdiagnosis was less than 10%[58] and this might decrease further with longer follow-up.[61]

Has Mammography Failed Because it Does Not Detect Fast-growing Aggressive Cancers?

A recent article raised still another argument against mammography screening by disparaging it because it is not perfect and does not detect the fast-growing aggressive cancers.[62] It is certainly not a new observation that mammography does not find all cancers and does not find all cancers early enough to effect a cure. This has been stated since screening began. The death rate from breast cancer has decreased by 30% since the institution of mammography screening. This is a remarkable achievement. However, it is fundamental to all periodic screening tests that they are unlikely to detect fast-growing aggressive cancers in time to prevent metastatic spread. This is the well-known effect of length bias sampling. Nevertheless, there are many cancers that are moderate and even slow growing which, if not

detected early, will be lethal years later. Finding a moderate growth cancer in a 45-year-old woman, and, as a result, preventing her from dying 7 years later at age 52 years, is no less a benefit than finding a fast-growing cancer in a 50-year-old woman and preventing her from dying at age 52 years.

Therapy Needs to be Tailored to the Individual and Her Tumor

There are no cures on the horizon. It was suggested by Esserman and colleagues[62] that care needs to be tailored to the virulence of the tumor and the host's response to it. There is no question that breast cancer is not a single malignancy. There are some breast cancers that have very low virulence and may not kill the individual, even if not treated. This is clear because, even before there was any screening or treatment of breast cancer, not all women died of their tumors. The suggestion that therapy needs to be tailored is far from new. For more than 40 years, efforts have been made to try to individualize therapy (the TNM grading system). No one has ever disputed that many women are overtreated for their breast cancers, both those presenting clinically and those detected with screening. The problem is that we are still unable to safely determine who can be treated minimally. Efforts continue to try to refine our ability to do this, but, because lives are a stake, only certain therapies can be safely tailored at this time. Furthermore, it is not the fault of mammography screening that therapy has not caught up to early detection. Mammography should not be faulted for finding cancers at a smaller size and earlier stage.

What Should be Done about Ductal Carcinoma in Situ?

Before mammography screening, only large palpable lesions of ductal carcinoma in situ (DCIS) were diagnosed and these made up only 2% to 5% of all breast cancers. DCIS now makes up 20% to 30% of cancers detected by screening mammography.[63] The treatment of these lesions continues to raise important unanswered questions. The debate about its proper treatment has not been resolved, and the relationship of these lesions to invasive cancer is also unclear. According to Page and colleagues,[64] even the most innocuous appearing of these lesions, if followed for 15 to 20 years can lead to death. Unfortunately, because surgeons and medical oncologists have not determined how best to treat these lesions, this has probably led to some overtreatment. Those who believe that DCIS is being overtreated should launch trials to investigate how best to treat these lesions, but it is dangerous to condemn mammography screening because, in addition to detecting invasive cancers earlier, it also finds DCIS.

Esserman and colleagues[41] suggested that finding DCIS by mammography has not led to a decline in the incidence of invasive cancers as would be expected if it is a precursor to invasive cancer. However, their argument is not supported by the facts. They correctly expect that if DCIS is a precursor lesion, then the incidence of invasive cancers should have dropped to less than the baseline incidence that was present before screening began. I believe that this is a correct expectation. However, they made 2 mistakes. There has indeed been a decrease in the incidence of invasive breast cancer. They accepted the unsubstantiated suggestion that the recent decline in incidence was to the result of the marked reduction in hormone use that accompanied the publication of data from the Women's Health Initiative linking the use of estrogen plus progesterone to a small increase in breast cancer risk.[65] That paper[66] argued that the decline in incidence began in 2003 when it clearly began in 1999, well before publication of the Women's Health Initiative paper. Zahl and Maehlen[67] clearly showed that decreasing hormone use has no effect on breast cancer incidence. Esserman and colleagues[41] also misjudged the baseline incidence. There has been a steady increase in incidence in the United States since 1940, and this increase was going on long before there was any screening. If the baseline incidence is projected appropriately, it appears that the present incidence may have dipped below baseline and this may well be because DCIS has been removed preventing invasive lesions from developing.

The USPSTF Drops a Health Care Bomb

In November 2009, the USPSTF caused major confusion by promulgating new guidelines for breast cancer screening.[68] These were actually the same guidelines promulgated (and then rescinded) by the National Cancer Institute in 1993. They recommended against mammography screening for women aged 40 to 49 years, and recommended that women aged 50 to 74 years be screened every 2 years instead of annually. There were no mammography screening experts on the Panel. There were no medical oncologists or surgical oncologists on the Panel. Although billed as an expert panel, they clearly had no expertise in mammography screening.

It is clear that the USPSTF did not understand mammography screening, and had not thought through the consequences of their guidelines. Arguing against CBE as well as teaching women to examine themselves, the Task Force was essentially telling women in their 40s to return to breast cancer detection at the level found in the 1950s and 1960s. These women would now have to wait until they could no longer ignore the lump in their breast and then seek treatment when it was likely too late. The Task Force admitted that their approach would result in unnecessary deaths that could be prevented by screening, but the guidelines would reduce the false-positive studies, which they decided was more important than saving lives.

The USPSTF made it clear, and this was dispassionately repeated in Dr Kerlikowske's accompanying editorial,[69] that screening every 2 years would mean that as many as 30% of the lives that could be saved with annual screening would be lost by switching to biennial screening.

What has been overlooked in the media coverage of these new guidelines is that the USPSTF guidelines denying screening mammography for women aged 40 to 49 years are unsupported by the science. As noted earlier, there are absolutely no data to support the use of the age of 50 years as anything but an arbitrary threshold when it comes to mammography screening. Instead of using the old dichotomous analysis around the age of 50 years, the task force used age grouping by decade that made cancer detection rates and benefit increase in steps jumping at age 50 years and again at age 60 years (Fig. 2). These jumps do not exist. They are artifacts of age grouping to make it appear that there are jumps when there are none.

The USPSTF also do not understand the RCT data. As noted earlier, the RCTs underestimate the benefit from screening because of noncompliance and contamination. The USPSTF chose to use a 15% decrease in breast cancer deaths, which is the lowest possible estimate (by including the CNBSS1), and they did not even acknowledge that this was an underestimate of benefit. The USPSTF, which had supposedly reviewed all the data, was clearly unaware of the decrease in deaths seen in Sweden and the Netherlands as a result, almost completely, of mammography screening and, instead of using direct data, the task force chose to use computer modeling focusing on a measure of the number of women needed to be screened to save one life (NNTS). Among women aged 40 to 49 years they calculated approximately 1900 women as the NNTS, whereas for women aged 50 to 59 years the NNTS was approximately

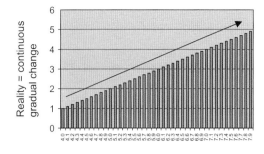

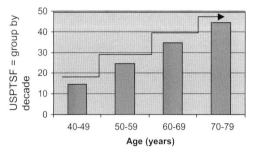

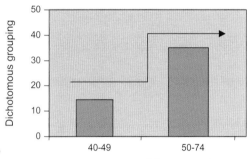

Fig. 2. Data grouping creates false impressions. Age grouping has been used to make data that actually change gradually with increasing age appear to change suddenly at the age of 50 years. In the upper graph the incidence increases by 0.1 each year. In the middle graph the same data are grouped by decade making it appear that there is a sudden jump at the age of 50 years and another at the age of 60 years. In the bottom graph the same data are grouped 40 to 49 years and compared with 50 years and older making it appear that there is a larger jump at the age of 50 years.

1300, and for women aged 60 to 74 years it was 300. The USPSTF has claimed that cost was not a factor in their calculations, but NNTS is clearly a surrogate for cost. Every woman gets screened only once each year, so that the NNTS is not important to her except as an estimate of risk. Furthermore, true cost-effectiveness analysis addresses additional issues such as the years of life saved, which the USPSTF clearly did not want to take into account because it has already been shown that screening annually beginning at the age of 40 years is cost-effective.[70]

The USPSTF ignored the studies listed earlier that showed at least a 30% reduction in deaths that occurs when screening is provided for the general public. Had they used the actual data instead of computer models, the NNTS of 1900 when a 15% benefit was used becomes 950 when a 30% reduction is used, and this would be well below the 1300 threshold that they set.

The USPSTF suggested, as had the ACP, that high-risk women in their 40s might be the only group that should be screened. As noted earlier, there are no data to support this approach. There is no evidence that screening only high-risk women will save lives and screening only high-risk women will miss the 75% to 90% of women who develop breast cancer each year because they are not at high risk.

SUMMARY

Enough is enough. The misinformation that opponents of screening have thrown up as impediments for women to participate in screening needs to stop. The age of 50 years is biologically meaningless. Its use as a threshold should be demonstrated with ungrouped data or it should cease to be a threshold. There is no reason to use computer modeling when direct data clearly show a benefit from mammography screening in the general population that has reduced deaths by 30% to 40%. There are no data that show that screening based on high risk will save lives, and it is clear that most women with breast cancer would be excluded from screening using this approach. The harms of screening have been overstated. In our practice the numbers vary, depending on the age of the woman, because the risk of breast cancer goes up steadily with increasing age. However, if 1000 women are screened, we recall approximately 80 women for additional evaluation. Among these false-positives, as defined by the USPSTF, in approximately 45 women (56%), a few extra images or an ultrasound examination will show that there is nothing to require any further work-up. In 25% (20/80) of these women the radiologist may want to have them return in 6 months just to be careful (<2% chance of malignancy). In approximately 15 (19%) women they will recommend a needle biopsy using local anesthesia. Approximately, 5 of these 15 women will be found to have breast cancer. False-positive mammograms are usually discussed without a frame of reference. There is a higher percentage of false-positives with cervical cancer screening yet there are only 11,000 new cases of invasive cervical cancer each year and fewer than 5000 deaths.

Mammography screening has been faulted for leading to overdiagnosis and overtreatment, but this is inappropriate. Any overdiagnosis is not the fault of mammography, but the inability, as yet, for the pathologists to determine the specific lethality of an individual's lesion. Similarly, overtreatment needs to be addressed by the therapists and is not the fault of mammography.

I would repeat again that it has never been suggested that mammography is a perfect test, nor the ultimate solution for breast cancer. It does not find all cancers and does not find all cancers early enough to effect a cure. However, it has now saved tens of thousands of lives. A decrease in the death rate of 30% translates to 15,000 to 20,000 lives saved by mammography screening each year. We all support intensive efforts to find a cure or to develop a safe way to prevent breast cancer, but these are not on the horizon. Rather than disparaging this lifesaving test, efforts should be directed toward adding to the success of mammography and improving our ability to detect early breast cancer. Those involved in therapy will continue their efforts to develop tailored treatments for the range of cancers detected by screening, but screening should not be withdrawn because of this range. The death rate from breast cancer, unchanged for 50 years, has been dramatically reduced with the use of screening mammograms. This is a remarkable achievement that should be applauded and not vilified. The unjustified attacks on mammography should cease and efforts should be made to build on its success while we continue intensive efforts to find the cure.

REFERENCES

1. White E, Lee CY, Kristal AR. Evaluation of increase in breast cancer incidence in relation to mammography use. J Natl Cancer Inst 1990;82:1546–52.

2. Kopans DB. Beyond randomized, controlled trials: organized mammographic screening substantially reduces breast cancer mortality. Cancer 2002;94:580–1.

3. Berry DA, Cronin KA, Plevritis SK, et al. Effect of screening and adjuvant therapy on mortality from breast cancer. N Engl J Med 2005;353:1784–92.

4. Tabar L, Vitak B, Tony HH, et al. Beyond randomized controlled trials: organized mammographic screening substantially reduces breast carcinoma mortality. Cancer 2001;91:1724–31.

5. Duffy SW, Tabar L, Chen H, et al. The impact of organized mammography service screening on breast carcinoma mortality in seven Swedish counties. Cancer 2002;95:458–69.

6. Otto SJ, Fracheboud J, Looman CW, et al. Initiation of population-based mammography screening in Dutch municipalities and effect on breast-cancer mortality: a systematic review. Lancet 2003;361:1411–7.

7. Feig S. Estimation of currently attainable benefit from mammographic screening of women aged 40–49 years. Cancer 1995;75:2412–9.

8. Cady abstract. Available at: http://www.asco.org/ASCOv2/Meetings/Abstracts?&vmview=abst_detail_view&confID=70&abstractID=40559<https://phsexchweb.partners.org/exchweb/bin/redir.asp?URL=http://www.asco.org/ASCOv2/Meetings/Abstracts?%26vmview=abst_detail_view%26confID=70%26abstractID=40559>. Accessed July 11, 2010.

9. Baker LH. Breast cancer detection demonstration project: five-year summary report. CA Cancer J Clin 1982;32(4):194–225.

10. Duffy SW, Tabar L, Smith RA. The mammographic screening trials: commentary on the recent work by Olsen and Gotzsche. CA Cancer J Clin 2002;52:68–71.

11. Kopans DB, Monsees B, Feig SA. Screening for cancer—when is it valid? Lessons from the mammography experience. Radiology 2003;229:319–27.

12. Shapiro S, Strax P, Venet L. Periodic breast cancer screening in reducing mortality from breast cancer. JAMA 1971;215:1777–85.

13. Bailar JC. Mammography: a contrary view. Ann Intern Med 1976;84:77–84.

14. Bhatia S, Robison LL, Oberlin O, et al. Breast cancer and other second neoplasms after childhood Hodgkin's disease. N Engl J Med 1996;334:745–51.

15. Mettler FA, Upton AC, Kelsey CA, et al. Benefits versus risks from mammography: a critical assessment. Cancer 1996;77:903–9.

16. Nystrom L, Andersson I, Bjurstam N, et al. Long-term effects of mammography screening: updated overview of the Swedish randomized trials. Lancet 2002;359:909–19.

17. Shapiro S, Venet W, Strax P, et al. Periodic screening for breast cancer: the health insurance plan project and its sequelae, 1963–1986. Baltimore (MD): The Johns Hopkins University Press; 1988.

18. Shapiro S, Venet W, Venet L, et al. Ten to fourteen-year effect of screening on breast cancer mortality. J Natl Cancer Inst 1982;69:349–55.

19. Chu KC, Smart CR, Tarone RE. Analysis of breast cancer mortality and stage distribution by age for the health insurance plan clinical trial. J Natl Cancer Inst 1988;80:1125–32.

20. Tabar L, Fagerberg CJ, Gad A, et al. Reduction in mortality from breast cancer after mass screening with mammography. Lancet 1985;1:829–32.

21. Shapiro S. Screening: assessment of current studies. Cancer 1994;74:231–8.

22. Miller AB, Baines CJ, To T, et al. Canadian National Breast Screening Study: 1. Breast cancer detection and death rates among women aged 40–49. Can Med Assoc J 1992;147:1459–76.

23. Miller AB, Howe GR, Wall C. The National Study of Breast Cancer Screening. Clin Invest Med 1981;4: 227–58.

24. Baines CJ, Miller AB, Kopans DB, et al. Canadian National Breast Screening Study: assessment of technical quality by external review. AJR Am J Roentgenol 1990;155:743–7.

25. Kopans DB. The Canadian screening program: a different perspective. AJR Am J Roentgenol 1990;155:748–9.

26. Yaffe MJ. Correction: Canada Study [letter]. J Natl Cancer Inst 1993;85:94.

27. Kopans DB, Feig SA. The Canadian National Breast Screening Study: a critical review. AJR Am J Roentgenol 1993;161:755–60.

28. Tarone RE. The excess of patients with advanced breast cancers in young women screened with mammography in the Canadian National Breast Screening Study. Cancer 1995;75:997–1003.

29. Kopans DB, Halpern E, Hulka CA. Statistical power in breast cancer screening trials and mortality reduction among women 40–49 with particular emphasis on The National Breast Screening Study of Canada. Cancer 1994;74: 1196–203.

30. Fletcher SW, Black W, Harris R, et al. Report of the International Workshop on Screening for Breast Cancer. J Natl Cancer Inst 1993;85:1644–56.

31. Testimony of Samuel Broder MD. House Committee on Government Operations. Misused science: the National Cancer Institutes elimination of mammography guidelines for women in their forties. Union Calendar No. 480. House report 103–863. October 20, 1994.

32. House Committee on Government Operations. Misused science: the National Cancer Institutes elimination of mammography guidelines for women in their forties. Union Calendar No. 480. House report 103–863. October 20, 1994.

33. Kerlikowske K, Grady D, Rubin SM, et al. Efficacy of screening mammography: a meta-analysis. JAMA 1995;273:149–53.

34. Lee Davis D, Love SM. Mammographic screening. JAMA 1994;271:152–3.

35. Harris R, Leininger L. Clinical strategies for breast cancer screening: weighing and using the evidence. Ann Intern Med 1995;122:539–47.

36. Harris R. Breast cancer among women in their forties: toward a reasonable research Agenda. J Natl Cancer Inst 1994;86:410–2.

37. Swanson GM. May we agree to disagree, or how do we develop guidelines for breast cancer screening in women? J Natl Cancer Inst 1994;86:901–3.

38. Black WC, Nease RF, Tosteson AN. Perceptions of breast cancer risk and screening effectiveness in women younger than 50 years of age. J Natl Cancer Inst 1995;87:720–31.

39. Rimer B. Putting the "informed" in informed consent about mammography. J Natl Cancer Inst 1995;87: 703–4.

40. Kopans DB. Bias in the medical journals: a commentary. AJR Am J Roentgenol 2005;185:176–82.

41. Kerlikowske K, Grady D, Barclay J, et al. Positive predictive value of screening mammography by age and family history of breast cancer. JAMA 1993;270:2444–50.

42. Sox H. Screening mammography in women younger than 50 years of age. Ann Intern Med 1995;122:550–2.

43. Stomper PC, D'Souza DJ, DiNitto PA, et al. Analysis of parenchymal density on mammograms in 1353 women 25–79 years old. AJR Am J Roentgenol 1996;167:1261–5.

44. Shapiro S. Evidence on screening for breast cancer from a randomized trial. Cancer 1977;39:2777–8.

45. de Koning HJ, Boer R, Warmerdam PG, et al. Quantitative interpretation of age-specific mortality reductions from the Swedish breast cancer-screening trials. J Natl Cancer Inst 1995;87:1217–23.

46. Fletcher SW. Breast cancer screening among women in their forties: an overview of the issues. J Natl Cancer Inst Monogr 1997;22:5–9.

47. Fletcher SW, Elmore JG. Mammographic screening for breast cancer. N Engl J Med 2003;348:1672–80.

48. Kopans DB. Informed decision making: age of 50 is arbitrary and has no demonstrated influence on breast cancer screening in women. Am J Roentgenol 2005;185:177–82.

49. Hendrick RE, Smith RA, Rutledge JH, et al. Benefit of screening mammography in women aged 40–49: a new meta-analysis of randomized controlled trials. J Natl Cancer Inst Monogr 1997;22:87–92.

50. Kolata G. Get a mammogram. No don't. Repeat. NY Times November 21, 2009. Available at: http://www.nytimes.com/2009/11/22/weekinreview/22kolata.html< https://phsexchweb.partners.org/exchweb/bin/redir.asp?RL=http://www.nytimes.com/2009/11/22/weekinreview/22kolata.html>. Accessed July 11, 2010.

51. Gotzsche PC, Olsen O. Is screening for breast cancer with mammography justifiable? Lancet 2000;355:129–34.

52. Olsen O, Gotzsche PC. Cochrane review on screening for breast cancer with mammography. Lancet 2001;358:1340–2.

53. Knottnerus JA. Report to the Minister of Health, Welfare, and Sport. The benefit of population screening for breast cancer with mammography. Health Council of the Netherlands. Publication no. 2002/03E.

54. International Agency for Research on Cancer. Press release no. 139, 19 March 2002. Available at: http://www.iarc.fr/en/media-centre/pr/2002/pr139.html <https://phsexchweb.partners.org/exchweb/bin/redir.asp?URL=http://www.iarc.fr/en/media-centre/pr/2002/pr139.html>. Accessed July 11, 2010.

55. Qaseem A, Snow V, Sherif K, et al. Screening mammography for women 40 to 49 years of age: a clinical practice guideline from the American College of Physicians. Ann Intern Med 2007;146:511–5.

56. Seidman H, Stellman SD, Mushinski MH. A Different perspective on breast cancer risk factors: some implications of nonattributable risk. Cancer 1982;32:301–13.

57. Kopans DB. Screening mammography for women age 40 to 49 years. Ann Intern Med 2007;147:740–1.

58. Zackrisson S, Andersson I, Janzon L, et al. Rate of over-diagnosis of breast cancer 15 years after end of Malmo mammographic screening trial: follow-up study. BMJ 2006;332:689–92.

59. Zahl PH, Maehlen J, Welch HG. The natural history of invasive breast cancers detected by screening mammography. Arch Intern Med 2008;168:2302–3.

60. Jørgensen KJ, Gøtzsche PC. Overdiagnosis in publicly organised mammography screening programmes: systematic review of incidence trends. BMJ 2009;339:b2587.

61. Duffy SW, Agbaje O, Tabar L, et al. Overdiagnosis and overtreatment of breast cancer: estimates of overdiagnosis from two trials of mammographic screening for breast cancer. Breast Cancer Res 2005;7:258–65.

62. Esserman L, Shieh Y, Thompson I. Rethinking screening for breast cancer and prostate cancer. JAMA 2009;302:1685–92.

63. Ernster VL, Barclay J, Kerliikowske K, et al. Incidence of and treatment for ductal carcinoma in situ of the breast. JAMA 1996;275:913–8.

64. Page DL, Dupont WD, Rogers LW, et al. Continued local recurrence of carcinoma 15–25 years after a diagnosis of low grade ductal carcinoma in situ of the breast treated only by biopsy. Cancer 1995;76:1197–200.

65. Writing Group for the Women's health Initiative Investigators. Risks and benefits of estrogen plus progestin in healthy postmenopausal women. Principal results from the women's health initiative randomized, controlled trial. JAMA 2002;288:321–33.

66. Ravdin PM, Cronin KA, Howlader N, et al. The decrease in breast-cancer incidence in 2003 in the United States. N Engl J Med 2007;356(16):1670–4.

67. Zahl PH, Maehlen J. A decline in breast-cancer incidence. N Engl J Med 2007;357:510–1.

68. U.S. Preventive Services Task Force. Screening for breast cancer: U.S. Preventive Services Task Force recommendation statement. Ann Intern Med 2009;151:716–26.

69. Kerlikowske K. Evidence-based breast cancer prevention: the importance of individual risk. Ann Intern Med 2009;151:750–2.

70. Rosenquist CJ, Lindfors KK. Screening mammography in women aged 40–49 years: analysis of cost-effectiveness. Radiology 1994;191:647–50.

The Use of Breast Imaging to Screen Women at High Risk for Cancer

Edward A. Sickles, MD

KEYWORDS

- Mammography • Breast MR imaging • Breast ultrasound
- Screening • Breast cancer • Women at high risk

Clinical experience and, more recently, genetic testing have identified a subset of women who are at substantially greater than average risk for developing breast cancer. The factors that define this group of women are diverse, ranging from previous biopsy showing cancer or high-risk lesions,[1–5] to strong family history of breast cancer,[6] to previous exposure to high doses of chest radiation.[7–11] Several underlying genetic abnormalities have been discovered among some women at high very risk that add another level of complexity.[12–21] Recent research has shown that breast density, as depicted at mammography, is a substantial independent risk factor for future breast cancer.[22–27]

Common to all women at high risk, by definition, is a greater likelihood of developing breast cancer. However, the cancers that occur in these women, especially those women with associated genetic abnormalities, tend to grow more rapidly,[28] tend to develop earlier in life,[13,17] tend to be more difficult to identify at mammography,[29–35] and may be less responsive to therapy.[36,37] This quadruple whammy creates a sense of urgency that has caused most health care providers to adopt an intuitive, rather than rigorously scientific, approach in devising strategies to identify cancers in women at high risk. This article discusses a major part of this effort: the use of 3 breast imaging modalities (mammography, magnetic resonance [MR] imaging, and ultrasound [US] examination) to screen asymptomatic women at high risk for breast cancer.

FACTORS THAT PLACE WOMEN AT HIGH RISK FOR DEVELOPING BREAST CANCER

There are a wide variety of risk factors associated with the future development of breast cancer. Only those that play a substantial role in guiding clinical-care decisions regarding screening with breast imaging are considered here. High risk may be defined in terms of relative risk (the risk of individuals with a given risk factor divided by the risk of individuals without the same factor). As such, relative risks of 3 of more are often considered clinically relevant.[38] Other measures of risk are expressed as the percentage of women expected to develop cancer in a given future interval (per year, in the next given number of years, from current age until a given future age, lifetime risk).

Previous Breast Biopsy

Women who have already undergone biopsy for lesions diagnosed as malignant (ie, women with a personal history of breast cancer) are known to be at considerably higher than average risk for developing 1 or more additional cancers. The likelihood of contralateral breast cancer diagnosis among women with a personal history of breast cancer is 5% to 10% in the first decade after initial diagnosis, with some evidence that this risk is higher in younger than in older women.[2] A slightly higher level of risk (but for recurrence or second primary cancer in the ipsilateral breast), 5% to 10% over 5 years and 10% to 15% over 10 years, is reported for women undergoing breast conservation as

Department of Radiology, Box 1667, UCSF Medical Center, San Francisco, CA 94143-1667, USA
E-mail address: edward.sickles@ucsfmedctr.org

Radiol Clin N Am 48 (2010) 859–878
doi:10.1016/j.rcl.2010.06.012
0033-8389/10/$ – see front matter © 2010 Elsevier Inc. All rights reserved.

treatment of a first cancer.[3] Overall risk decreases in the second and subsequent decades after initial cancer diagnosis, at least partially because of decreased frequency of ipsilateral recurrence, but the risk during the first decade is high. However, all these risks are partially ameliorated if the patient is undergoing either systemic chemotherapy or chemoprevention.

Substantial risk also is imparted by a previous biopsy diagnosis (personal history) of epithelial ovarian cancer, especially for women younger than 50 years and within 10 years of the diagnosis of ovarian cancer.[39]

Women who carry a biopsy diagnosis of lobular carcinoma in situ (LCIS) also are at considerably higher than average risk. Invasive cancers are more frequently lobular than ductal carcinoma, and are ipsilateral more frequently than contralateral to the LCIS, occurring at or near the site of LCIS diagnosis when ipsilateral.[5] The rate of development of subsequent invasive carcinoma is estimated at 0.5% to 1% per year for LCIS, also reported as a 10% to 20% risk over 15 to 20 years and a 6- to 10-fold relative risk.[4] Similar levels of high risk are reported for women who have a previous biopsy diagnosis of atypia. For both atypical lobular hyperplasia (ALH) and atypical ductal hyperplasia (ADH), in a study involving an average follow-up of 17 years, the relative risk of future invasive carcinoma is 4.2 for ALH and 4.3 for ADH, risks that are essentially doubled for women who also have a first-degree maternal relative with breast cancer (ALH 8.4, ADH 9.7).[1]

Family History of Breast Cancer

There is an abundance of evidence demonstrating significant associations between a family history of breast cancer and subsequent development of breast cancer.[6] As expected, these associations are strongest when first-degree relatives are involved. The future breast cancer risk to age 80 years of a 20-year-old woman with no family history is 7.8%, but the same woman has a risk of 13.3% with 1 first-degree relative and 21.1% with 2 first-degree relatives.[6] Increased risk is imparted by either a maternal or paternal family history, although the infrequency of breast cancer among men causes most strong family history to involve mothers, sisters, and daughters. Among women who have a strong family history, risk is highest at young ages, and, for women of a given age, the risk is greater the younger the family member was when diagnosed with breast cancer.[6] Despite the high relative risk at young ages, the absolute incidence of cancer is low, so the magnitude of this risk is tempered. For this reason, most women with positive family history who develop breast cancer do so at either middle or old age. Substantial risk also is imparted by a family history of epithelial ovarian cancer.[40]

Previous Mediastinal Radiation Therapy

Chest radiation therapy before age 30 years, primarily involving mantle irradiation for Hodgkin disease, is associated with an increased risk for developing breast cancer (latent period after treatment: mean 15–18 years, range 7–34 years).[7,8,39] The frequency of subsequent breast cancer before age 40 years is reported to range from 31% to 50%.[7,9,10,39] The relative risk of subsequent breast cancer diagnosis is highly dependent on age at irradiation, ranging from 136 for age at exposure less than 15 years, to 19 for ages 15 to 24 years, to 7 at ages 25 to 29 years, to 0.7 (no elevated risk) at ages 30 years and older.[9] Risk also is directly proportional to radiation dose.[39]

GENETIC ABNORMALITIES ASSOCIATED WITH A HIGH RISK OF DEVELOPING BREAST CANCER

Genetic abnormalities are believed to account for 5% to 10% of all cases of breast cancer.[18] Women who are known or suspected carriers of *BRCA1* or *BRCA2* mutations are at especially high risk for developing breast (and ovarian) cancer, with an estimated breast cancer risk by age 70 years ranging from 46% to 87% for *BRCA1* mutation carriers (average 65%, 95% confidence interval 44%–78%) and 37% to 84% for *BRCA2* mutation carriers (average 45%, 95% confidence interval 31%–56%).[12,13,17] Risks that are estimated from families with multiple cancer cases are at the high end of the observed range, approximately 85% risk for *BRCA1* and 65% for *BRCA2*.[12,13,17] The risk imparted by both mutations is expressed at younger ages than in the general population.[13,17] In one study involving *BRCA1* mutation carriers, the risk is reported as 3% by age 30 years, 19% by 40 years, and 51% by 50 years.[12] However, the relative risk associated with *BRCA1*, but not *BRCA2*, mutation declines significantly with advancing age,[13,17] which likely accounts for the general observation that risk is expressed at somewhat younger ages for *BRCA1* than for *BRCA2* mutation carriers.[17] The overall effect of this difference in relative risk is limited by the more substantial contribution imparted by increasing absolute incidence of breast cancer with advancing age, because the differences in relative risk occur primarily during years in which there is low absolute incidence.

There are also hereditary cancer predisposition syndromes associated with specific genetic abnormalities and an increased risk of breast cancer. Elevated risk is attributed to mutations of the *PTEN* gene in Cowden and Bannayan-Riley-Ruvalcaba syndrome, the *TP53* gene in Li-Fraumeni syndrome, the *MSH2* and *MLH1* genes in Muir-Torre syndrome, and the *STK11* gene in Peutz-Jeghers syndrome.[14–16,18–21] The rarity of these syndromes precludes the calculation of reliable risk estimates for these syndromes.

Several sophisticated mathematical models have been developed to predict breast cancer risk based on family history and other factors. These models are used for risk assessment of individual patients, to decide whether to recommend genetic testing for *BRCA* gene mutations, to predict which patients may benefit from chemoprevention and/or high-risk screening, and by some investigators to determine study eligibility for research interventions designed for patients at high risk. Because these models are derived from different data sets, use different risk-calculating algorithms, and vary in the age to which they calculate cumulative breast cancer risk, each model indicates a somewhat different level of risk for the same woman. If more than 1 model is used to estimate risk for a given woman, it has been recommended to use the highest level of estimated risk.[41]

The Gail model, first and perhaps still the most widely used, is based on a woman's age, the number of first-degree relatives with breast cancer, age at menarche, age at first live birth, the number of previous breast biopsies (including presence/absence of atypia), and race/ethnicity (www.cancer.gov/bcrisktool/, accessed December 20, 2009).[42] This is the only model validated for use among African American women as well as white women. However, this risk model omits consideration of age at diagnosis of first-degree relatives, any data on second-degree relatives, and paternal family history, limiting the value of the model as an estimator of risk associated with family history. The Claus model is based on more comprehensive family history data, including maternal and paternal family history, first- and second-degree relatives, as well as age at diagnosis of these relatives' cancers, albeit omitting family history data on ovarian cancer (www.palmgear.com/index.cfm?fuseaction=software.showsoftware&prodID=29820, accessed December 20, 2009).[43] Both of these models provide estimates of breast cancer risk, but do not specifically predict likelihood of the presence of *BRCA1* or *BRCA2* mutations. However, there are other models that do provide estimates for *BRCA* gene mutations. The BRCAPRO model is based on both personal history and comprehensive family history data of breast and ovarian cancer (first- and second-degree relatives), as well as Ashkenazi Jewish ancestry (www4.utsouthwestern.edu/breasthealth/cagene/default.asp, accessed December 20, 2009).[44] The BOADICEA model incorporates data on family history of breast, ovarian, prostate, and pancreatic cancer, and also includes estimates of both breast and ovarian cancer risk (www.srl.cam.ac.uk/genepi/boadicea/boadicea_home.html, accessed December 20, 2009).[45] The Tyrer-Cuzick model uses not only comprehensive data on family history and Ashkenazi Jewish ancestry but also data on menstrual and reproductive history, previous biopsy showing either LCIS or atypia, height, and body mass index (www.ems-trials.org/riskevaluator, accessed December 20, 2009).[46]

Although breast imaging facilities routinely collect most of the data required by the various models for calculating breast cancer and *BRCA* gene mutation risk, radiologists generally have neither training nor expertise in using the models, performing the calculations, and interpreting the results. Therefore, many find it helpful to partner with a nearby high-risk clinic, staffed by health care professionals who specialize in risk assessment and genetic counseling. However, for many women, the radiologists who interpret their breast imaging examinations may be more aware of the likelihood that they may be at high risk for future breast cancer than any of their other health care providers. For this reason, it is advisable for radiologists to develop a basic understanding of risk assessment, to know whether a given request for high-risk screening is appropriate.

MAMMOGRAPHIC BREAST DENSITY ASSOCIATED WITH A HIGH RISK FOR DEVELOPING BREAST CANCER

There is a growing body of evidence of an independent association between breast density as depicted at mammography and subsequent risk of developing breast cancer. Observational studies have shown a statistically significant increase in relative risk for progressively increasing categories of breast density.[22–27] In the United States and in many other countries, breast density is usually described according to the 4 categories defined in the Breast Imaging Data and Reporting System (BI-RADS) of the American College of Radiology (ACR): almost entirely fatty (0%–24%), scattered areas of fibroglandular density (25%–50%), heterogeneously dense (51%–75%), and extremely dense (>75%).[47] The most frequently described result is that the relative risk of women having extremely dense breasts ($\geq$75% dense) is 4 to 6 times that of women with almost entirely fatty breasts (0%, <1%, or <10% dense).[22–27]

However, these seemingly high levels of risk may be misleading. All the breast cancer risk factors described earlier are present in only a small minority of women, so it is clinically relevant to consider absence of these risk factors as representing average risk. This is not the case for mammographic breast density. Fewer than 10% of screening mammography examinations in the United States are categorized during image interpretation as showing almost entirely fatty breasts, and fewer than 10% of examinations are interpreted as showing the breasts to be extremely dense.[48] Therefore, more than 80% of screening examinations show breasts with scattered areas of fibroglandular density or heterogeneously dense breasts. The relative risk for the heterogeneously dense compared with the scattered areas category is less than 1.5 in all studies.[22–27] Compared with breasts of average density (those approximately 50% dense, at or near the threshold between the scattered areas and heterogeneously dense categories), the relative risk for heterogeneously dense breasts is less than 1.2 in all studies, and the relative risk for extremely dense breasts is less than 2.1.[22–27]

BREAST IMAGING APPROACHES TO SCREENING ASYMPTOMATIC WOMEN AT HIGH RISK FOR CANCER

In devising strategies to screen asymptomatic women at high risk for breast cancer, the following types of evidence should be assessed, in order of decreasing quality and reliability: systematic reviews and meta-analyses of randomized controlled trials (RCTs), individual RCTs, nonrandomized intervention studies (cohort and case-control studies), observational studies, nonexperimental studies (case series), and expert opinion.[49] The only high-quality evidence supporting recommendations for routine periodic cancer screening using breast imaging come from the several RCTs of screening mammography performed in the United States and Europe, involving nearly 500,000 subjects.[50–57] All but 1 of these RCTs demonstrated a statistically significant reduction in breast cancer mortality among the populations invited to screening. Overall, based on a recent meta-analysis of the RCTs, there was a 20% reduction in breast cancer mortality among the women invited to screening.[58] However, none of the RCTs were designed to study screening mammography among women of any age at high

risk. Therefore, screening strategies for these women must be based on less–scientifically rigorous evidence. Given the clinical context that there is a known subset of women at very high risk (hence, sufficiently high disease prevalence and incidence), coupled with the combination of rapid tumor growth, early age at diagnosis, lower than usual sensitivity of screening mammography, and possible poor response to therapy, most health care providers are willing to accept more intuitive approaches to screening, based on observational studies, case series, and expert opinion.

Within the past few years, several national medical organizations have developed guidelines and recommendations for screening women at high risk using breast imaging. First was the American Cancer Society (ACS), which published guidelines for screening with MR imaging as an adjunct to mammography in 2007.[59] More recently, the National Comprehensive Cancer Network (NCCN) issued parallel guidelines,[60] followed by recommendations for mammography, MR imaging, and US made jointly by the Society of Breast Imaging (SBI) and the ACR.[61] There are only minor differences in the guidelines and recommendations of these several organizations, although those of the SBI/ACR are more comprehensive. This article discusses separately the roles of mammography, MR imaging, and US in screening women at high risk, primarily because the strengths and limitations of these imaging modalities differ considerably, resulting in different recommendations for their use.

Mammography

As stated earlier, screening mammography is the only breast imaging modality validated by multiple RCTs and meta-analyses to reduce breast cancer mortality. Most national medical organizations in the United States, weighing this and other benefits against the several harms of screening (false-positive–induced anxiety, inconvenience, cost, and occasional morbidity, as well as overdiagnosis), have endorsed the routine annual use of mammography beginning at age 40 years. These organizations include the ACS, NCCN, SBI, ACR, the American College of Obstetricians and Gynecologists (every 1–2 years at ages 40–49 years), and the American College of Surgeons. The widespread use of screening mammography in the past several decades has contributed substantially to the nearly 30% reduction in breast cancer mortality observed in the United States.[56,62,63]

Given that routine screening mammography is already recommended in almost all (if not all) countries that have widely available mammographic service (annually, starting at age 40 years in the United States), the primary screening mammography issue for women at high risk is whether to lower the age at which screening should begin, and if so, to what age.

There are theoretic advantages and limitations to screening mammography in women less than the age of 40 years. Potential advantages include the long life expectancy of younger women and the low frequency of comorbidity. Reduction in breast cancer mortality in younger women, in the absence of substantial comorbidity, by definition would add many quality-adjusted life years (QALY), the most frequently used metric in assessing cost-effectiveness. If one is willing to infer the existence of some mortality reduction, by extrapolation from RCT data involving older women, as well as the observation of similar cancer detection rates in screening women at high risk aged 30 to 39 years versus women at average risk aged 40 to 49 years (**Table 1**), then there would be substantial benefit.

Potential limitations to screening mammography in women less than the age of 40 years include the reduced frequency of breast cancer, somewhat reduced sensitivity of mammography, slightly increased radiation risk, and the suggestion of an increase in recall rate. However, the recall rate issue seems to be spurious, because the apparent overall increase in recall rate among women less than 40 years of age disappears when examinations are segregated by availability of previous examinations for comparison; absence of previous examinations is the strongest factor producing increased recall rate,[64] and younger women are more likely to have baseline examinations (**Table 2**).

The risk of radiation oncogenesis imparted at mammography is exceptionally small, because of the very low doses imparted at mammography and the relative insensitivity of the mature breast to the carcinogenic effects of ionizing radiation. At the usual lower age limit for screening (age 40 years), estimates of radiation risk are tiny, and are considered minor in comparison with the proven benefits of breast cancer mortality reduction.[65] However, at younger ages, especially less than 30 years, the breast seems to be more radiosensitive, not only as demonstrated by the age-dependent risk among women with Hodgkin disease who received chest radiation therapy before the age of 30 years,[9] but also among Japanese atomic bomb survivors, women receiving radiation therapy for postpartum mastitis, fibroadenomatosis, and other benign breast conditions, as well as women exposed to high cumulative doses of chest radiation when undergoing repeated fluoroscopic monitoring of artificial pneumothorax as treatment of tuberculosis.[65] In the age range 30 to 39 years, for which benefit is presumed but not proven and for which radiation risk is only slightly higher than at age 40 years and older, expert opinion indicates that benefit substantially exceeds risk, so concerns about radiation oncogenesis should not limit the acceptability of screening mammography in women at high risk for future breast cancer.[61] Benefit/risk ratios are somewhat less favorable for women in their 20s, but, among this age cohort, it is observed that more than half of the benefit and less than half of the radiation risk is found in women aged 25 to 29 years, so expert opinion supports the acceptability of screening mammography down to age 25 years, but only for those women at the highest levels of future breast cancer risk.[61]

The sensitivity of screening mammography has also been shown to be age-dependent, lower in younger than in older women, and lowest for women younger than 40 years.[66,67] The major explanation for this reduced sensitivity is the tumor-masking effect of dense fibroglandular tissue, which is present more frequently in younger women. For the subset of women at very high risk younger than 40 years who have also undergone screening MR imaging, the sensitivity of mammography is very low indeed, principally because of the

Table 1			
Cancer detection rates for screening mammography at ages 30 to 39 years for women at high risk and at ages 40 to 49 years for all women			
Age Range (y)	Examinations	Cancers	Cancer Detection Rate (/1000)
30–39	3252	11	3.4
40–49	65,209	216	3.3

Data are from the screening mammography practice at the University of California San Francisco (UCSF) Medical Center, from 1985 to 2009. At UCSF, screening mammography is recommended at ages 30 to 39 years only for women at high risk.

Table 2
Recall rates for screening mammography at less than 40 years of age for women at high risk and at ages 40 to 70 years and older than 70 years for all women, depending on whether interpreted in comparison with previous examination(s)

Age Range (y)	Examinations	Recalls	Recall Rate (%)
All examinations			
<40	4727	336	7.11
40–70	108,087	6245	5.78
>70	27,730	1266	4.57
Total	140,544	7847	5.58
Examinations interpreted in comparison with previous examination(s)			
<40	1450	53	3.66
40–70	86,489	3784	4.38
>70	24,426	918	3.76
Total	112,365	4755	4.23
Examinations interpreted without comparison with previous examination(s)			
<40	3277	283	8.64
40–70	21,598	2461	11.39
>70	3304	348	10.53
Total	28,179	3092	10.97

Data are from the screening mammography practice at the UCSF Medical Center, from 1997 to 2009. At UCSF, screening mammography is recommended at less than 40 years of age only for women at high risk. Recalls = all abnormal interpretations (BI-RADS assessment categories 0, 4, or 5). Recall rate = number of recalls divided by number of examinations. When considering all examinations, the recall rate seems to be lower for women less than 40 years of age than for older women, but, after accounting for whether examinations were interpreted in comparison with previous examination(s), this difference in recall rate is no longer present. A likely explanation is that a greater proportion of women less than 40 years of age are undergoing baseline examinations, at which there are no previous examinations and at which the recall rate is known to be significantly and substantially higher. This explanation, based on less extensive data, initially was proposed in Sickles EA. Successful methods to reduce false-positive mammography interpretations. Radiol Clin North Am 2000;38(4):693–700.

many mammographically and clinically occult cancers that are identified at MR imaging.[41] However, despite lower sensitivity (all women <40 years of age) or very much lower sensitivity (women <40 years of age who also undergo screening MR imaging), there still is presumed benefit in screening with mammography, because some mammographically visible cancers (especially ductal carcinoma in situ [DCIS] presenting as a small group of microcalcifications) are not depicted at MR imaging.[41] Furthermore, the ongoing switch among radiology practices from the use of screen film to digital mammography is likely to result in improved sensitivity in screening women at high risk younger than 40 years, because the use of digital mammography has been shown to result in superior performance (including higher sensitivity) for women aged less than 50 years who are pre- or perimenopausal and who have dense breasts.[68,69]

This leaves the observed low frequency of breast cancer as the principal limitation to screening women less than 40 years of age. In the United States, fewer than 7% of all breast cancers are found in women younger than 40 years.[70] Described in other terms, the likelihood of breast cancer diagnosis in the next 10 years for an 30-year-old woman at average risk is only 0.4% (1 in 250).[38] The efficacy of screening is reduced if there is a low prior probability of disease in the screened population, and this is a major reason why screening mammography is not recommended for women at average risk in their 30s. However, given the proven efficacy and widely accepted use of screening mammography for women at average risk beginning at 40 years of age, it seems reasonable to screen women at high risk at any age less than 40 years if their current risk is either equal to or greater than that of a 40-year-old woman at average risk, because these women have a sufficiently high prior probability of disease.

Ultimately, the decision about when to begin high-risk screening mammography depends on the balance between benefits and harms. In terms of benefit, women with the full spectrum of breast cancer risk discussed earlier (except for the lower risk levels imparted by dense breasts alone) can be expected to have risk levels in their 30s exceeding that of a 40-year-old woman at average risk, so it is reasonable to support high-risk screening mammography in this decade. Because breast cancer is exceedingly rare among women less than the 30 years of age,[70] except for BRCA mutation carriers and in other exceptional circumstances, age 30 years seems to be the appropriate lower age limit for screening mammography among women at high risk. For known carriers of the BRCA1 mutation, breast cancer risk is sufficiently high at age 20 years to possibly justify screening,[41] but concerns about radiation risk among such young women suggest that, instead, the beginning age for screening mammography should not be before age 25 years.[61] The breast cancer risk of BRCA2 mutation carriers also is sufficiently high to support the start of screening mammography at age 25 years.[41]

Among the guidelines and recommendations recently issued by national medical organizations in the United States, those made jointly by the SBI and ACR specifically list the indications for screening mammography in women at high risk. The ACS and NCCN guidelines discuss screening mammography only by inference, in that they involve screening MR imaging as an adjunct to mammography (hence the assumption that mammography is also recommended). The ACS and NCCN did not consider the indications for screening mammography in women at high risk other than those who should also undergo screening MR imaging. The more comprehensive SBI/ACR recommendations are listed in Table 3, with footnotes indicating the inferred guidelines of the ACS and NCCN.

MR Imaging

RCTs, cohort studies, and case-control studies have not been performed to assess the efficacy of screening MR imaging to reduce breast cancer mortality. Therefore, the efficacy of screening MR imaging must be estimated based on less robust data, and it must be remembered that, at best, such data provide inferential evidence rather than scientific proof.

There are several prospective observational studies of screening MR imaging as an adjunct to mammography. This article discusses those

Table 3
Recommendations on periodic high-risk screening mammography made by national medical organizations in the United States

Indication	Age to Start (y)
BRCA mutation carriers[a,b]	25–30[c]
Untested first-degree relatives of BRCA mutation carriers[a,b]	25–30[c]
Lifetime breast cancer risk 20% or greater[a,b,d]	Variable[e]
Chest radiation therapy between age 10 and 30 y[a,b]	Variable[f]
Personal history of breast cancer (invasive carcinoma, DCIS)	At diagnosis
Previous breast biopsy showing LCIS[b]	At diagnosis
Previous breast biopsy showing ADH or ALH	At diagnosis
Personal history of invasive ovarian carcinoma	At diagnosis
Mother or sister with early-onset breast cancer	Variable[e]

These are the recommendations of the SBI and ACR.[61] The recommendations involve annual screening and continue to the age at which routine screening mammography is recommended for women at average risk, which, in the United States, is 40 years according to these and many other national medical organizations.

[a] Recommendations attributed to the ACS, by inference, in that they involve screening MR imaging as an adjunct to mammography.[59] These recommendations include women with Li-Fraumeni, Cowden, and Bannayan-Riley-Ruvalcaba syndromes and their first-degree relatives (not recommended by SBI/ACR).

[b] Recommendations attributed to the NCCN, by inference, in that they involve screening MR imaging as an adjunct to mammography.[60] These recommendations include women with Li-Fraumeni, Cowden, and Bannayan-Riley-Ruvalcaba syndromes and their first-degree relatives (not recommended by SBI/ACR).

[c] Age 30 years but not before age 25 years.

[d] As defined by a risk-assessment model that is largely dependent on family history (Gail model excluded).

[e] Age 30 years (but not before age 25 years), or 10 years earlier than age at diagnosis of youngest affected relative, whichever is later.

[f] Eight years after radiation therapy, but not before age 25 years.

studies involving nonoverlapping patient populations in which multiple rounds of screening were performed and in which at least 10 cancers were detected at screening. In chronologic sequence by date of publication, these include the Dutch multi-institution study reported by Kriege and colleagues,[29] the single-institution Canadian study reported by Warner and colleagues,[30] the United Kingdom multi-institution study reported by Leach and colleagues,[31] the single-institution German study reported by Kuhl and colleagues,[32] the multi-institution Italian study reported by Sardanelli and colleagues,[33] the multi-institution Norwegian study reported by Hagen and colleagues,[34] and the Austrian single-institution study reported by Riedl and colleagues.[35]

Interstudy comparisons are of limited value because the eligibility criteria for entry into these various studies differ substantially, as do other important aspects of study design, including that some, but not all, of the studies also involve supplemental screening with US. However, because all the studies involve patient populations heavily weighted with women at high risk, it is reasonable to analyze study findings in combination as well as individually (**Table 4**). When doing so, several observations are clear. The sensitivity of screening MR imaging is substantially higher than that of either mammography or US (or the combination of mammography and US); almost all detectable cancers are identified at screening with the combination of mammography and MR imaging; most of the malignancies detected only at MR imaging are small, node-negative, invasive cancers; and screening MR imaging results in a low interval cancer rate (see **Table 4**).

The superior ability of screening MR imaging to detect clinically occult breast cancer is especially apparent in the subset of women at very high risk involving carriers of *BRCA* mutations,[71] in whom screening with mammography alone results in limited success.[29,72–74] In this select patient population, the disparity in sensitivity between MR imaging and mammography is greater, and the cancers detected at MR imaging are small, frequently node-negative, with few interval cancers.[71]

The sensitivity of mammography combined with MR imaging permits detection of virtually all detectable cancers. As shown in **Table 4**, the sensitivity of screening MR imaging across all studies is 81%, which is increased to 92% by its use in combination with screening mammography. Given the interval cancer rate of approximately 6% across all studies, the incremental benefit of further adding screening US seems to be minimal. In the American College of Radiology Imaging Network (ACRIN) high-risk screening study, supplemental screening MR imaging was provided to 627 self-selected women shortly after completion of the third and final screening round involving mammography and US.[75] The addition of prevalence MR imaging screening doubled the number of cancers detected in this incidence screening round (from 8 to 16); only 2 of the 16 cancers would have been missed had screening been limited to mammography and MR imaging.[75] It is now widely accepted that, if screening includes both mammography and MR imaging in a given woman at high risk, there is no need for additional US screening.[41]

In clinical practice, some breast imaging centers perform screening mammography and MR imaging concurrently, whereas others prefer to stagger the examinations every 6 months (for example, mammography in October and MR imaging in April). The theoretic advantage of staggered examinations is the potential for detection 6 months earlier of cancers that would be visible at both examinations; this amounts to approximately 25% to 30% of detectable cancers (see **Table 4**). However, there are also practical advantages to concurrent screening; in addition to increased patient convenience, it may be helpful to compare a borderline abnormal MR imaging examination with concurrently performed mammography to establish the benignity of the MR imaging finding(s). Given the absence of data comparing the efficacies of concurrent and staggered approaches, either is considered acceptable. In my practice, we provide staggered screening to our patients at high risk, except for those for whom examinations on 2 separate days would be inconvenient.

Insofar as the success of supplemental screening MR imaging is dependent on limitations to the success of screening mammography among women at high risk, one would expect superior MR imaging performance among women with denser breasts. However, in a population of *BRCA* mutation carriers screened with both modalities, the sensitivities of MR imaging versus mammography are reported as 86% versus 18% for women with primarily dense (>50% dense) breasts, and 94% versus 33% for women with primarily fatty (≤50% dense) breasts.[76] Therefore, supplemental MR imaging screening seems to have benefit that is independent of mammographic breast density.

As discussed earlier, the decision about whether to recommend high-risk screening depends on the balance between benefits and harms. For MR imaging, the observed benefits of increased sensitivity, detection of small node-negative cancers, and a low interval cancer rate seem to be substantial, although these permit only the inference of reduced breast cancer mortality. The observed harms of screening MR imaging include false-positive interpretations (resulting in recall for additional breast imaging work-up but not cancer diagnosis), a high percentage of probably benign assessments (resulting in short-interval follow-up MR imaging examinations that rarely lead to cancer diagnosis), and recommendations for biopsy (that do not produce a cancer diagnosis). **Table 4** displays the frequencies of false-positive results for screening MR imaging, as best can be determined from the source articles (which do not describe false-positive outcomes in as much detail as true-positive outcomes). All but 1 of the studies of screening MR imaging also reports at least 1 calculation of specificity, albeit with variable definitions of false-positive examinations. Specificity is uniformly reported to be lower for screening MR imaging than for screening mammography, indicating poorer performance.[29–33,35] Furthermore, the overall frequencies of probably benign assessments (8%) and biopsies performed for MR imaging–detected abnormalities (4%), shown in **Table 4**, are considerably higher than those observed for screening mammography among women at average risk.[77]

However, these unfavorable false-positive results are balanced, at least somewhat, by the additional report that the likelihood of malignancy (positive predictive value) among lesions undergoing biopsy based on screening MR imaging is acceptably high (41%, see **Table 4**), being somewhat higher than that reported for screening mammography in women at average risk (25%).[77] Such a higher positive predictive value in screening women at high risk might be expected, because of the greater prior probability of cancer.

The other factor that limits the effect of the high false-positives reported for screening MR imaging is that false-positive MR imaging rates are reported to be substantially lower at incidence screening than at the initial prevalence screen.[30] This likely occurs not only because of the learning process for screening MR imaging interpretation such that increased experience leads to fewer false-positives (as already shown for mammography),[78] but also because false-positive rates generally are lower when current examinations are compared with previous examinations.[64]

Most health care providers seem willing to consider that the inferred benefits of screening MR imaging (substantial numbers of additional cancers detected) outweigh the observed harms of high false-positives. This is mirrored by the same national medical organizations that recommend screening mammography for women at high risk also recommending supplemental screening with MR imaging.[59–61] The ACS, the first organization to develop screening MR imaging guidelines, recommends screening MR imaging only for women at very high risk (several specific risk factors, as well as lifetime risk estimated to be at least 20% using risk assessment models that are largely dependent on family history). The ACS recommends against screening MR imaging for women at a lifetime risk of less than 15% (the woman at average risk has a lifetime risk of approximately 12% when estimated at age 20 years). The ACS states that current evidence is insufficient to recommend either for or against screening MR imaging for women at high risk at a lifetime risk between 15% and 20%, with further clarification that screening decisions should be made on a case-by-case basis and that payment should not be a barrier.[59] The joint SBI/ACR recommendations and the NCCN guidelines are similar to those of the ACS (details are given in **Table 5**).

The guidelines and recommendations of all these national organizations use estimates of lifetime risk, which decreases with advancing age despite breast cancer incidence progressively increasing. As a result, the lifetime risk of a 60-year-old woman, for example, may be substantially lower than her risk at age 30 years, whereas her risk of breast cancer diagnosis in the next several years may be considerably higher at age 60 years than at 30 years. The net effect is that a woman's lifetime risk inaccurately estimates the (perhaps more clinically relevant) shorter-term risk that she and her health care provider often consider in deciding on screening MR imaging. As a result, some have proposed that a shorter term than lifetime risk may provide a more appropriate basis for screening guidelines.[41] In this regard, a 10-year interval of risk may be the most useful, because this time period is sufficiently long to indicate substantial benefit (assuming the presence of benefit), but it is also sufficiently short to overcome the limitations inherent in lifetime estimates of risk. Based on data derived from the Claus risk assessment model, Berg[41] asserts that the use of a 5% 10-year-risk threshold for recommending screening MR imaging identifies groups of women similar to those who have a lifetime risk estimated to be at least 20%.

Despite the ACS suggestion that payment should not be a barrier in deciding on screening MR imaging, the examination indeed is expensive in comparison with mammography and US, especially when annual examinations are

Table 4
Prospective studies of screening MR imaging involving multiple screening rounds, in which at least 10 cancers were identified

Country	Women/Screening Examinations	Cancers[a]	Invasive Cancers	Node Positive[b]	Cancers Detected at Mammography[c]
Netherlands	1909/4169	45	39	5 (13)	18 (40)
Canada	236/457	22	16	2 (13)	8 (36)
United Kingdom	649/1881	35	29	5 (17)	14 (40)
Germany	529/1452	43	34	5 (15)	14 (33)
Italy[h]	278/377	15	11	1 (9)	9 (60)
Norway[i]	491/867	21	18	6 (26)	9 (43)
Austria	327/672	27	16	2 (13)	13 (48)
Total	4419/9875	208	163	26 (16)	85 (41)

Cancers Detected at:

Country	US[c]	MR Imaging[c]	Mammography + US[c]	Mammography + MR Imaging[c]	Interval Cancers[c]
Netherlands	—	32 (71)	—	40 (89)	4 (9)
Canada	7 (32)	17 (77)	12 (55)	20 (91)	1 (5)
United Kingdom	—	27 (77)	—	33 (94)	2 (6)
Germany	17 (40)	39 (91)	21 (49)	40 (93)	1 (2)
Italy[h]	9 (60)	13 (87)	10 (67)	15 (100)	0
Norway[i]	—	17 (81)	—	18 (86)	2 (10)
Austria	11 (41)	23 (85)	13 (48)	25 (93)	2 (7)
Total	44 (41)	168 (81)	56 (52)	191 (92)	12 (6)

Country	Recalls[d]	MR Imaging False-positives		PPV$_3$ (Biopsy Performed)[g]
		Probably Benign[e]	Biopsy Performed[f]	
Netherlands	177 (4)	275 (7)	56 (1)	32 (57)
Canada	58 (13)	24 (5)	32 (7)	17 (53)
United Kingdom	202 (11)	169 (9)	77 (4)	27 (35)
Germany	—	167 (12)	78 (5)	39 (50)
Italy[h]	—	—	24 (6)	13 (54)
Norway[i]	—	—	—	—
Austria	—	—	101 (15)	23 (23)
Total	437 (7)	635 (8)	368 (4)	151 (41)

[a] Breast cancers only, including both screen-detected and interval cancers. All studies report data for only the most advanced cancer diagnosed (1 cancer per woman).

[b] Number of node-positive invasive cancers (%).

[c] Number of cancers (% of all cancers). The percentage calculation represents sensitivity.

[d] Number of MR imaging examinations assessed as BI-RADS category 0, 4, or 5 (% of examinations).

[e] Number of MR imaging examinations assessed as BI-RADS category 3 (% of examinations).

[f] Number of MR imaging examinations assessed as BI-RADS category 0, 3, 4, or 5 for which fine-needle aspiration, core, or surgical biopsy subsequently was performed (% of examinations).

[g] PPV, positive predictive value. Number of cancers detected at MR imaging (number of cancers detected at MR imaging divided by the number of biopsies performed for MR imaging–detected abnormalities,[f] expressed as %).

[h] Three of 18 cancers are excluded because either mammography, US, or MR imaging was not performed.

[i] Four of 25 cancers are excluded because either mammography or MR imaging was not performed.

Table 5
Recommendations on periodic high-risk screening MR imaging made by national medical organizations in the United States

Indication	Age to Start (y)
BRCA mutation carriers	30
Untested first-degree relatives of *BRCA* mutation carriers	30
Lifetime breast cancer risk 20% or greater	30
Chest radiation therapy between age 10 and 30 y	Variable

These are the recommendations of the SBI and ACR.[61] The recommendations involve annual screening, and continue to the age at which routine screening mammography stops because of limited life expectancy, substantial comorbidity, or unwillingness to undergo additional testing (including biopsy), if recommended, and cancer treatment, if appropriate. The ACS and NCCN also recommend screening MR imaging for women with Li-Fraumeni, Cowden, and Bannayan-Riley-Ruvalcaba syndromes and their first-degree relatives, starting at age 30 years. The NCCN also recommends screening MR imaging for women with a biopsy diagnosis of LCIS (starting at diagnosis), based on 1 single-institution study that demonstrates cancer detection in 5 of 135 women.

Data from Port ER, Park A, Borgen PI, et al. Results of MR imaging screening for breast cancer in high-risk patients with LCIS and atypical hyperplasia. Ann Surg Oncol 2007;14(3):1051–7.

planned. A recent cost-effectiveness study reported acceptable cost per QALY-gained data (<$100,000) for annual screening MR imaging, but only for women at highest risk (known *BRCA1* mutation carriers from 35–59 years of age and known *BRCA2* mutation carriers from 40–49 years of age).[79] This same study reports the cost-effectiveness in QALY gained for screening mammography for the even wider age range of 25 to 69 years as being highly favorable, only $18,952 and $28,421 for *BRCA1* and *BRCA2* carriers, respectively; the study also reports that the incremental effect of adding screening MR imaging from ages 25 to 29 years to any range of older women adds more than $300,000 per QALY gained.[79]

Comparison of the data in **Tables 3** and **5** shows a large discrepancy in the groups of women recommended for screening mammography and MR imaging, according to SBI/ACR guidelines. The basic difference is that women in the intermediate-risk group (several specific risk factors and 15%–20% lifetime risk) are recommended for screening mammography at ages 30 to 39 years, but not routinely for screening MR imaging at any age (only on a case-by-case basis). There are several reasons to recommend screening mammography among these women: inference of a benefit in mortality reduction from extrapolation of RCT results, mammography for women in this group yields a similar cancer detection rate to that for women at average risk in their 40s (see **Table 1**), and women in this group have a breast cancer risk equal to or greater than that of a 40-year-old woman at average risk. Screening MR imaging is not routinely recommended in these

women, at least in part because, compared with mammography, it has more frequent false-positives, is more expensive, takes longer to perform and interpret, requires an intravenous injection, and has more frequent intolerances (reports from 2 high-risk screening studies indicate MR imaging nonparticipation rates of 9% and 42%).[80,81]

US

As with screening MR imaging, RCTs, cohort studies, and case-control studies have not been completed to assess the efficacy of screening US to reduce breast cancer mortality. Therefore, the efficacy of screening US also must be estimated based on less robust data, and, at best, such data provide inferential evidence rather than scientific proof.

However, there are several single-institution observational studies of screening US as an adjunct to mammography. The eligibility criteria for entry into these studies differ substantially, as do other important aspects of study design. Nonetheless, because the studies each involve patient populations heavily weighted with women at high risk, it is reasonable to analyze study findings in combination. Berg[38] has summarized the outcomes reported in these studies, comprising almost 50,000 examinations (see Table 2 in Ref.[38]). Overall, the incremental cancer detection rate provided by screening US is 3.6 per 1000 examinations, 94% of the cancers are invasive, more than 70% are 1 cm in size or smaller, and 86% are node-negative.[38] However, the potential effect of the encouraging results reported in these several studies is limited by several aspects of experimental design: performance of each study at only a single institution or breast imaging practice, US interpretive criteria used in each study not fully described, only 1 round of screening US performed (1 of the studies included multiple rounds of screening but did not separately report outcomes at prevalence and incidence screening), interpretation of screening US examinations not done independently of mammography, false-positive outcomes reported incompletely, and interval cancer rates not reported at all.

To overcome these deficiencies, as well as to provide more complete evidence on the efficacy of screening US, ACRIN has conducted a multi-institution prospective study involving 3 rounds of screening.[82] The first screening round resulted in incremental cancer detection outcomes that were strikingly similar to those reported for the several previous single-institution studies, albeit with high false-positive rates.[83] Preliminary results from the 2 incidence screening rounds were presented recently, showing similar cancer detection rates, but somewhat lower false-positive rates than those observed at prevalence screening.[84,85]

There are particularly pertinent data from the 4 screening MR imaging studies among women at high risk that also include screening US (discussed earlier), 1 of which is a multi-institution study. Outcomes are summarized in **Table 4**. Overall, these studies show modest incremental rates of cancer detection and sensitivity for screening US beyond what is detected at mammography, similar to the results reported for the several single-institution US-only studies and for the multi-institution ACRIN study. However, these studies also show that screening US performance in detecting cancer is far inferior to that of screening MR imaging (at false-positive rates similar to those of MR imaging), and that screening US provides no substantial incremental increase in cancer detection beyond that achieved by the combination of screening mammography and MR imaging (see **Table 4**). Therefore, screening MR imaging seems to be more effective than screening US as an adjunctive examination to mammography for women at very high risk, leading to the suggestion that screening US should be considered only if MR imaging is unavailable, impractical, or poorly tolerated by a given woman.

Although MR imaging is the preferred examination to screen women at very high risk, some have proposed the use of screening US for those women in the so-called intermediate-risk group of women (those with a personal history of breast cancer, previous biopsy diagnosis of LCIS or atypia, or a family history from which lifetime risk of breast cancer is estimated at 15%–20%) who, after consideration on a case-by-case basis, do not undergo screening MR imaging.[41] Despite its limited efficacy compared with MR imaging, there are several reasons why screening US might be considered in this scenario. It is more readily available, less expensive, better tolerated, and does not require intravenous injection. However, when used as in almost all the reported observational studies, as a physician-performed examination using a hand-held transducer, screening US is a more time-consuming examination for the interpreting physician than MR imaging, one that may become a major time sink. In the ACRIN study, the median duration of a physician-performed screening US examination was 19 minutes.[83] For this reason, many breast imaging practices have decided not to provide screening US services for this, or any other, indication.

Even more problematic when considering workforce issues is the consideration of whether screening US should be offered to all women with mammographically dense breasts. There already is evidence among women at intermediate risk demonstrating incremental cancer detection beyond that achieved by screening mammography, albeit at much higher false-positive rates.[83,86–92] However, as discussed earlier, the presence of dense breasts alone may not impart enough risk to justify screening (because the added risk beyond that of women with average-density breasts is not particularly high). For women with dense breasts with no other substantial risk factors, who are at only slightly higher than average risk, why not simply consider the use of screening US for purposes of incremental cancer detection?[61] Given the extremely large number of women who might be screened (approximately half of women undergoing screening mammography have heterogeneously or extremely dense breasts, increasing to 90% if women with scattered areas of fibroglandular density also are included),[48] this might be reasonable if the magnitude of incremental cancer detection is similar to that demonstrated for intermediate risk and women at very high risk (not yet known), if false-positive rates are acceptably low (not yet known), if the cost of examination is acceptably low (similar to that of screening mammography), and if workforce issues are solved by automated rather than physician-performed hand-held approaches to screening US (encouraging results are already reported for one automated US screening device).[93] Among women with primarily fatty breasts, screening US as an adjunct to mammography has been shown to be ineffective in incremental cancer detection.[38,89–91] So, until sufficient evidence is reported to justify the use of screening US for all women with dense breasts, perhaps the better way to consider this issue is that, for now, fatty breasts are a contraindication to screening US.

Two large-scale studies involving screening US are already underway that may provide the necessary evidence on the usefulness of screening US for women with dense breasts. An RCT has been started in Japan, designed to study 50,000 women with screening mammography and handheld US performed by a technologist or a physician and then interpreted by a physician (and 50,000 controls with screening mammography only).[94] The defined study population is women aged 40 to 49 years, because this is the age range in Japan at which breast cancer incidence peaks, and because a high percentage of Japanese women in this age range have dense breasts. The primary end points of this trial are sensitivity and specificity, so data on both incremental cancer detection and false-positives should be forthcoming. The rate of advanced cancers will also be measured, because this has been demonstrated in the screening mammography RCTs to be a surrogate for reduction in breast cancer mortality.[58] However, this trial has several limitations: the screening interval is 2 years, despite evidence that screening mammography at age 40 to 49 years is more effective with annual screening[58,95]; the study population being so different from those in Western countries may limit the generalization of study outcomes; and the study likely is underpowered to provide follow-up data on breast cancer deaths because of the low breast cancer risk of native Japanese women, and also because women with fatty breasts are not excluded from the study.

The second study is a nonrandomized multi-institution effort involving multiple annual screening rounds, conducted primarily in the United States, using a matched-pair design similar to that of the ACRIN study, assessing the performance of screening mammography alone versus the combination of screening mammography and US. However, this is a much larger-scale study than the ACRIN study (approximately 25,000 women with dense breasts), with no emphasis on recruiting an especially high-risk population of women with dense breasts, using automated rather than hand-held US, and involving US scanning of only the dense portions of the breasts.

Interpretation of both mammography and US examinations is done using the standard batch-reading approach used for screening examinations, with mammography and US examinations read independently by different radiologists. The primary study end point is sensitivity; the rate of advanced cancers is also measured. Study strengths include use of a more workforce-efficient, purely screening approach to US, and large-scale multi-institution design in a population of women likely to be representative of all women with dense breasts in Western countries. Study limitations are non-randomized experimental design and inability to study breast cancer deaths as an end point.

One other issue concerning screening US deserves discussion. Almost all current data comparing the performance of mammography alone with that of mammography plus US involves screen-film mammography.[30,32,33,86–92] However, digital mammography is currently in the process of replacing screen-film mammography, largely because of research that shows superior performance of digital mammography for women younger than 50 years, who are pre- or perimenopausal, and who have dense breasts.[68,69] As indicated earlier, the improved performance of adjunctive screening with US is observed primarily in women with dense breasts,[38,89–91] most of whom also are younger than 50 years and pre- or perimenopausal. Therefore, it is likely that the gradual but steady switch from screen film to digital mammography is resulting in improved mammography performance and, consequently, in diminished benefit for supplemental screening with US. However, the potentially limiting effect of digital mammography on screening US performance, not incorporated into most of the data produced by the already reported studies, is indeed factored into the currently ongoing hand-held US study in Japan and the automated US study in the United States, because the mammography component in both these studies involves digital mammography alone.

Other Imaging Modalities

Breast imaging modalities other than mammography, MR imaging, and US have also been used for purposes of cancer detection. Nuclear medicine imaging, initially using standard gamma cameras,[96,97] but more recently with higher-resolution breast-specific equipment,[98] and also with positron emission scanning,[99] has been performed principally in the diagnostic setting, although there is 1 preliminary report suggesting possible efficacy for screening women at high risk.[100] Breast-specific computed tomography (CT) scanning, initially studied in the late 1970s using prototype equipment that then was abandoned,[101,102] is now being investigated with renewed interest. Several research groups are developing dedicated breast CT scanners, and a preliminary report indicates some degree of incremental cancer detection beyond that provided by mammography.[103] Most promising in this regard is the use of contrast-enhanced CT scanning, which, theoretically, may provide similar cancer detection ability to that currently achieved by screening MR imaging.[104] Thermography, although widely evaluated in the 1970s and found to be ineffective for screening,[105,106] continues to be modified and, presumably, improved; the most recent adaptations of thermographic imaging have not been tested extensively. Breast transillumination,[107–109] electrical impedance spectroscopy,[110,111] near infrared spectroscopy,[110,112] and microwave imaging[110,113] also have yet to demonstrate screening efficacy. In summary, current screening applications involving any of these modalities are considered investigational.

Future Developments

Active research is underway involving new applications of mammography, MR imaging, and US technology. For mammography, several tomosynthesis approaches are being developed that promise to increase the detection of some cancers currently not depicted in dense breasts using either screen-film or digital imaging, simultaneously substantially reducing the frequency of false-positive screening outcomes by verifying the benignity of most recalled lesions that are determined to represent summation artifact (superimposition of normal breast structures) at diagnostic mammography.[114–116] For MR imaging, new applications using either diffusion imaging[117,118] or spectroscopy[119–122] may permit early cancer detection without the need for intravenous contrast injection. For both MR imaging and US, studies of the differential elasticity of benign and malignant breast structures may permit earlier detection of some cancers that currently are not depicted.[123–125] If 1 or more of these currently investigational applications eventually demonstrates screening efficacy, especially efficacy of considerable magnitude, the current balance of usefulness among mammography, MR imaging, and US may change, perhaps substantially.

SUMMARY

Although there currently is no evidence of reduced breast cancer mortality for screening women at high risk with mammography, MR imaging, or US, the presumptive evidence of early cancer detection provided by numerous observational studies has led to the publication of guidelines and recommendations for the selective use of these imaging modalities. In general, annual screening mammography is recommended for women of appropriately high risk beginning at age 30 years, supplemental screening with MR imaging is recommended for a subset of women at very high risk, and screening US is suggested for women for whom MR imaging is appropriate but unavailable, impractical, or poorly tolerated. The use of screening US remains controversial among women who have no substantial risk factors other than dense breasts.

REFERENCES

1. Page DL, Dupont WD, Rogers LW, et al. Atypical hyperplastic lesions of the female breast: a long-term follow-up study. Cancer 1985;55(11):2698–708.
2. Fowble B, Hanlon A, Freedman G, et al. Second cancers after conservative surgery and radiation for stages I-II breast cancer: identifying a subset of women at increased risk. Int J Radiat Oncol Biol Phys 2001;51(3):679–90.
3. Dershaw DD. Breast imaging and the conservative treatment of breast cancer. Radiol Clin North Am 2002;40(3):501–16.
4. Arpino G, Laucirica R, Elledge RM. Premalignant and in situ breast disease: biology and clinical implications. Ann Intern Med 2005;143(6):446–57.
5. Li CI, Malone KE, Saltzman BS, et al. Risk of invasive breast carcinoma among women diagnosed with ductal carcinoma in situ and lobular carcinoma in situ. Cancer 2006;106(10):2104–12.
6. Collaborative Group on Hormonal Factors in Breast Cancer. Familial breast cancer: collaborative reanalysis of individual data from 52 epidemiological studies including 58,209 women with breast cancer and 101,986 women without the disease. Lancet 2001;358(9291):1389–99.
7. Dershaw DD, Yahalom J, Petrek JA. Breast carcinoma in women previously treated for Hodgkin disease: mammographic evaluation. Radiology 1992;184(2):421–3.
8. Yahalom J, Petrek JA, Biddinger PW, et al. Breast cancer in patients irradiated for Hodgkin's disease: a clinical and pathological analysis of 45 events in 37 patients. J Clin Oncol 1992;10(11):1674–81.

9. Hancock SL, Tucker MA, Hoppe RT. Breast cancer after treatment of Hodgkin's disease. J Natl Cancer Inst 1993;85(1):25–31.

10. Bhatia S, Robison LL, Oberlin O, et al. Breast cancer and other second neoplasms after childhood Hodgkin's disease. N Engl J Med 1996;334(12):745–51.

11. Travis LB, Hill DA, Dores GM, et al. Breast cancer following radiotherapy and chemotherapy among young women with Hodgkin disease. JAMA 2003; 290(4):465–75.

12. Easton DF, Ford D, Bishop DT, et al. Breast and ovarian cancer incidence in BRCA1-mutation carriers. Am J Hum Genet 1995;56(1):265–71.

13. Ford D, Easton DF. The genetics of breast and ovarian cancer. Br J Cancer 1995;72(4):805–12.

14. Propeck PA, Warner T, Scanlan KA. Sebaceous carcinoma of the breast in a patient with Muir-Torre syndrome. AJR Am J Roentgenol 2000; 174(2):541–2.

15. Chen J, Lindblom A. Germline mutation screening of the STK11/LKB1 gene in familial breast cancer with LOH on 19p. Clin Genet 2000;57(5):394–7.

16. Srivastava A, McKinnon W, Wood ME. Risk of breast and ovarian cancer in women with strong family histories. Oncology (Williston Park) 2001; 15(7):889–902.

17. Antoniou A, Pharoah PD, Narod S, et al. Average risks of breast and ovarian cancer associated with BRCA1 or BRCA2 mutations detected in case series unselected for family history: a combined analysis of 22 studies. Am J Hum Genet 2003;72(5):1117–30.

18. Garber JE, Offit K. Hereditary cancer predisposition syndromes. J Clin Oncol 2005;23(2):276–92.

19. Newman BD, Maher JF, Subauste JS, et al. Clustering of sebaceous gland carcinoma, papillary thyroid carcinoma and breast cancer in a woman as a new cancer susceptibility disorder: a case report. J Med Case Reports 2009;3:6905.

20. Hobert JA, Eng C. PTEN hamartoma tumor syndrome: an overview. Genet Med 2009;11(10): 687–94.

21. Clements A, Robison K, Granai C, et al. A case of Peutz-Jeghers syndrome with breast cancer, bilateral sex cord tumor with annular tubules, and adenoma malignum caused by STK11 gene mutation. Int J Gynecol Cancer 2009;19(9):1591–4.

22. Boyd NF, Byng JW, Jong A, et al. Quantitative classification of mammographic densities and breast cancer risk: results from the Canadian National Breast Screening Study. J Natl Cancer Inst 1995;87(9):670–5.

23. Byrne C, Schairer C, Wolfe J, et al. Mammographic features and breast cancer risk: effects with time, age, and menopause status. J Natl Cancer Inst 1995;87:1622–9.

24. Ursin G, Ma H, Wu AH, et al. Mammographic density and breast cancer in three ethnic groups. Cancer Epidemiol Biomarkers Prev 2003;12(4):332–8.

25. Vacek PM, Geller BM. A prospective study of breast cancer risk using routine mammographic breast density measurements. Cancer Epidemiol Biomarkers Prev 2004;13(5):715–22.

26. Boyd NF, Martin LJ, Sun L, et al. Body size, mammographic density, and breast cancer risk. Cancer Epidemiol Biomarkers Prev 2006;15(11): 2086–92.

27. Boyd NF, Guo H, Martin LJ, et al. Mammographic density and the risk and detection of breast cancer. N Engl J Med 2007;356(3):227–36.

28. Tilanus-Linthorst MM, Kriege M, Boetes C, et al. Hereditary breast cancer growth rates and its impact on screening policy. Eur J Cancer 2005; 41(11):1610–7.

29. Kriege M, Brekelmans CTM, Boetes C, et al. Efficacy of MRI and mammography for breast-cancer screening in women with a familial or genetic predisposition. N Engl J Med 2004; 351(5):427–37.

30. Warner E, Plewes DB, Hill KA, et al. Surveillance of BRCA1 and BRCA2 mutation carriers with magnetic resonance imaging, ultrasound, mammography, and clinical breast examination. JAMA 2004;292(11):1317–25.

31. Leach MO, Boggis CRM, Dixon AK, et al. Screening with magnetic resonance imaging and mammography of a UK population at high familial risk of breast cancer: a prospective multicentre cohort study (MARIBS). Lancet 2005;365(9473):1769–78.

32. Kuhl CK, Schrading S, Leutner CC, et al. Mammography, breast ultrasound, and magnetic resonance imaging for surveillance of women at high familial risk for breast cancer. J Clin Oncol 2005;23(33): 8469–76.

33. Sardanelli F, Podo F, D'Agnolo G, et al. Multicenter comparative multimodality surveillance of women at genetic-familial high risk for breast cancer (HIBCRIT study): interim results. Radiology 2007; 242(3):698–715.

34. Hagen AI, Kvistad KA, Maehle L, et al. Sensitivity of MRI versus conventional screening in the diagnosis of BRCA-associated breast cancer in a national prospective series. Breast 2007;16(4): 367–74.

35. Riedl CC, Ponhold L, Flöry D, et al. Magnetic resonance imaging of the breast improves detection of invasive cancer, preinvasive cancer, and premalignant lesions during surveillance of women at high risk for breast cancer. Clin Cancer Res 2007;13(20):6144–52.

36. Robson M, Levin D, Federici M, et al. Breast conservation therapy for invasive breast cancer in

Ashkenazi women with BRCA gene founder mutations. J Natl Cancer Inst 1999;91(24):2112–7.

37. Foulkes WD, Chappuis PO, Wong N, et al. Primary node negative breast cancer in BRCA1 mutation carriers has a poor outcome. Ann Oncol 2000; 11(3):307–13.

38. Berg WA. Beyond standard mammographic screening: mammography at age extremes, ultrasound, and MR imaging. Radiol Clin North Am 2007;45(5):895–906.

39. Travis LB, Curtis RE, Boice JD Jr, et al. Second malignant neoplasms among long-term survivors of ovarian cancer. Cancer Res 1996;56(7):1564–70.

40. Lee JS, John EM, McGuire V, et al. Breast and ovarian cancer in relatives of cancer patients, with and without BRCA mutations. Cancer Epidemiol Biomarkers Prev 2006;15(2):359–63.

41. Berg WA. Tailored supplemental screening for breast cancer: what now and what next? AJR Am J Roentgenol 2009;192(2):390–9.

42. Gail MH, Brinton LA, Byar DP, et al. Projecting individualized probabilities of developing breast cancer for white females who are being examined annually. J Natl Cancer Inst 1989; 81(24):1879–86.

43. Claus EB, Risch N, Thompson WD. Autosomal dominant inheritance of early-onset breast cancer. Cancer 1994;73(3):643–51.

44. Berry DA, Iversen ES Jr, Gudbjartsson DF, et al. BRCAPRO validation, sensitivity of genetic testing of BRCA1/BRCA2, and prevalence of other breast cancer susceptibility genes. J Clin Oncol 2002; 20(11):2701–12.

45. Antoniou AC, Cunningham AP, Peto J, et al. The BOADICEA model of genetic susceptibility to breast and ovarian cancers: updates and extensions. Br J Cancer 2008;98(8):1457–66.

46. Tyrer J, Duffy SW, Cuzick J. A breast cancer prediction model incorporating familial and personal risk factors. Stat Med 2004;23(7):1111–30.

47. D'Orsi CJ, Bassett LW, Berg WA, et al. Breast imaging reporting and data system – mammography: ACR BI-RADS® – mammography. 4th edition. Reston (VA): American College of Radiology; 2003. p. 179–89.

48. D'Orsi CJ, Sickles EA, Bassett LW, et al. Breast imaging reporting and data system – mammography: ACR BI-RADS® – mammography. 5th edition. Reston (VA): American College of Radiology, in press.

49. Harbour R, Miller J. A new system for grading recommendations in evidence based guidelines. Br Med J 2001;323(7308):334–6.

50. Shapiro S, Venet W, Strax P, et al. Periodic screening for breast cancer: the health insurance plan project and its sequelae, 1963–1986. Baltimore (MD): Johns Hopkins University Press; 1988.

51. Alexander FE, Anderson TJ, Brown HK, et al. 14 years of follow-up from the Edinburgh randomised trial of breast-cancer screening. Lancet 1999; 353(9168):1903–8.

52. Tabár L, Vitak B, Chen HH, et al. The Swedish two-county trial twenty years later: updated mortality results and new insights from long-term follow-up. Radiol Clin North Am 2000;38(4):625–51.

53. Miller AB, To T, Baines CJ, et al. Canadian National Breast Screening Study-2: 13-year results of a randomized trial in women aged 50–59 years. J Natl Cancer Inst 2000;92(18):1490–9.

54. Nyström L, Andersson I, Bjurstam N, et al. Long-term effects of mammography screening: updated overview of the Swedish randomized trials. Lancet 2002;359(9310):909–19.

55. Miller AB, To T, Baines CJ. The Canadian National Breast Screening Study-1: breast cancer mortality after 11 to 16 years of follow-up. Ann Intern Med 2002;137(5 Part 1):305–12.

56. Otto SJ, Fracheboud J, Looman CWN, et al. Initiation of population-based mammography screening in Dutch municipalities and effect on breast-cancer mortality: a systematic review. Lancet 2003; 361(9367):1411–7.

57. Bjurstam N, Bjorneld L, Warwick J, et al. The Gothenburg breast screening trial. Cancer 2003; 97(10):2387–96.

58. Smith RA, Duffy SW, Gabe R, et al. The randomized trials of breast cancer screening: what have we learned? Radiol Clin North Am 2004;42(5):793–806.

59. Saslow D, Boetes C, Burke W, et al. American Cancer Society guidelines for breast screening with MRI as an adjunct to mammography. CA Cancer J Clin 2007;57(2):75–89.

60. Lehman CD, Smith RA. The role of MRI in breast cancer screening. J Natl Compr Canc Netw 2009; 7(10):1109–15.

61. Lee CH, Dershaw DD, Kopans D, et al. Breast cancer screening with imaging: recommendations from the Society of Breast Imaging and the ACR on the use of mammography, breast MRI, breast ultrasound, and other technologies for the detection of clinically occult breast cancer. J Am Coll Radiol 2010;7(1):18–27.

62. Jemal A, Siegel R, Ward E, et al. Cancer statistics, 2009. CA Cancer J Clin 2009;59(4):225–49.

63. Age-adjusted United States death rates by year (female breast - invasive cancer). SEER cancer statistics review 1975–2006. Available at: seer. cancer.gov/csr/1975_2006/results_single/sect_04_ table.08.pdf. Accessed December 20, 2009.

64. Sickles EA. Successful methods to reduce false-positive mammography interpretations. Radiol Clin North Am 2000;38(4):693–700.

65. Rothenberg LN, Feig SA, Haus AG, et al. A guide to mammography and other breast imaging

procedures: NCRP report no. 149. Bethesda (MD): National Council on Radiation Protection and Measurements; 2004. p. 252–66.

66. Kerlikowske K, Grady D, Barclay J, et al. Effect of age, breast density, and family history on the sensitivity of first screening mammography. JAMA 1996;276(1):33–8.

67. Rosenberg RD, Hunt WC, Williamson MR, et al. Effects of age, breast density, ethnicity, and estrogen replacement therapy on screening mammographic sensitivity and cancer stage at diagnosis: review of 183,134 screening mammograms in Albuquerque, New Mexico. Radiology 1998;209(2):511–8.

68. Pisano ED, Gatsonis C, Hendrick E, et al. Diagnostic performance of digital versus film mammography for breast-cancer screening. N Engl J Med 2005;353(17):1773–83.

69. Pisano ED, Hendrick RE, Yaffe MJ, et al. Diagnostic accuracy of digital versus film mammography: exploratory analysis of selected population subgroups in DMIST. Radiology 2008;246(2): 376–83.

70. Age distribution of incidence cancers (female breast - invasive). SEER cancer statistics review 1975–2006. Available at: seer.cancer.gov/csr/1975_2006/results_single/sect_01_table.10_2pgs.pdf. Accessed December 20, 2009.

71. Causer PA, Jong RA, Warner E, et al. Breast cancers detected with imaging screening in the BRCA population: emphasis on MR imaging with histopathologic correlation. Radiographics 2007; 27(Suppl 1):S165–82.

72. Brekelmans CTM, Seynaeve C, Bartels CCM, et al. Effectiveness of breast cancer surveillance in BRCA1/2 gene mutation carriers and women with high familial risk. J Clin Oncol 2001;19(4): 924–30.

73. Møller P, Borg Å, Evans DG, et al. Survival in prospectively ascertained familial breast cancer: analysis of a series stratified by tumour characteristics, BRCA mutations and oophorectomy. Int J Cancer 2002; 101(6):555–9.

74. Komenaka IK, Ditkoff B-A, Joseph K-A, et al. The development of interval breast malignancies in patients with BRCA mutations. Cancer 2004; 100(10):2079–83.

75. Berg WA, Zhang Z, Cormack JB, et al. Supplemental yield and performance characteristics of screening MRI after combined ultrasound and mammography: ACRIN 6666 American College of Radiology Imaging Network. In: Programs and abstracts of the 95th Scientific Assembly and Annual Meeting of the Radiological Society of North America. Chicago, November 29 to December 4, 2009. p. 103.

76. Bigenwald RZ, Warner E, Gunasekara A, et al. Is mammography adequate for screening women with inherited BRCA mutations and low breast density? Cancer Epidemiol Biomarkers Prev 2008; 17(3):706–11.

77. Rosenberg RD, Yankaskas BC, Abraham LA, et al. Performance benchmarks for screening mammography. Radiology 2006;241(1):55–66.

78. Miglioretti DL, Gard CC, Carney PA, et al. When radiologists perform best: the learning curve in screening mammogram interpretation. Radiology 2009;253(3):632–40.

79. Plevritis SK, Kurian AW, Sigal BM, et al. Cost-effectiveness of screening BRCA1/2 mutation carriers with breast magnetic resonance imaging. JAMA 2006;295(20):2374–84.

80. Sardanelli F, Podo F, Santoro F, et al. Compliance for mammography, ultrasound, and contrast-enhanced MRI during a multicenter surveillance of women at high risk for breast cancer. In: Programs and abstracts of the 95th Scientific Assembly and Annual Meeting of the Radiological Society of North America. Chicago, November 29 to December 4, 2009. p. 102.

81. Berg WA, Blume JD, Adams AM, et al. Reasons women at elevated risk of breast cancer refuse breast MR imaging screening: ACRIN 6666. Radiology 2010;254(1):79–87.

82. Berg WA. Rationale for a trial of screening breast ultrasound: American College of Radiology Imaging Network (ACRIN) 6666. AJR Am J Roentgenol 2003; 180(5):1225–8.

83. Berg WA, Blume JD, Cormack JB, et al. Combined screening with ultrasound and mammography vs mammography alone in women at elevated risk of breast cancer. JAMA 2008; 299(18):2151–63.

84. Berg WA, Zhang Z, Cormack JB, et al. Screening breast ultrasound as a supplement to mammography: yield of annual screening in ACRIN 6666 American College of Radiology Imaging Network. In: Programs and abstracts of the 95th Scientific Assembly and Annual Meeting of the Radiological Society of North America. Chicago, November 29 to December 4, 2009. p. 100–1.

85. Berg WA, Zhang Z, Marques H, et al. False positives induced by annual screening US added to mammography: ACRIN 6666 American College of Radiology Imaging Network. In: Programs and abstracts of the 95th Scientific Assembly and Annual Meeting of the Radiological Society of North America. Chicago, November 29 to December 4, 2009. p. 102.

86. Gordon PB, Goldenberg SL. Malignant breast masses detected only by ultrasound: a retrospective review. Cancer 1995;76(4):626–30.

87. Buchberger W, Niehoff A, Obrist P, et al. Clinically and mammographically occult breast lesions: detection and classification with high-resolution sonography. Semin Ultrasound CT MR 2000;21(4):325–36.

88. Kaplan SS. Clinical utility of bilateral whole-breast US in the evaluation of women with dense breast tissue. Radiology 2001;221(3):641–9.

89. Kolb TM, Lichy J, Newhouse JH. Comparison of the performance of screening mammography, physical examination, and breast US and evaluation of factors that influence them: an analysis of 27,825 patient evaluations. Radiology 2002; 225(1):165–75.

90. Leconte I, Feger C, Galant C, et al. Mammography and subsequent whole-breast sonography of nonpalpable breast cancers: the importance of radiologic breast density. AJR Am J Roentgenol 2003;180(6):1675–9.

91. Crystal P, Strano SD, Shcharynski S, et al. Using sonography to screen women with mammographically dense breasts. AJR Am J Roentgenol 2003; 181(1):177–82.

92. Corsetti V, Ferrari A, Ghirardi M, et al. Role of ultrasonography in detecting mammographically occult breast carcinoma in women with dense breasts. Radiol Med 2006;111(3):440–8.

93. Kelly KM, Dean J, Comulada WS, et al. Breast cancer detection using automated whole breast ultrasound and mammography in radiographically dense breasts. Eur Radiol 2010;20(3):734–42.

94. Ohuchi N, Suzuki A, Sakurai Y, et al. Current status and problems of breast cancer screening. Japan Medical Association Journal 2009;52(1):45–9.

95. Duffy SW, Day NE, Tabár L, et al. Markov models for breast tumor progression: estimates from empirical screening data and implications for screening. In: Programs and abstracts of the NIH Consensus Development Conference on Breast Cancer Screening for Women Ages 40–49. Bethesda (MD); 1997. p. 91–2.

96. Khalkhali I, Villanueva-Meyer J, Edell SL, et al. Diagnostic accuracy of ^{99m}Tc-sestamibi breast imaging: multicenter trial results. J Nucl Med 2000;41(12):1973–9.

97. Khalkhali I, Baum JK, Villanueva-Meyer J, et al. [99m]Tc sestamibi breast imaging for the examination of patients with dense and fatty breasts: multicenter study. Radiology 2002;222(1):149–55.

98. Brem RF, Floerke AC, Rapelyea JA, et al. Breast-specific gamma imaging as an adjunct imaging modality for the diagnosis of breast cancer. Radiology 2008;247(3):651–7.

99. Berg WA, Weinberg IN, Narayanan D, et al. High-resolution fluorodeoxyglucose positron emission tomography with compression ("positron emission mammography") is highly accurate in depicting primary breast cancer. Breast J 2006;12(4):309–23.

100. Brem RF, Rapelyea JA, Zisman G, et al. Occult breast cancer: scintimammography with high-resolution breast-specific gamma camera in women at high risk for breast cancer. Radiology 2005;237(1):274–80.

101. Chang CHJ, Sibala JL, Fritz SL, et al. Specific value of computed tomographic breast scanner (CT/M) in diagnosis of breast disease. Radiology 1979; 132(3):647–52.

102. Gisvold JJ, Reese DF, Karsell PR. Computed tomographic mammography (CTM). AJR Am J Roentgenol 1979;133(6):1143–9.

103. Lindfors KK, Boone JM, Nelson TR, et al. Dedicated breast CT: initial clinical experience. Radiology 2008;246(3):725–33.

104. Lindfors KK. Breast CT. In: Programs and abstracts of the 9th Postgraduate Course of the Society of Breast Imaging. Colorado Springs (CO), 2009.

105. Moskowitz M, Milbrath J, Gartside P, et al. Lack of efficacy of thermography as a screening tool for minimal and stage I breast cancer. N Engl J Med 1976;295(5):249–52.

106. Moskowitz M. Screening for breast cancer: how effective are our tests? A critical review. CA Cancer J Clin 1983;33(1):26–39.

107. Gisvold JJ, Brown LR, Swee RG, et al. Comparison of mammography and transillumination light scanning in the detection of breast lesions. AJR Am J Roentgenol 1986;147(1):191–4.

108. Monsees B, Destouet JM, Totty WG. Light scanning versus mammography in breast cancer detection. Radiology 1987;163(2):463–5.

109. Monsees B, Destouet JM, Gersell D. Light scan evaluation of nonpalpable breast lesions. Radiology 1987;163(2):467–70.

110. Poplack SP, Paulsen KD, Hartov A, et al. Electromagnetic breast imaging: average tissue property values in women with negative clinical findings. Radiology 2004;231(2):571–80.

111. Zheng B, Zuley ML, Sumkin JH, et al. Detection of breast abnormalities using a prototype resonance electrical impedance spectroscopy system: a preliminary study. Med Phys 2008;35(7):3041–8.

112. Pogue BW, Poplack SP, McBride TO, et al. Quantitative hemoglobin tomography with diffuse near-infrared spectroscopy: pilot results in the breast. Radiology 2001;218(1):261–6.

113. Meaney PM, Fanning MW, Raynolds T, et al. Initial clinical experience with microwave breast imaging in women with normal mammography. Acad Radiol 2007;14(2):207–18.

114. Poplack SP, Tosteson TD, Kogel CA, et al. Digital breast tomosynthesis: initial experience in 98 women with abnormal digital screening

mammography. AJR Am J Roentgenol 2007; 189(3):616–23.

115. Rafferty EA. Digital mammography: novel applications. Radiol Clin North Am 2007;45(5):831–43.

116. Gur D, Abrams GS, Chough DM, et al. Digital breast tomosynthesis: observer performance study. AJR Am J Roentgenol 2009;193(2): 586–91.

117. Yoshikawa MI, Ohsumi S, Sugata S, et al. Comparison of breast cancer detection by diffusion-weighted magnetic resonance imaging and mammography. Radiat Med 2007;25(5): 218–23.

118. Park MJ, Cha ES, Kang BJ, et al. The role of diffusion-weighted imaging and the apparent diffusion coefficient (ADC) values for breast tumors. Korean J Radiol 2007;8(5):390–6.

119. Bartella L, Morris EA, Dershaw DD, et al. Proton MR spectroscopy with choline peak as malignancy marker improves positive predictive value for breast cancer diagnosis: preliminary study. Radiology 2006;239(3):686–92.

120. Bartella L, Thakur SB, Morris EA, et al. Enhancing nonmass lesions in the breast: evaluation with proton (^{1}H) MR spectroscopy. Radiology 2007; 245(1):80–7.

121. Sardanelli F, Fausto A, Di Leo G, et al. In vivo proton spectroscopy of the breast using the total choline peak integral as a marker of malignancy. AJR Am J Roentgenol 2009;192(6):1608–17.

122. Tozaki M, Fukuma E. ^{1}H MR spectroscopy and diffusion-weighted imaging of the breast: are they useful tools for characterizing breast lesions before biopsy? AJR Am J Roentgenol 2009; 193(3):840–9.

123. McKnight AL, Kugel JL, Rossman PJ, et al. MR elastography of breast cancer: preliminary results. AJR Am J Roentgenol 2002;178(6):1411–7.

124. Itoh A, Ueno E, Tohno E, et al. Breast disease: clinical application of US elastography for diagnosis. Radiology 2006;239(2):341–50.

125. Ginat DT, Destounis SV, Barr RG, et al. US elastography of breast and prostate lesions. Radiographics 2009;29(7):2007–16.

Cost-Effectiveness of Mammography, MRI, and Ultrasonography for Breast Cancer Screening

Stephen Feig, MD

KEYWORDS

- Breast cancer • MRI • Mammography • Ultrasound

The cost-effectiveness of screening can be described using several different parameters: the *cost per breast cancer detected* is calculated by dividing the total cost of a screening program by the number of cancers detected. The program cost = (cost per mammogram + [cost × frequency of imaging workup for screen-detected abnormalities] + [cost × frequency of image-guided biopsy]) × number of women screened.

The *cost per breast cancer death averted* is calculated by (1) dividing screening program costs by the difference in breast cancer mortality between study and control groups found in randomized screening trials (RCTs), such as the Swedish Two-County Trial, or in service screening studies, such as the Swedish Seven-County Study[1,2] or (2) the expected differences in breast cancer deaths based on size and stage of detected tumors versus those in a comparable nonscreened population.

The *cost per year of life expectancy gained* is calculated by dividing the screening program costs by the expected number of years of life gained among screened women. The years of life gained through screening can be calculated by (1) subtracting the lifespan of patients with breast cancer in the control group from the lifespan of patients with breast cancer in the study group observed in RCT's or service screening studies or (2) expected gain in lifespan based on the size and stage of detected tumors versus those in comparable nonscreened population.

A cost analysis of the US National Breast and Cervical Cancer Early Detection Program found that in 2003 and 2004, the median cost of screening mammography was $94 and the cost per cancer detected was $10,566. For cervical cancer, these costs were $56 and $13,340, respectively. This program provides screening for medically underserved low-income women aged 40 to 64 years for breast cancer and aged 18 to 64 years for cervical cancer.[3]

Screening program costs depend on screening protocols. Annual screening finds most cancers earlier than biennial screening but doubles the cost.[4] Screening with craniocaudal and mediolateral oblique (MLO) mammographic views detects 3% to 11% (mean 7%) more cancers but is costlier than screening using bilateral MLO views alone.[5]

Digital mammography detects more cancers in women younger than 50 years with dense breasts but is more expensive than conventional mammography.[6,7] Tosteson and colleagues[7] estimated that substitution of digital mammography for film mammography is not cost-effective, because Medicare reimbursement for screening with digital mammography is 60% more than film mammography ($135.29 vs $85.65), and overall detection rates are not increased except in women with dense breasts. However, restricting digital screening mammography to women with dense breasts is neither practical for a breast imaging facility nor acceptable to most patients.

Department of Radiological Sciences, UC Irvine Medical Center, 101 The City Drive South, Orange, CA 92868, USA
E-mail address: sfeig@uci.edu

Radiol Clin N Am 48 (2010) 879–891
doi:10.1016/j.rcl.2010.06.002
0033-8389/10/$ – see front matter

SCREENING MAMMOGRAPHY

The cost per cancer detected is always lower in older populations, because screening detection rates parallel the natural cancer incidence, thus increasing with age. The cost per life saved and cost per year of life expectancy gained progressively decreases from age 40 years until age 70 years but then increases as a result of the lower normal life expectancy among older women. Assuming a 30% reduction in breast cancer mortality through annual screening mammography, Rosenquist and Lindfors[8] estimated that the cost per year of life expectancy saved was $26,000, $16,000, $15,000, $20,000, and $35,000 for women aged 40 to 49, 50 to 59, 60 to 69, 70 to 79, and 80 to 85 years at detection, respectively. Although population costs per year of life expectancy gained are higher for screening women in their 40s, the average woman with breast cancer detected by screening during that decade stands to gain more years of life expectancy than her older counterpart with breast cancer detected by screening during a later decade of life.

Many investigators have calculated the cost-effectiveness of screening women in their 40s. Their estimates have varied because of the different assumptions for benefits and costs and the different methods of calculation. Using data from the Breast Cancer Detection Demonstration Projects conducted in the United States in the 1970s, Moskowitz and Fox,[9,10] Eddy,[11] and Feig[12] independently derived estimates for the cost-effectiveness of screening women aged 40 to 49 years that were similar to or lower than those of Rosenquist and Lindfors. A study published by Salzmann and colleagues[13] in 1997 claiming that screening women aged 40 to 49 years is not cost-effective is no longer valid, because they used a 16% mortality reduction for screening women aged 40 to 49 years, which is too low.

Calculations by Rosenquist and Lindfors assumed a cost of $84 for a conventional mammogram in 1994 dollars. Current 2010 Medicare reimbursement is approximately $82 for conventional screening mammography and $130 for digital screening mammography. Recent service screening studies performed with conventional mammography have found a 40% to 45% mortality reduction for screened women aged 40 to 74 years.[2,14] However, even if the current costs per year of life expectancy saved are higher than those used by Rosenquist and Lindfors, they are still lower than the $100,000 per year of life threshold deemed to be acceptably cost-effective for other preventive medical procedures and tests.[15]

A subsequent study by Rosenquist and Lindfors estimated that annual screening mammography beginning at age 40 years and continuing until age 79 years would cost $18,800 per year of life expectancy saved.[16] The assumption for screening benefit in that study was that annual screening would reduce breast cancer deaths by 36% for cancers detected in women aged 40 to 49 years and by 45%, in women aged 50 to 79 years. Their estimate for the cost-effectiveness of screening mammography is in the same general range as that for other commonly accepted interventions, such as screening for cervical cancer and osteoporosis (**Table 1**). The cost per year of life gained from annual screening mammography is higher than that for screening for colorectal cancer but is much lower than that for the use of seat belts and airbags in automobiles.[17] Several other investigations found that annual and biennial screenings are cost-effective for all ages studied.[9,10,18,19] Annual screening is more effective but less cost-effective. Addition of computed-aided detection to the screening protocol increases the mean cost per year of life saved by 19% but is still within the accepted range for cost-effectiveness.[20]

COSTS OF SCREENING RECALL AND BIOPSY

In a low-cost screening project in Southern California in 1986 reported by Cyrlak,[21] the costs of screening mammograms accounted for less than one-third of total screening program costs, with diagnostic imaging workups, surgical consultations, and biopsies for benign disease representing the major induced costs of screening. In this study, 18% of women were recalled from screening for additional imaging workup or clinical evaluation. Among 72 biopsied patients, only 12 were found to have malignancy, that is, a biopsy positive predictive value (PPV) of 17% (12 of 72).

Screening costs can be reduced without sacrificing early detection if radiologists achieve the clinical outcome values recommended by the US Agency for Health Care Policy and Research (now renamed the Agency for Health Care Research and Quality).[22] These desirable values include a screening recall rate of 10% or less and a PPV when biopsy is recommended (PPV_2) of 25% to 40%. These values are further described in the American College of Radiology (ACR) Breast Imaging Reporting and Database (BI-RADS) Atlas.[23] A recent survey of screening results at Breast Cancer Surveillance Consortium (BCSC) sites throughout the United States found a mean recall rate of 9.7% (12.3% on initial screen and 8.8% in subsequent screens). This means that nearly half of all sites had recall rates higher than the recommended upper limit of 10%. Results from BCSC sites are believed to represent practice

Table 1
Median cost per life-year saved for annual mammographic screening of women aged 40 to 79 years and other selected types of lifesaving interventions

Intervention	Median Cost per Year of Life Saved ($)
Colorectal screening	3000
Cholesterol screening	6000
Cervical cancer screening	12,000
Antihypertensive drugs	15,000
Osteoporosis screening	18,000
Mammography screening	18,800
Coronary artery bypass surgery	26,000
Automobile seat belts and air bags	32,000
Hormone replacement therapy	42,000
Renal dialysis	46,000
Heart transplant	54,000
Cholesterol treatment	154,000

Data on non-mammographic interventions *from* Tengs TO, Adams M, Pliskin J, et al. Five hundred life-saving interventions and their cost-effectiveness. Risk Anal 1995;15:369–90.

Cost-effectiveness estimate for screening mammography *from* Rosenquist CJ, Lindfors KK. Screening mammography beginning at age 40 years: a reappraisal of cost-effectiveness. Cancer 1998;82:2235–40.

throughout the country. BCSC sites also reported that their PPV$_2$ at screening was 25.0%, just at the lower limit of the recommended range.[24] Radiologists having clinical outcome values that differ substantially from the recommended values should consider additional training to modify their interpretive thresholds.[25]

Screen-detected lesions appropriately categorized as probably benign (BI-RADS 3) should have a less than 2% likelihood of malignancy. These lesions may be safely followed up at 6 months, 12 months, and annually thereafter, rather than biopsied. Adoption of this concept over the past 20 years has reduced the number of false-positive biopsy results, a potentially large component of screening costs.[26] False-positive callbacks for additional mammographic views and/or ultrasonography are another potentially large component of screening costs.

Widespread implementation in the United States of image-guided core biopsy instead of open surgical biopsy has occurred since 1990. At most facilities, these biopsies now represent of the majority for screen-detected lesions.[27–29] Costs of image-guided core biopsy are 16% to 33% of those for an open excisional biopsy.[30–37] Use of needle core biopsy instead of surgical biopsy can reduce the cost per year of life saved by screening by 23% ($20,770 to $15,934).[38]

In contrast with the screening program conducted in Southern California in 1986,[21] the one conducted in New Hampshire a decade later

showed that 68% of its costs were from screening and only 32% of the costs were from consequent diagnostic imaging, biopsy, and surgical consultation.[39] This probably reflects a lower screening callback rate, substitution of short-term follow-up of probably benign lesions for biopsy, image-guided core biopsy instead of surgical biopsy for initial histologic diagnosis, and fewer surgical consults. Results from the 1996 to 2000 study of Poplack and colleagues[39] are similar to contemporary studies by Lidbrink and colleagues[40] and Elmore and colleagues[41] in which additional costs of evaluating false-positive results can add up to one-third of the total cost of screening all women.

Yet, even during the years 1996 to 2000, excisional biopsies represented 65% of all diagnostic costs versus 31% for stereotactic and ultrasound-guided biopsies.[29] It has been estimated that more than one million breast biopsies are performed in the United States yearly, but fewer than 25% prove to be malignant. Use of image-guided core biopsies instead of open surgical biopsies for all lesions would be equivalent to a cost reduction of about $1.5 billion.[42]

SCREENING MAMMOGRAPHY RESULTS, GUIDELINES, AND CONTROVERSIES: ROLE OF COST-EFFECTIVENESS

Screening controversies have been recurrent since 1975, when screening began to be widely used in the United States. With long-term follow-up, screening trials have demonstrated convincingly greater proof of benefit. Since 1997, annual screening for all women aged 40 years and older has been recommended by the American Cancer Society (ACS) and the ACR.[43,44] Currently, about 51% of all women in this age group report that they have had a mammogram in the past year and 67%, in the past 2 years.[45] The most recent screening controversy erupted in November 2009 with the publication of a series of papers in the Annals of Internal Medicine accompanied by issuance of new screening guidelines from the United States Preventive Services Task Force (USPSTF).[46–48]

The new USPSTF guidelines advise against any screening for women in their 40s except for those at very high risk.[46] Gross underestimation of the benefits for screening women in their 40s and unwarranted concern regarding callbacks and false-positive biopsy results in that age group were used as justification.[48] The USPSTF underestimated the mortality reduction for women offered screening in their 40s as 15%, rather than the 30% shown in the Swedish randomized trials.[49] More correctly, the benefit from service screening of women aged 40 to 49 years should be 48%, as found in the Swedish Two-County Study, 40%, in the British Columbia study, and/or 30%, in the study in 2 Northern Swedish counties.[2,14,50] The USPSTF then arbitrarily determined that the number needed to invite (NNI) to screening in their 40s to prevent one death from breast cancer was too small to justify screening average-risk women in that age group. Although monetary cost of screening was not mentioned per se in their report, it is clear that NNI is a code word for financial cost-effectiveness.

The USPSTF should not have included results from the National Breast Screening Study of Canada (NBSS) in the 40- to 49-year and 50- to 59-year age group estimates because of major problems in design and execution of the NBSS.[50] Because of a fatal flaw in the NBSS protocol, women presenting with late-stage breast cancer to screening centers were preferentially enrolled in the NBSS study group rather than being equally enrolled in study and control groups. This resulted in an excess of late-stage breast cancers and breast cancer deaths in the study group. Additionally, NBSS mammograms were often technically deficient, even by the standards of the 1980s, when the trial was conducted, a conclusion confirmed by numerous outside consultants invited by NBSS to evaluate mammographic image quality.[51] If the USPSTF had not included NBSS results in their meta-analysis, their calculated mortality reduction among 39- to 59-year-old women would have been 26% to 30% instead of 15%.

A second major change in screening recommendations was directed at women aged 50 to 75 years,[47] where the USPSTF recommended biennial instead of annual screening. Their rationale for less frequent screening of older women was their estimate that biennial screening could achieve 81% (range 67%–99%) of the benefit of annual screening while halving the number of mammograms and biopsies.[48] The USPSTF ignored other mathematical models, such as the one by Michaelson and colleagues,[52] which estimate that annual screening will double the benefit of biennial screening. Again, cost seems to be the unspoken rationale for their recommendations.

Reduced Treatment Costs Through Detection of Earlier Disease

It is well established that the costs of initial care, continuing care, and terminal care for patients with breast cancer increase according to the stage at diagnosis. Treatment and management costs become progressively greater for in situ, local, regional, and distant metastatic breast cancer.[53] A 4-year follow-up study by Legoretta and colleagues[54] of 200 women with newly diagnosed breast cancer in 1989 among 180,000 women enrolled in a health maintenance organization in Southeastern Pennsylvania found that the mean cumulative costs for stage 0, I, II, and stages III and IV were $18,900, $23,200, $28,800, and $55,000, respectively.[54] Of the total cohort of 200 patients, 116 (58%) were initially detected through mammographic screening. Among these screening-detected cancers, 74% (n = 86) were stage 0 or I; 24% (n = 28), stage II; and 2% (n = 2), stage III or IV. Among the 84 nonscreened patients with breast cancer, 31% (n = 26) were stage 0 or I; 52% (n = 44), stage II; and 17% (n = 14), stage III or IV. The mean cumulative treatment costs over 4 years were $31,000 for patients with breast cancer who had not undergone screening and $23,000 for those who had.

Several studies have compared the cost of screening with the savings from decreased treatment costs. In a Norwegian service screening program, breast cancer mortality was reduced by 30% among women offered screening biennially between ages 50 and 69 years. Norum[55] estimated that 33% of the screening costs were offset by the consequent lower treatment costs. Another screening program in Nijmegan and Utrecht in the Netherlands also offered biennial screening to women aged 50 to 70 years beginning in the late 1980s.[56] Breast cancer deaths were initially reduced by 12% at an attendance rate of 70%. Van der Maas and colleagues[19] also found that 33% of the cost of screening was offset by the decreased need for advanced care. In a longer-term follow-up analysis, de Koning and colleagues[57] found that breast cancer mortality reduction was 23%. After program start-up costs had ended, as much as 47% of the remaining annual program cost was offset by the lower cost of treatment.[57–59]

A study at the Jackson Memorial Hospital/ University of Miami by Zavertnik and colleagues[60] compared stage of disease, 5-year survival rates, and treatment costs before and after implementation of a screening mammography program in Dade County Florida in 1987. Comparing 1990 with 1983 to 1988, the frequency of in situ disease increased from 2.7% to 33.3% and local disease, from 30.4% to 38.1%; whereas regional disease decreased from 46.2% to 28.6% and distant metastatic disease, from 20.7% to 0%. The 5-year survival rate increased from 50% to 74%. Treatment costs were $5000 per case for in situ, local, and regional disease and $80,000 per case for distant and recurrent disease. The total cost for screening and treatment in the early detection program was $2,424,532. The estimated cost of treatment without the screening program was $2,594,029. Thus, the investigators calculated that the screening program saved $169,497 ($2,594,029 − $2,424,532), a savings of $14.28 per mammogram performed or $2872.83 per patient whose breast cancer was diagnosed and treated. Even greater improvement in stage at diagnosis was reported after 1990, equivalent to savings of $46.89 per mammogram performed or $9745.83 per patient whose cancer was diagnosed and treated.

In a similar type study, Glenn[61] used Brooke Army Medical Center (BAMC) patient data and Department of Defense Tumor Registry data to compare breast cancer staging distribution at BAMC during the period before 1980 when there was no screening and 1994 to 1995 when there was increased screening. Costs of treatment for each stage were calculated using 1994 current procedural terminology and diagnosis-related group codes in the BAMC Medical Expense Reporting System (MEPRS). A theoretical population of 100,000 women with 500 breast cancers per year was assumed. The total cost of breast care, including screening, workup, diagnosis, and treatment, was $16.6 million for no screening (pre-1980) versus $10.5 million for the 1994 to 1995 screening years. The total cost per patient was $166 for no screening (pre-1980) versus $105 for the 1994 to 1995 screening years. The investigator

concluded that cost-efficient screening involves high front-end costs, but these are more than offset in the long run by dollars saved through lower treatment costs.

Using breast cancer detection rates and mortality reduction results from the Health Insurance Plan of New York (HIP) randomized trial, which screened women aged 40 to 64 years with annual mammography and clinical examination in the 1960s, Moskowitz[62] applied 1987 screening and treatment costs to compare the total costs for 65,000 screens performed at HIP versus no screening.[11] Screening costs included mammography, time off from work to attend screening, and induced costs, such as ultrasonography, additional mammography, aspiration, and false-positive biopsy results. When the costs avoided were limited to those for treatment of more advanced disease for the 37 women whose lives were saved through screening, these costs were $2,220,000 compared with screening costs of $4,072,200. However, when the avoided costs also included costs for short-term disability, long-term disability, and employee replacement, the total cost of not screening was $5,570,160, thus, far exceeding the costs of screening. Therefore, the net effect on a health-care system engendered by the HIP screening program using 1987 costs would be a gain of about $1,497,960 ($5,570,160 − $4,072,200). Strictly speaking, cost-effectiveness compares the costs for a given intervention with the costs of no intervention.[62] When the ratio of the cost of the intervention is less than one, it is clearly cost-effective. The cost-effectiveness ratio calculated by Moskowitz[62] for HIP screening was 0.73. Strictly speaking, the cost per death averted and the cost per year of life gained are measures of cost-benefit rather than cost-effectiveness. Using 1987 costs, Moskowitz found that the cost per year of life saved in HIP was $3770.[11]

MAGNETIC RESONANCE IMAGING SCREENING OF VERY HIGH-RISK WOMEN: RESULTS AND GUIDELINES

Unlike mammography, no randomized trial has ever been conducted to evaluate whether magnetic resonance imaging (MRI) screening can reduce breast cancer mortality. However, since 2004, 9 nonoverlapping series with a total of 4485 very high-risk women screened with mammography and MRI found that 36% (70 of 192) of cancers were detected by mammography and an additional 56% (108 of 192) were identified only by MRI for a combined screening sensitivity of 92.7% (4157 of 4485).[63–71] Eligibility criteria for these trials were largely a projected lifetime risk of 20% to 25% or the presence of BRCA1 or 2 mutation in the patient or a first-degree relative.[72]

On the basis of these trial results, in 2007, the ACS recommended annual screening MRI as a supplement to annual screening mammography for women at very high risk of breast cancer.[73]

These included women who:

- BRCA1 or 2 mutation or are untested first-degree relatives of a BRCA carrier
- lifetime risk of 20% to 25% or more using a breast cancer risk model, such as BRCAPRO(BRCA probability), Tyrer-Cuzick, BOADICEA(Breast and Ovarian Analysis of Disease Incidence and Carrier Estimation Algorithm), Gail, or Claus.

Based on expert consensus opinion, the ACS also recommended annual mammography and annual MRI screening for the following women:

- History of receiving radiation to the chest between age 10 and 30 years, usually for treatment of Hodgkin disease
- Those with Li-Fraumeni, Cowden, or Bannayen-Riley-Ruvalcaba syndromes or their first-degree relatives.

The ACS found insufficient evidence to recommend or not recommend annual MRI for women having a lifetime risk of 15% to 20% or those at increased risk because of biopsy-proven lobular carcinoma in situ (LCIS); atypical lobular hyperplasia (ALH); atypical ductal hyperplasia (ADH); heterogeneously or extremely dense breasts on mammography; or their personal history of invasive carcinoma or in situ ductal carcinoma (DCIS). The ACS recommended against screening MRI for women at less than 15% lifetime risk.

In 2008, the National Comprehensive Cancer Network recommended that women with BRCA1 or 2 mutation begin screening MRI at age 25 years.[74]

In 2010, the Society of Breast Imaging and the American College of Radiology made the following recommendations for screening high-risk women[75]:

- BRCA1 or 2 carriers or their first-degree relatives should begin annual mammography and annual MRI by age 30 years but not before 25 years
- Women with a 20% or higher lifetime risk of breast cancer should begin annual mammography and annual MRI by age 30 years (but not before 20 years) or 10 years before the age that their youngest affected

first-degree relative developed breast cancer, whichever is later.

- Women having a history of chest irradiation between ages 10 and 30 years should begin annual mammography and annual MRI eight years after treatment but not before age 25 years.
- For women with a history of breast cancer (invasive cancer or DCIS), ovarian cancer, biopsy-proven lobular neoplasia (ALH or LCIS), or ADH, annual mammography and annual MRI should also be considered from the time of diagnosis.

MRI SCREENING OF VERY HIGH-RISK WOMEN: COST-EFFECTIVENESS

Several studies have evaluated the cost-effectiveness of screening MRI. Plevritis and colleagues[76] estimated that the cost per quality-adjusted life year (QALY) for annual screening with mammography and MRI relative to screening with mammography alone between ages 35 and 54 years was $55,420 for women with a BRCA1 mutation and $130,695, for BRCA2. For women with dense breasts, estimated cost per QALY was $41,183 for BRCA1 carriers and $98,454 for BRCA2. Higher cancer rates and more aggressive cancers in BRCA1 compared with BRCA2 carriers and lower sensitivity of mammography in women with dense breasts can explain these differences.

A recent study by Lee and colleagues[77] compared 3 different annual screening strategies starting at age 25 years for a BRCA1 carrier: combined screening with mammography and MRI, MRI alone, and mammography alone. Compared with an estimated 533 breast cancer deaths among 1000 women having clinical surveillance alone, the estimated number of breast cancer deaths was 446 for mammography alone, 438 for MRI alone, and 415 for MRI and mammography combined. Although combined screening was the most effective in reducing deaths, it had the slightly higher cost at $110,973 per QALY compared with $108,641 and $100,336 per QALY for screening with MRI alone and mammography alone, respectively.

MRI SCREENING OF MODERATELY HIGH-RISK WOMEN: COST-EFFECTIVENESS

Using results from the Magnetic Resonance Imaging Breast Screening Study (MARIBS) conducted in the UK, Griebsch and colleagues[78] found that the incremental cost of adding MRI screening to mammographic screening for women having a 50% likelihood of BRCA1 or 2 was $50,911 per cancer detected. For known mutation carriers, the cost was $27,544 per cancer detected. A further analysis of the UK MRI screening data found that the incremental cost of screening 40- to 49-year-old women with mammography and MRI versus mammography alone was $14,005 per QALY for a BRCA carrier having a 31% ten-year breast cancer risk. For 40- to 49-year-old non-BRCA carriers, the cost per QALY was $53,320 and $96,379 for those with a 12% and 6% ten-year risk, respectively. For 30- to 39-year-old women, the incremental cost was $24,275 for BRCA1 carriers (10-year risk of 11%) and $70,054 for high-risk non-BRCA carriers (10-year risk of 5%).[78] These estimates were based on costs within the UK National Health Service. Current UK policy is to offer screening MRI to women aged 30 to 39 years at familial risk, having a 10-year risk of more than 8%. For women aged 40 to 49 years, screening MRI is offered to those at a 10-year risk of 20% or more. For women aged 40 to 49 years with dense breasts having lower mammographic sensitivity, screening MRI is offered to those with a 10-year risk of 12% or more.[79]

A model to evaluate the cost-effectiveness of screening high-risk women with MRI and mammography versus mammography alone was developed by Taneja and colleagues.[80] These investigators estimated that among 10,000 women age 40 years with BRCA1 or 2 mutations, 400 (4% prevalence) would have clinically undiagnosed breast cancer. Among these, 361 would be detected by MRI and mammography combined, 290 by MRI alone, and 160 by mammography alone. For these women, the incremental cost per QALY gained through screening with MRI and mammography versus mammography alone was estimated at $25,270. For non-BRCA women with an annual breast cancer prevalence of 3%, 2%, or 1%, the incremental cost per QALY gained was calculated as $73,813, $154,045, and $315,210, respectively. The authors concluded that MRI is cost-effective for BRCA carriers and also for other very high-risk women, albeit at the higher end ($100,000) of the generally accepted range for those with a prevalence of 2.5% to 3.0%.

IMPACT OF RISK ASSESSMENT MODELS AND FUTURE TECHNICAL ADVANCES ON COST-EFFECTIVENESS OF MRI SCREENING

Because the cost of MRI is more than $1000 compared with about $100 for mammography, accurate determination of individual breast cancer risk is essential for a cost-effective MRI screening program. By age 70 years, the lifetime risk of breast cancer is 65% for BRCA1 carriers and 45% for BRCA2 carriers[81] compared with a cumulative lifetime risk of 12% by age 80 years for a woman with no known risk factors.[82] All current risk models are inaccurate for predicting breast cancer risk for the vast majority of women, who are non-BRCA carriers. The prevalence of BRCA1 mutations is estimated to be between 1:500 and 1:1000 in the general population.[83] The ACS estimated the lifetime risk for 5 hypothetical women using 3 risk models: BRCAPRO, Claus, and Tyrer-Cuzick to determine whether they met the 20% or greater lifetime risk level set by ACS MRI screening guidelines.[73] Among them, 2 women qualified according to only one of the 3 models; 2, according to two of the 3 models; and only one, according to all 3 models.[73] According to Amir and colleagues,[84] risk models may underestimate risk by as much as 50% in observed populations. Using women from their own practice, these investigators found that the ratios of expected to observed breast cancers were 0.48 for the Gail model, 0.56 for the Claus model, 0.49 for the Ford model, and 0.81 for the Tyrer-Cuzick model. Although the Tyrer-Cuzick model was more accurate than the other 3 models, it underestimated risk by 19%.[84]

Compared with a woman with no known risk factor, the relative risk of developing breast cancer is increased in women with: a personal history of breast cancer (8–10x overall; 3–4x for a second primary)[85,86]; two or more family members with breast cancer (2.9x)[82]; a mother diagnosed before age 50 years (2.4x)[87]; a sister diagnosed before age 50 years (3.2x)[87]; a personal history of biopsy-proven LCIS (8–12x),[88] ADH (4–5x),[89] or ALH (3x)[90]; and dense breasts on mammography (4–6x).[91] Development of a single model to more accurately predict breast cancer risk through incorporation of all of these family and personal risk factors is much needed. Conducting clinical studies to determine MRI-only detection rates for women in the 15% to 20% lifetime risk group is also needed. Such data could be used to better determine the cost-effectiveness of MRI for each projected risk level. It has also been suggested by Berg[92] that 10-year risk may be more accurate than lifetime risk.

In the future, evolving MRI techniques, such as diffusion-weighted imaging, spectroscopy, and noncontrast perfusion imaging might reduce examination time and eliminate the need for intravenous contrast injection, so that breast MRI could be performed faster and at lower cost.[93] If successful, these techniques would improve the cost-effectiveness of MRI and allow cost-effective screening of greater numbers of women.

SCREENING ULTRASONOGRAPHY: TARGET POPULATIONS

Among the 9 series of very high-risk women screened with MRI and mammography, 4 also included ultrasonography. These 4 series found that the sensitivity of mammography and ultrasonography combined was only 52%, compared with a 92.7% sensitivity for mammography and MRI combined.[64,67–69] This observation that the sensitivity of MRI is much higher than that of ultrasonography is substantiated by the clinical experience that most MRI-detected cancers cannot be localized for ultrasound-guided biopsy but require MRI-guided biopsy instead.[94]

The main indication for screening ultrasonography is women with dense fibroglandular breast tissue in whom mammographic detection rates are lower.

Although ultrasonography is a less sensitive screening examination than MRI, combined screening with mammography and ultrasonography has been found to substantially increase detection rates beyond those from mammography alone. The lower sensitivity of mammography for cancer detection in dense breasts first noted in the 1970s[95] persists to a lesser degree in more recent studies.[96–101] Dense breasts, usually defined as breasts having 50% or greater dense tissue, are more common among younger women. The prevalence of dense breasts among women age 30 to 39, 40 to 49, 50 to 59, and 60 to 69 was found to be 62%, 56%, 38%, and 27%, respectively by Stomper and colleagues.[102] Thus, the number of women with dense breasts who might benefit from supplementary screening with breast ultrasonography far exceeds the estimated 1.4 million American women who would qualify for supplementary screening with breast MRI according to ACS MRI screening guidelines.[73]

NONBLINDED ULTRASONOGRAPHIC SCREENING TRIALS

Between 1995 and 2003, 42,836 women with generally dense breast tissue were screened with mammography and ultrasonography using hand-held high-resolution transducers (7.5–10.0 MHz) in 6 published series.[103–110] Interpretations were nonblinded to those of the other modality. A review of these studies by Feig[111] found that cancer detection rates with ultrasonography alone ranged from 2.7 to 9.0 per 1000 (mean = 3.5 per 1000). Mean tumor size was 1.0 cm for ultrasonography-only lesions. PPVs for biopsies and aspirations performed by ultrasonography alone ranged from 6.6% to 18.0% (mean = 11.4%). For 4 series that separately analyzed results for core biopsies of solid lesions, PPV for ultrasonography alone ranged from 11.8% to 20.5%. The detection rate of 3.5 per 1000 for ultrasonography alone is extremely encouraging because at BCSC Centers considered generally representative of clinical practice in the United States, the detection rate at mammographic screening is 4.4 per 1000 examinations.[24] The mean tumor size of 1.0 cm for ultrasonography-only cancers is also encouraging because it more than fulfills the US Agency for Health Care Policy and Research (AHCPR) recommendation that 30% or more of mammographic screening-detected cancers be minimal (<1 cm invasive or DCIS) and that 50% or more be Stage 0 or I.[112] However, because AHCPR recommends a PPV_2 of 25% to 40% for screening mammography, the frequency of false-positive biopsies for ultrasonography-only lesions is greater than that expected for screening mammography.[112,113]

BLINDED ULTRASONOGRAPHIC SCREENING TRIALS

Because nonblinded studies may be subject to reader bias, the ACR Imaging Network (ACRIN) initiated ACRIN Trial 6666 to determine if results from the prior 6 nonblinded ultrasonographic screening studies could be duplicated under a more scientifically rigorous protocol. Radiologist readers of mammography and ultrasonography were each masked to results from the other modality. Following initial screening of 2809 very high-risk women having dense breasts, Berg and colleagues[114] diagnosed 41 cancers: 12 on mammography alone, 12 on ultrasonography alone, 8 on mammography and ultrasonography, and 9 on neither modality. The diagnostic yield was 7.6 cancers per 1000 women on mammography versus 11.8 cancers per 1000 women for combined screening with mammography and ultrasonography, for a supplementary yield of 4.2 cancers per 1000 women. Although the 95% confidence interval was wide, 1.1 to 7.2 per 1000, the results of this study suggest that among women with dense breasts, supplementary ultrasonographic screening is associated with a 50% increase in cancer detection. Median size of ultrasonography-detected cancers was 1 cm. The study also confirms findings from prior studies that false-positive biopsy rates are higher on ultrasonography than on mammography. At ACRIN 6666, the PPV_2 was 8.9% for ultrasonography versus 22.6% for mammography and 11.2% for combined ultrasonographic and mammographic screening.

The value of screening ultrasonography was further corroborated in another blinded study of hand-held ultrasonography by Corsetti and colleagues[115] in Italy. An initial negative mammographic assessment was confirmed at subsequent review by 4 internal radiologists and an external expert radiologist. Among 9157 women with negative mammographic assessments and dense breasts, ultrasonography alone found 4.0 cancers per 1000 women. The overall incremental cancer detection rate for ultrasonography was 20.6% for all women, 41.3% for those younger than 50 years, and 13.5% for those older than 50 years. This study suggests that the most cost-effective strategy would result from using ultrasonography as a supplementary screening modality in younger women with dense breasts. Among cancers detected by ultrasonography alone by Corsetti and colleagues, 65% were less than 1 cm and 27% were 1 to 2 cm. The proportion of minimal cancers (invasive <1 cm or DCIS) was higher for detection by ultrasonography alone than for mammographic detection: 65% versus 36%. PPV for ultrasonography-only biopsies was 37.5%, much higher than in the other ultrasonography screening studies. Corsetti and colleagues estimated that the cost per cancer detected by ultrasonography alone was $18,900 to $19,760, higher than the cost of $6350 per mammography-detected cancer. This higher cost of ultrasonography is because it increased the detection rate by 20.6% while approximately doubling the overall cost of screening.

AUTOMATED ULTRASONOGRAPHIC SCREENING

The length of time for the US screening examination is another limitation and was clocked at 19 minutes in the ACRIN trial, moderately higher than the estimated examination times in other studies of ultrasonographic screening performed using hand-held transducers. Thus, total radiologist time for performance, interpretation, and report dictation for ultrasonographic screening could be 25 to 30 minutes. By comparison, the time for interpretation of screening mammography was measured as 5 minutes by Enzmann and colleagues.[116] Screening with hand-held ultrasonography performed by a radiologist may be a time-consuming and expensive endeavor and would lose money for a facility at the current Medicare reimbursement rate of $80 for diagnostic ultrasonography. More importantly, neither Medicare nor most other insurers currently pay for screening ultrasonography. Radiologist staff shortages are another consideration, because a radiologist may be able to complete only 2 to 3 hand-held ultrasonographic screening examinations per hour versus interpretation of 20 to 50 screening mammograms per hour depending on whether automatic reporting systems are used.

One way to decrease the cost of breast ultrasonographic screening would be through the use of an automated whole-breast ultrasound scanner (ABUS). Potential advantages would be elimination of a radiologist or even an ultrasonography technologist to perform the study, standardization of an examination that is notoriously operator-dependant, and reduction in examination time. Several automated ultrasound scanners have been developed and are under clinical investigation.[117] In one study of automated breast ultrasonography, Kelly and colleagues[118] screened 6425 women with dense breasts and/or elevated risk of breast cancer. In this nonblinded study, ultrasonography alone found a prevalence of 3.6 cancers per 1000 women, similar to that in studies performed with hand-held units. Among cancers detected by ultrasonography alone, 64% were 1 cm or less and 91% were 2 cm or less, generally smaller sizes than found with mammographic screening at the BCSC.[24] Biopsy PPV for ABUS was 38.4%, higher than that for the ACRIN trial and similar to the 39.0% PPV for mammography in the ABUS population. The use of ABUS as a supplementary screening modality doubled the cancer detection rate from 3.6 per 1000 for mammography alone to 7.2 per 1000 for combined screening. At these incremental detection rates and at a cost of $300 per screening with ultrasonographic examination used by the investigators, ABUS would be only one-third as cost-effective as mammography but still within the generally acceptable range for cost-effectiveness and currently more cost-effective than MRI for most populations.

SUMMARY

Screening mammography performed annually on all women beginning at age 40 years has reduced breast cancer deaths by 30% to 50%. The cost per year of life saved is well within the range for other commonly accepted medical interventions. Various studies have estimated that reduction in treatment costs through early screening detection may be 30% to 100% or more of the cost of screening. MRI screening is also cost-effective for very high-risk women, such as BRCA carriers, and others at 20% or greater lifetime risk. Further studies are needed to determine whether MRI is cost-effective for those at moderately high (15%–20%) lifetime risk. Future technical advances could make MRI more cost-effective than it is today.

Automated whole breast ultrasonography will probably prove cost-effective as a supplement to mammography for women with dense breasts.

REFERENCES

1. Tabar L, Vitak B, Chen H-H, et al. The Swedish Two County Trial twenty years later. Radiol Clin North Am 2000;38:625–52.
2. Tabar L, Yen M-F, Vitak B, et al. Mammography service screening and mortality in breast cancer patients: 20-year follow-up before and after introduction of screening. Lancet 2003;361: 1405–10.
3. Ekwueme DU, Gardner JG, Subramanian S, et al. Cost analysis of the National Breast and Cervical Cancer Early Detection Program, selected states, 2003–2004. Cancer 2008;112:626–35.
4. Feig SA. Increased benefit from shorter screening mammography intervals for women ages 40–49 years. Cancer 1997;80:2035–9.
5. Feig SA. Estimation of currently attainable benefit from mammographic screening of women aged 40–49 years. Cancer 1995;75:2412–9.
6. Pisano ED, Gatsonis C, Hendrick E, et al. Diagnostic performance of digital versus film mammography for breast-cancer screening. N Engl J Med 2005;353:1773–83.
7. Tosteson AN, Stout NK, Fryback DG, et al. Cost-effectiveness of digital mammography in breast cancer screening. Ann Intern Med 2008;148:1–10.
8. Rosenquist CJ, Lindfors KK. Screening mammography in women aged 40–49 years: analysis of cost-effectiveness. Radiology 1994;191:647–50.
9. Moskowitz M, Fox SH. Cost analysis of aggressive breast cancer screening. Radiology 1979; 130:253–6.
10. Moskowitz M. Costs of screening for breast cancer. Radiol Clin North Am 1987;25:1031–7.
11. Eddy DM. Screening for breast cancer. Ann Intern Med 1989;111:389–99.
12. Feig SA. Mammographic screening of women aged 40–49 years: benefit, risk, and cost considerations. Cancer 1995;76:2097–106.
13. Salzmann P, Kerlikowske K, Phillips K. Cost-effectiveness of screening mammography of women aged 40–49 years of age. Ann Intern Med 1997; 127:955–65.
14. Coldman A, Phillips N, Warren L, et al. Breast cancer mortality after screening mammography in British Columbia women. Int J Cancer 2006;120: 1076–80.
15. Gold M, Siegel J, Russell L, et al. Cost-effectiveness in health and medicine. New York: Oxford University Press; 1996.
16. Rosenquist CJ, Lindfors KK. Screening mammography beginning at age 40 years: a reappraisal of cost-effectiveness. Cancer 1998;82:2235–40.
17. Tengs TO, Adams M, Pliskin J, et al. Five hundred life-saving interventions and their cost-effectiveness. Risk Anal 1995;15:369–90.
18. Brown ML. Sensitivity analysis in the cost-effectiveness of breast cancer screening. Cancer 1992;69:1963–7.
19. Van der Maas PJ, de Koning HJ, Van Inveld M, et al. The cost-effectiveness of breast cancer screening. Int J Cancer 1989;43:1055–60.
20. Lindfors KK, McGahan MC, Rosenquist CJ, et al. Computer aided detection: a cost-effective study. Radiol 2006;238:710–7.
21. Cyrlak D. Induced costs of low-cost screening mammography. Radiology 1988;168:661–3.
22. Bassett LW, Hendrick RG, Bassford TL, et al. Clinical practice guidelines number 13: quality determinants of mammography. Rockwell (MD): US Department of Health and Human Services; 1999. p. 83.
23. D'Orsi CJ, Bassett LW, Berg WA, et al. Breast imaging reporting and data system: ACR BI-RADS. 4th edition. Reston (VA): American College of Radiology; 2003. p. 229–51.
24. Rosenberg RD, Yankaskas BC, Abraham LA, et al. Performance benchmarks for screening mammography. Radiology 2006;241:55–66.
25. Carney PA, Sickles EA, Monsees B, et al. Identifying minimally acceptable interpretive performance criteria for screening mammography. Radiology 2010;255:354–61.
26. Leung JWT, Sickles EA. The probably benign assessment. Radiol Clin North Am 2007;45:773–90.
27. March DE, Raslavicus A, Coughlin BF, et al. Use of core biopsy in the United States. Am J Roentgenol 1997;169:697–701.
28. Zannis VJ, Aliano KM. The evolving practice pattern of the breast surgeon with disappearance of open biopsy for nonpalpable lesions. Am J Surg 1998;176:525–8.
29. Crowe JP, Rim A, Patrick R, et al. A prospective review of the decline of excisional breast biopsy. Am J Surg 2002;184:353–5.
30. Yim JH, Barton P, Weber B, et al. Mammographically detected breast cancer: benefits of stereotactic core versus wire localization biopsy. Ann Surg 1996;223:688–700.
31. Pitre B, Baron PL, Baron LF, et al. Efficacy of stereotactic needle biopsy in the evaluation of mammographic abnormalities. Surg Forum 1995;46:625–7.
32. Schmidt RA. Stereotactic breast biopsy. CA Cancer J Clin 1994;44:172–91.
33. Howisey RL, Acheson MBG, Rowbotham RK, et al. A comparison of Medicare reimbursement and results for various imaging-guided breast biopsy techniques. Am J Surg 1997;173:395–8.

34. Lind DS, Minter R, Steinbach B, et al. Stereotactic core biopsy reduces the reexcision rate and the cost of mammographically detected cancer. J Surg Res 1998;78:23–6.

35. Rubin E, Mennemeyer ST, Desmond RA, et al. Reducing the cost of diagnosis of breast cancer. Cancer 2001;91:324–32.

36. Cross MJ, Evans WP, Peters GN, et al. Stereotactic breast biopsy as an alternative to open excisional biopsy. Ann Surg Oncol 1995;2:195–200.

37. Hillner BE, Bear HD, Fajardo LL. Estimating the cost-effectiveness of stereotactic biopsy for non-palpable breast abnormalities: a decision analysis model. Acad Radiol 1996;3:351–60.

38. Lindfors KK, Rosenquist CJ. Needle core biopsy guided with mammography: a study of cost-effectiveness. Radiology 1994;190:217–22.

39. Poplack SP, Carney PA, Weiss JE, et al. Screening mammography: costs and use of screening-related services. Radiology 2005;234:79–85.

40. Lidbrink E, Elfving J, Frisell J, et al. Neglected aspects of false positive findings of mammography in breast cancer screening: analysis of false positive cases from the Stockholm trial. BMJ 1996; 312:273–6.

41. Elmore JG, Barton MB, Moceri VM, et al. Ten-year risk of false positive screening mammograms and clinical breast examinations. N Engl J Med 1998; 338:1089–96.

42. Nields MW. Cost-effectiveness of image-guided core needle biopsy versus surgery in diagnosing breast cancer. Acad Radiol 1996;3(Suppl 1): S138–40.

43. Smith RA, Saslow D, Sawyer KA, et al. American Cancer Society guidelines for breast cancer screening: update 2003. CA Cancer J Clin 2003; 53:141–69.

44. Feig SA, D'Orsi CJ, Hendrick RE, et al. American College of Radiology Guidelines for breast cancer screening. AJR Am J Roentgenol 1998;171:29–33.

45. American Cancer Society. Cancer prevention and early detection facts and figures 2009. Atlanta (GA): American Cancer Society; 2009.

46. US Preventive Services Task Force. Screening for breast cancer: US preventive services task force recommendation statement. Ann Intern Med 2009;151:716–26.

47. Nelson HD, Tyne K, Naik A, et al. Screening for breast cancer: an update for the US preventive services task force. Ann Intern Med 2009;151: 727–37.

48. Mandelblatt JS, Cronin KA, Bailey S, et al. Effects of mammography screening under different screening schedules: model estimates of potential benefits and harms. Ann Intern Med 2009;151:738–47.

49. Hendrick RE, Smith RA, Rutledge JH, et al. Benefit of screening mammography in women ages 40–49:a new meta-analysis of randomized controlled trials. J Natl Cancer Inst Monogr 1997;22:87–92.

50. Jonsson H, Bordas P, Wallin H, et al. Service screening with mammography in Northern Sweden: effects on breast cancer mortality annual updates. J Med Screen 2007;1:87–93.

51. Kopans DB, Feig SA. The Canadian National Breast Screening Study: a critical review. AJR Am J Roentgenol 1993;161:755–60.

52. Michaelson JS, Halpern E, Kopans DB. Breast cancer: computer simulation method for estimating optimal intervals for screening. Radiology 1999; 212:551–60.

53. Taplin SH, Barlow W, Urban N, et al. Stage, age, comorbidity, and direct costs of colon, prostate, and breast cancer care. J Natl Cancer Inst 1995; 87:417–26.

54. Legorreta AP, Brooks RJ, Liebowitz AN, et al. Costs of breast cancer treatment: a 4-year longitudinal study. Arch Intern Med 1996;156:2197–201.

55. Norum J. Breast cancer screening by mammography in Norway. Is it cost effective? Ann Oncol 1999;10:197–203.

56. Otto SJ, Fracheboud J, Looman CW, et al. Initiation of population-based mammography screening in Dutch municipalities and effect on breast cancer mortality: a systematic review. Lancet 2003;361: 1411–7.

57. de Koning HJ, van Ineveld BM, van Oortmarssen GJ, et al. Breast cancer screening and cost-effectiveness; policy alternatives, quality of life considerations and the possible impact of uncertain factors. Int J Cancer 1991;49:531–7.

58. de Koning HJ, van Ineveld BM, de Haes JC, et al. Advanced breast cancer and its prevention by screening. Br J Cancer 1992;65:950–5.

59. de Koning HJ, Coebergh JW, van Dongen JA. Is mass screening for breast cancer cost-effective? Eur J Cancer 1996;32A(11):1835–9.

60. Zavertnik JJ, McCoy CB, Robinson DS, et al. Cost-effective management of breast cancer. Cancer 1992;69:1979–84.

61. Glenn ME. Can treatment dollars saved through earlier breast cancer diagnosis offset increased costs of mammography screening? The BAMC experience. Radiology 1997;205(P):142–3.

62. Moskowitz M. Cost-benefit determinations in screening mammography. Cancer 1987;60: 1680–3.

63. Kriege M, Brekelmans CT, Boetes C, et al. Efficacy of MRI and mammography for breast cancer screening in women with a familial or genetic predisposition. N Engl J Med 2004;351:427–37.

64. Kuhl CK, Schrading S, Leutner CC, et al. Mammography, breast ultrasound, and magnetic resonance imaging for surveillance of women at

high familial risk for breast cancer. J Clin Oncol 2005;23:8469–76.

65. Leach MO, Boggis CR, Dixon AK, et al. Screening with magnetic resonance imaging and mammography of a UK population at high familial risk of breast cancer: a prospective multicentre cohort study (MARIBS). Lancet 2005;365:1769–78.

66. Lehman CD, Blume JD, Weatherall P, et al. Screening women at high risk for breast cancer with mammography and magnetic resonance imaging. Cancer 2005;103:1898–905.

67. Sardanelli F, Podo F, D'Agnollo G, et al. Multicenter comparative multimodality surveillance of women at genetic-familial high risk for breast cancer (HIBCRIT study); interim results. Radiology 2007;242:698–715.

68. Warner E, Plewes DB, Hill KA, et al. Surveillance of BRCA1 and BRCA2 mutation carriers with magnetic resonance imaging, ultrasound, mammography, and clinical breast examination. JAMA 2004;292:1317–25.

69. Lehman CD, Issacs C, Schnall MD, et al. Cancer yield of mammography, MRI and US in high-risk women: prospective multi-institution breast cancer screening study. Radiology 2007;244:381–8.

70. Hagen AI, Kvistad KA, Maehle L, et al. Sensitivity of MRI versus conventional screening in the diagnosis of BRCA-associated breast cancer in a national prospective series. Breast 2007;16:367–74.

71. Hartman AR, Daniel BL, Kurian AW, et al. Breast magnetic resonance image screening and ductal lavage in women at high genetic risk for breast carcinoma. Cancer 2004;100:479–89.

72. Warner E, Messersmith H, Causer P, et al. Systematic review: using magnetic resonance imaging to screen for breast cancer. Ann Intern Med 2008;148:671–9.

73. Saslow D, Boetes C, Burke W, et al. American Cancer Society guidelines for breast screening with MRI as and adjunct to mammography. CA Cancer J Clin 2007;57:75–89.

74. Bevers TB, Anderson BO, Bonaccio E, et al. Breast cancer screening and diagnosis. J Natl Compr Canc Netw 2009;7:1060–96.

75. Lee CH, Dershaw DD, Kopans D, et al. Breast cancer screening with imaging: recommendations from the Society of Breast Imaging and the ACR on the use of mammography, breast MRI, breast ultrasound, and other technologies for the detection of clinically occult breast cancer. J Am Coll Radiol 2010;7:18–27.

76. Plevritis SK, Kurian AW, Sigal BM, et al. Cost-effectiveness of screening BRCA 1/2 mutation carriers with breast magnetic resonance imaging. JAMA 2006;295:2374–84.

77. Lee JM, McMahon PM, Kong CY, et al. Cost-effectiveness of breast MRI imaging and screen-film mammography for screening BRCA 1 gene mutation carriers. Radiology 2010;254:793–800.

78. Griebsch I, Brown J, Boggis C, et al. Cost-effectiveness of screening with contrast enhanced magnetic resonance imaging versus x-ray mammography of women at high familial risk of breast cancer. Br J Cancer 2006;95:801–10.

79. National Institute for Clinical Excellence (NICE), National Collaborating Centre for Primary Care. Familial breast cancer – the classification and care of women at risk of familial breast cancer in primary, secondary, and tertiary care. Available at: http://www.nice.org.uk. Accessed January 5, 2010.

80. Taneja C, Edelsberg J, Weycker D, et al. Cost effectiveness of breast cancer screening with contrast- enhanced MRI in high-risk women. J Am Coll Radiol 2009;6:171–9.

81. Easton DF, Ford D, Bishop DT. Breast and ovarian cancer incidence in BRCA1-mutation carriers. Breast cancer linkage consortium. Am J Hum Genet 1995;56:265–71.

82. Collaborative Group on Hormonal Factors in Breast Cancer. Familial breast cancer: collaborative reanalysis of individual data from 52 epidemiological studies including 58,209 women with breast cancer and 101,986 women without the disease. Lancet 2001;358:1389–99.

83. Petrucelli N, Daly MB, Culver JOB, et al. BRCA1 and BRCA2 hereditary breast/ovarian cancer. Gene reviews. Available at: http://www.genetests.org/querydz=brcal. Accessed January 5, 2010.

84. Amir E, Evans DG, Shenton A, et al. Evaluation of breast cancer risk assessment packages in the family history evaluation and screening programme. J Med Genet 2003;40:807–14.

85. Fisher B, Anderson S, Redmond CK, et al. Reanalysis and results after 12 years of follow-up in a randomized clinical trial comparing total mastectomy with lumpectomy with or without irradiation in the treatment of breast cancer. N Engl J Med 1995;333:1456–61.

86. Fisher B, Anderson S, Bryant J, et al. Twenty-year follow-up of a randomized trial comparing total mastectomy, lumpectomy, and lumpectomy plus irradiation for the treatment of invasive breast cancer. N Engl J Med 2002;347:1233–41.

87. Easton DF. Familial risks of breast cancer. Breast Cancer Res 2002;4:179–81.

88. Frykberg ER. Lobular carcinoma in situ of the breast. Breast J 1999;5:296–303.

89. Dupont WD, Parl FF, Hartmann WH, et al. Breast cancer risk associated with proliferative breast disease and atypical hyperplasia. Cancer 1993;71:1258–65.

90. Page DL, Schuyler PA, Dupont WD, et al. Atypical lobular hyperplasia as a unilateral predictor of

breast cancer risk: a retrospective cohort study. Lancet 2003;361:125–9.

91. Boyd NE, Guo H, Martin LJ, et al. Mammographic density and the risk and detection of breast cancer. N Engl J Med 2007;356:227–36.

92. Berg WA. Tailored supplementary screening for breast cancer: what now and what next? AJR Am J Roentgenol 2009;192:390–9.

93. Hendrick RE. Breast MRI: fundamental and technical aspects. New York: Springer Verlag; 2008.

94. La Trenta LR, Menell JH, Morris EA, et al. Breast lesions detected with MR imaging: utility and histopathologic importance of identification with US. Radiology 2003;227:856–61.

95. Feig SA, Shaber GS, Patchefsky A, et al. Analysis of clinically and mammographically occult breast tumors. AJR Am J Roentgenol 1977;128:403–8.

96. Kerlikowske K, Grady D, Barclay J, et al. Effect of age, breast density, and family history on the sensitivity of first screening mammography. JAMA 1996; 276:33–8.

97. Rosenberg RD, Hunt WC, Williamson MR, et al. Effects of age, breast density, ethnicity, and estrogen replacement therapy on screening mammographic sensitivity and cancer stage at diagnosis: review of 183, 134 screening mammograms in Albuquerque, New Mexico. Radiology 1998;209:511–8.

98. van Gils CH, Otten JD, Verbeeck AL, et al. Effect of mammographic breast density on breast cancer screening performance: a study in Nijmegen, the Netherlands. J Epidemiol Community Health 1998;52:267–71.

99. Mandelson MT, Oestreicher N, Porter PL, et al. Breast density as a predictor of mammographic detection: comparison of interval and screen-detected cancers. J Natl Cancer Inst 2000;92:1081–7.

100. Ma I, Fischell C, Wright B, et al. Case control study of factors associated with failure to detect breast cancer by mammography. J Natl Cancer Inst 2000;92:1081–7.

101. Jackson VP, Hendrick RE, Feig SA, et al. Imaging the radiographically dense breast. Radiology 1993;188:297–301.

102. Stomper PC, D'Souza DJ, DiNitto PA, et al. Analysis of parenchymal density on mammograms of 1353 women 25–79 years old. AJR Am J Roentgenol 1996;167:1261–5.

103. Gordon PB, Goldenberg SL. Malignant breast masses detected only by ultrasound: a retrospective review. Cancer 1995;76:626–30.

104. Kolb TM, Lichy J, Newhouse JH. Occult cancer in women with dense breast: detection with screening US-diagnostic yield and tumor characteristics. Radiology 1998;207:191–9.

105. Buchberger W, DeKoekkoek-Doll P, Springer P, et al. Incidental findings on sonography of the

106. Buchberger W, Niehoff A, Orbist A, et al. Clinically and mammographically occult breast lesions; detection and classification with high-resolution sonography. Semin Ultrasound CT MR 2000;21:325–36.

107. Kaplan SS. Clinical utility of bilateral whole-breast US in the evaluation of women with dense breast tissue. Radiology 2001;221:641–9.

108. Kolb TM, Lichy J, Newhouse JH. Comparison of the performance of screening mammography physical examination, and breast US and evaluation of factors that influence them: an analysis of 27,825 patient evaluation. Radiology 2002;225: 165–75.

109. Leconte I, Feger C, Galant C, et al. Mammography and subsequent whole-breast sonography of nonpalpable breast cancers: the importance of radiologic breast density. AJR Am J Roentgenol 2003;180:1675–9.

110. Crystal P, Strano S, Shcharynski S, et al. Using sonography to screen women with mammographically dense breasts. AJR Am J Roentgenol 2003; 181:177–82.

111. Feig SA. Current status of screening US. Breast imaging: RSNA categorical course in diagnostic radiology. Oak Brook (IL): Radiological Society of North America Inc; 2005. p. 143–54.

112. Bassett LW, Hendrick RE, Bassford TL, et al. Clinical practice guideline number 13: quality determinants of mammography. AHCPR Publication 95-0632. Rockville (MD): US Department of Health and Human Services, Agency for Health Care Policy and Research, Public Health Service; 1994. p. 83.

113. Feig SA. Auditing and benchmarks in screening and diagnostic mammography. Radiol Clin North Am 2007;45:791–800.

114. Berg WA, Blume JD, Cormack JB, et al. Combined screening with ultrasound and mammography versus mammography alone in women at elevated risk of breast cancer. JAMA 2008;299(18):2151–63.

115. Corsetti V, Houssami N, Ferrari A, et al. Breast screening with ultrasound in women with mammography-negative dense breasts: evidence on incremental cancer detection and false positives, and associated cost. Eur J Cancer 2008; 44:539–44.

116. Enzmann DR, Anglada PM, Haviley C, et al. Providing professional mammography services: financial analysis. Radiology 2001;219:467–73.

117. Chou YH, Tiu C-M, Chen J, et al. Automated full-field breast ultrasonography: the past and the present. J Med Ultrasound 2007;15(1):31–44.

118. Kelly KM, Dean J, Comulada WS, et al. Breast cancer detection using automated whole breast ultrasound and mammography in radiographically dense breasts. Eur Radiol 2010;20:734–42.

breast clinical significance and diagnostic workup. AJR Am J Roentgenol 1999;173:921–7.

The Basics and Implementation of Digital Mammography

Margarita L. Zuley, MD

KEYWORDS

- Digital mammography • Breast imaging • Basics
- Implementation

Digital mammography has been widely accepted by the breast imaging community in the last few years, with more than half of all units in the country now digital. Most are direct ray (DR) units, which completely replace screen film units and have a built-in digital detector. A small fraction are computed ray (CR) units, which are add-on digital conversion detectors that replace the screen film cassette system in a screen film unit. The earliest comparative trials, known as the Colorado-Massachusetts study published in 2002[1] and the Oslo I trial[2] published in 2003 showed only minimal inferiority that was not statistically significant of digital mammography compared with screen film. These 2 studies were quickly followed with 2 more prospective studies and several retrospective studies, all of which showed at least equivalence of the 2 technologies[3–9] for breast cancer detection. Indeed, several of these studies have shown improved detection with digital mammography in younger women who have dense breasts and in the detection of malignant calcifications. However, the recall rate of digital mammography has been higher than screen film mammography when the study results are pooled[7,10] and so the positive predictive value of digital and screen film mammography at this point is similar. All of these studies were completed in the early days of the digital technology and so such results are impressive in that this relatively new technology has been shown to be at least comparable with its seasoned and highly optimized predecessor. Since those studies were completed, vendors have continued to work to optimize the digital equipment both for improved lesion detection and characterization, as well as improved ease of use.

Although the digital technique has many similarities to screen film in that it is a low-dose exposure to the breast and many of the requirements for an optimal image are the same, such as correct compression and positioning, the digital mammogram is constructed in a different way from screen film images. Having an understanding of how the images are created and how the different variables influence image quality is important to the radiologist for both diagnostic reasons and quality assurance purposes. Another component of using digital mammography is learning how to optimize the workflow efficiencies that digital imaging offers. This article discusses the technical basics of the digital mammogram to assist in understanding and troubleshooting the images as well as implementation choices to maximize the potential efficiencies.

DETECTORS

The first part of the digital imaging chain is the acquisition unit. From a technical point of view, the efficient use of the x-ray beam and the resultant quality of the image is dictated by the materials of the system and the method by which the x-ray beam information is recorded. There are several types of technology deployed in digital detectors.[11–14] Detectors are classified as either direct or indirect capture. In indirect capture, the energy from the x-ray beam is converted by an x-ray scintillator first into light and then into a digital

Magee-Womens Hospital of UPMC, Breast Imaging Department, 300 Halket Street, 3rd Floor, Pittsburgh, PA 15213, USA
E-mail address: zuleyml@upmc.edu

Radiol Clin N Am 48 (2010) 893–901
doi:10.1016/j.rcl.2010.06.003

signal. This is similar to how the image is produced with screen film mammography. Charge couple devices (CCD), photostimulable phosphors, and amorphous silicon are types of indirect digital detectors currently in use. Direct capture units do not have this light conversion step; instead the substrate used is a photoconductive material that is able to directly convert the x-ray photons into an electrical charge. Amorphous selenium detectors are direct capture as are crystal silicon detectors that use photon counting technology. With every alteration of the x-ray beam, noise is introduced into the images and information is lost; in theory then, direct capture units have the advantage of potentially using more of the primary beam than indirect systems. With this variability in detector technology there are differences in the clinical images produced. However, no study to date has shown that any system has a clinical advantage to detect cancer over another system.

SPATIAL RESOLUTION

All systems capture the exposure onto a digital matrix that is comprised of a grid of detector elements, or dels. The spatial resolution of a system is determined in large part by the size and spacing of the dels (dels are also called pixels and the distance between the center of 2 adjacent dels is called pixel pitch). The smallest structure that can be resolved by the detector turns out to be one that is twice the size of a del. This is called the Nyquist frequency of the detector.[12,15] So for a detector with a 70-μm pixel pitch, the smallest resolvable structure is 140 μm. The term frequency is used because shapes can be viewed as a series of waveforms; fine shapes like spicules are considered high-frequency shapes, and more coarse shapes such as a round 2-cm mass have lower spatial frequency. In screen film mammography, spatial resolution is defined by how many line pairs could be resolved per millimeter of film. Now we must translate our understanding of spatial resolution to pixel pitch and dels. It so happens that half of the pixel pitch in millimeters (mm, not micrometers) is equal to the line pair resolution. So, for the same 70-μm detector, the line pair resolution would be 0.5 x 7 mm = 3.5 line pairs/mm. For comparison, screen film systems have a requirement to have a minimum of 11 or 13 line pairs/mm depending on the orientation of the x-ray tube.[16]

Pixel pitch is only part of the determination of spatial resolution as it is also dependent on the focal spot size, the spread of the signal in the detector, and motion. Each of these variables is evaluated by its modulation transfer function (MTF). In essence, the MTF simply describes how precisely any shape is transmitted through the system.[15] Another way to think of MTF is that it describes how much of the original contrast is lost in the system for each exposure.[12] The MTF of any system is the average of its MTF for each variable. Most systems have a nearly perfect MTF (of 1) for large shapes and a lower MTF as shapes become more fine MTF gives some but not all of the indication of system efficiency. The other important parameter is the detective quantum efficiency (DQE), which takes into account not only the spatial resolution (and thus considers pixel pitch and MTF) of a system but also the signal to noise ratio (SNR).[17] DQE basically describes what percentage of the beam (or signal) produces an image versus how much is lost as noise in the system. Digital systems have higher DQEs than screen film units and so with digital mammography has come a reduction in dose to patients without loss of information.

ANALOG TO DIGITAL UNITS

Once the energy from the beam is captured in the detector, the signal is converted into an image. All detectors have a matrix into which the signal from the acquisition is stored. The matrix is divided into rows and columns of pixels (dels). As the x-ray energy is collected in the pixels, the information is stored as analog to digital units (ADU). Essentially, each time an electron reaches a pixel, it is counted as an ADU. Therefore, the denser the patient tissue overlying any one pixel, the lower the ADU count of that pixel. For each exposure, an ADU map is created on the matrix. This ADU map is converted into a gray scale image. The size of each pixel and the size of the matrix vary between equipment. As mentioned earlier, pixel pitch describes the distance from the center of one pixel to the center of the adjacent pixels. Currently available systems have pixel pitches of 50, 70 or 100 μm. One system, the Fischer Senoscan, (no longer produced) had a slit scanner technology, and acquired images at both 50 and 25 μm. Although there are detectable differences in the clinical images from these different pixel pitches, no study to date has definitively shown any one of all the available units to be optimal, or even better for cancer detection than another. The first full-field digital system approved by the US Food and Drug Administration (FDA) in 2000, the General Electric Senographe D (General Electric, Inc Buc, France), had a relatively small 18 × 23 cm detector that resulted in a fair proportion of patients requiring more than 1 image per mammographic view to image the entire breast. Since that first device, the detectors have become larger, so that now, only large breasts require this additional imaging.

Most systems have an automatic exposure control (AEC) that determines the optimal imaging parameters, such as kilovolt peak (kVp), and milliamps (mA). Unlike screen film mammography where the AEC is used primarily to control image brightness, the AEC in digital mammography is used mainly to ensure that the radiation exposure is optimized for appropriate SNR.[18] This feature works by having a very low-dose fast test exposure given to the patient before the diagnostic exposure which generates a test ADU map that allows the system to evaluate one or more areas for determination of the correct exposure. The AEC uses this information along with the compressed breast thickness to determine the correct exposure parameters. The exposure results in a for-processing dataset, which is a set of images with processing algorithms applied to them that correct for detector artifacts but are still not suitable for interpretation. (This is also the dataset that is sent to computer-aided detection (CAD) devices for algorithm application, if CAD is used at the facility.) The for-processing dataset also has additional processing algorithms applied to it to convert it into an image that is suitable for interpretation. These are called for-presentation images and it is these images that are then sent to an image archiver for future display and interpretation.

PROCESSING ALGORITHMS

To convert the digital signals captured during an exposure into a readable mammographic view, multiple types of processing algorithms are applied. The first category of processing is detector correction algorithms designed to remove any inhomogeneities in the detector that may be perceived on the final image. Two examples are masking of dead pixels and flat-field calibration. The second type of processing is used to generate a diagnostic image. These are applied to the for-processing dataset and include thickness equalization (also called peripheral equalization) and contrast enhancement algorithms. Thickness equalization refers to a process whereby the areas of breast tissue containing high ADU counts, such as the subcutaneous fat and retroglandular fatty areas, are enhanced so that they can be easily seen at display. Contrast enhancement algorithms bring out the differences in ADU counts between adjacent pixels or groups of pixels by making those differences larger. Some methodologies include unsharp masking, MUSICA filters, and CLAHE filters. This processing enhances calcifications

and fine details like the spicules on a cancer and are meant to aid visibility because of the lower MTF of the systems for these high-frequency structures. Most manufacturers do not reveal all or, in some cases, any of the processing schemes that they use to generate an image. Some vendors have options of processing algorithms, whereas others only offer 1 set of algorithms. For those vendors that offer choices, typically a facility will choose a default algorithm and then if another one is desired, it can be done at the acquisition workstation, as long as the original for-processing dataset is still available there. For example, if a radiologist is reading a study and notices an area of tissue that looks more conspicuous compared with the older images, but the radiologist is not sure if the change is simply a result of the processing of the image, they can have the image reprocessed with a different algorithm to see if the change on the mammogram is real.

In the beginning of digital mammography, most vendors applied the processing algorithms to the images at the diagnostic workstation, but this forced users to buy both the vendor-specific acquisition units and their workstations. Now that all necessary processing occurs at the acquisition unit, facilities can make their mammogram unit and display workstation decisions separately. Some vendors now offer the option to further manipulate the image display on the diagnostic workstation to try and match the appearance of mammograms that are from different full-field digital mammography (FFDM) units. Although there is no trial to date conclusively showing that one type of processing algorithm is superior to another for detection of masses or calcifications, a few preliminary studies suggest that not all algorithms perform equally well,[19–22] and some may offer better agreement between readers for both mass and calcifications.[22] it is to be hoped that the current situation of vendors maintaining secrecy over their processing algorithms will change in that vendors will be forced by radiologists to reveal some of the processing so that the effects on the image can be better appreciated and advances in both production and interpretation of images can be made.

DYNAMIC RANGE

The bit depth of a system describes how many shades of gray are available for viewing. Most digital systems collect 12 to 14 bits of data, but through processing and transfer some of this information is lost and so at display, only 8 to 10 bits of data are available to the radiologist. This is the dynamic range of the image. The manufacturers apply look-up tables (LUT) to the images to optimize presentation of this information. Those LUTs may follow a linear or nonlinear (like an H and D curve) shape across the dynamic range. One LUT is not better than the other. Each manufacturer chooses which works best with the processing algorithms to produce a quality image. Workstations should be able to apply the correct LUT to the images. Some workstations cannot apply all curve shapes and so the images will be slightly degraded. These workstations should be summarily rejected. To ensure that the workstation follows such rules, it should comply with the Integrating the Healthcare Enterprise (IHE) Mammography Image Profile.[23] This profile specifies the technical parameters necessary to correctly display digital mammograms from all vendors.

PADDLES

Just as with screen film mammography, there are multiple paddles for imaging with digital systems. In screen film mammography, almost all paddles are rigid so that the paddle is parallel to the imaging surface throughout. This allows for consistent compression thickness across the breast. With digital imaging these rigid paddles are still commonly used but there are also flexible paddles that have a spring at the chest wall side so that the paddle has more even compressive force across the breast tissue. The processing algorithms can correct for any differences in thickness with these paddles and so many facilities prefer them. Even though digital mammography is widely believed to display calcifications better than screen film, magnification should be used to better characterize calcifications and so magnification paddles are available, as are various spot compression paddles.

COMPUTER-AIDED DETECTION (CADE) AND COMPUTER-AIDED DIAGNOSIS (CADX)

CAD devices produce their marks from the for-processing information, not the for-presentation information and so they are not influenced by processing algorithms. Two separate algorithms are applied: one for calcifications and the second for masses, just as was the case with screen film. CADe refers to those algorithms that simply mark areas to be reviewed without providing any information regarding likelihood of malignancy. There are new algorithms that go a bit further and actually convey some additional information through variable sizing of marks and lesion metrics, such as likelihood of malignancy of similar lesions that were used to train the system. These are called

CADx devices. The Food and Drug Administration has guidance documents for vendors that clearly explain the differences between CADx and CADe devices.[24] Both methods of marking findings should still be used in the FDA approved method as for screen film. These marking methods are meant to be adjunctive to the radiologist's interpretation and not intended to cause the radiologist to dismiss any lesion that was seen without the aid of the CAD marks.

ARTIFACTS

Artifacts in digital mammography can arise from a detector failure, a processing failure, corrupted calibration files, extraneous objects in between the x-ray target and detector, or a failure of the components such as the grid or the plate transporter in a CR unit. Aside from dust and debris on the surface of the detector or paddles, detector artifacts are the most commonly seen artifacts and include ghosting, dead pixels, and flat-field inhomogeneities. Ghosting is the result of latent charge remaining in the detector from previous exposures and is specific to and one of the weaknesses of using amorphous selenium direct detectors and photostimulable phosphor plates in CR imaging. Both substrates retain charge and need to be cleared. In busy practices, by the end of the day it is not uncommon to see some ghosting from previous exposures (**Fig. 1**), especially the outlines from the smaller paddles and as the detector or

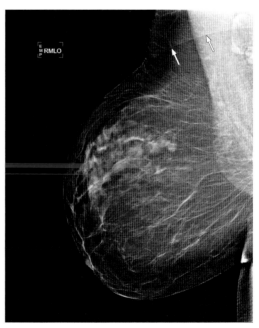

Fig. 1. This mediolateral oblique view demonstrates a ghosting artifact (*arrows*).

plates age. For the phosphor plates, the charge can generally be cleared by putting the plate through the cassette reader, which uses laser technology to clear it. For amorphous selenium, a flat field can be done and the detector recalibrated to overcome the ghosting or, in some instances, the detector must be replaced.

All digital detectors can have dead pixels. A few are of no clinical concern and they appear as bright white dots on the image. Generally, when there are more than 3 dead pixels in a centimeter, the vendor will replace the detector if it is under a service contract. A row of dead pixels is seen as a straight thin white line (**Fig. 2**). One of the quality control tests is to evaluate the system for these. Many detectors are constructed as groups of arrays with associated amplifiers that are smaller than the matrix. These arrays are placed in the detector housing to create the matrix. Occasionally, 1 array may appear different than the adjacent ones and this background inhomogeneity can be visible to the radiologist.[25] If an exposure is done at high dose or a display has little dynamic range, these arrays are visible in the background of the image (**Fig. 3**). A flat-field image using an acrylic slab will identify these and a flat-field recalibration will generally correct it. Stitching lines are thin gaps between adjacent arrays and appear as thin faint white lines. These lines are not often seen because they

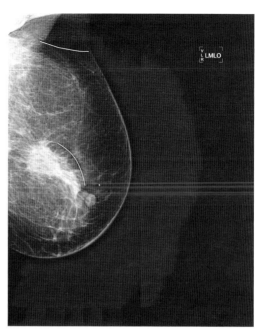

Fig. 3. In the dark parts of this image outside the breast, there are adjacent blocks that are different shades of gray. These are the arrays in the detector.

are corrected in flat-field calibration but that are generally acceptable because they are no more than 1 pixel wide. If a horizontal thin white line is seen repeatedly on clinical images the other possibility is that there is a row of dead pixels (see **Fig. 2**, as mentioned earlier), a situation that may require detector replacement.

Processing algorithms occasionally fail and this can create artifacts. Typically, these are seen as dark straight lines in the for-presentation images only (**Fig. 4**). To differentiate from a detector problem, the for-processing images should be reviewed if available or a flat-field image should be acquired and not processed. If this is a processing algorithm artifact, this test should not show the artifact. Occasionally, when the quality control technologist performs the unit calibration, the collimator is not properly aligned and this will produce either a dark or white vertical band at the chest wall side of the image (**Fig. 5**). To eliminate this artifact, the system must have a flat-field recalibration after the collimator position is corrected.[26] If the grid is not fully engaged, the gantry grid lines can be seen. In addition, there can be the rare event of a vibration artifact from the cooling fan, which causes alternating horizontal white and dark lines on an image. If a vibration artifact is seen, the service engineer may have to replace the detector or the fan. In the case of CR, if the cassette transporter fails, the image may not be read out entirely

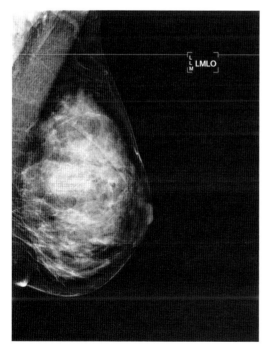

Fig. 2. The white horizontal line in this image is caused by a dead row of pixels in the detector.

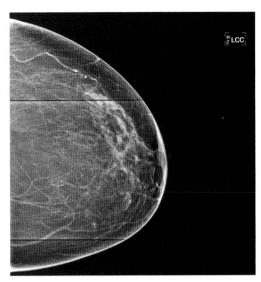

Fig. 4. The dark horizontal bands on this image are caused by a processing algorithm failure.

and it may appear that the patient was poorly positioned.

DIAGNOSTIC WORKSTATION CONSIDERATIONS

Because digital mammography has been regulated by the FDA as a class III device, vendors

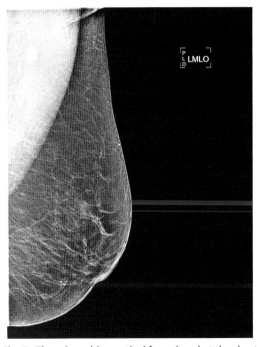

Fig. 5. There is a white vertical fuzzy band at the chest wall side of this image that is present because the paddle was not properly aligned when the flat-field calibration was done. This is a collimation artifact.

have been required to develop acquisition and processing algorithms that produce images that are not inferior to screen film mammography. Class III devices are those that have not yet been proved to be safe and effective for patient use in the eyes of the FDA and so they are strictly regulated. This regulation on FFDM first included the entire digital imaging chain from acquisition to display to print, however, the FDA has removed the printer and the workstation from this requirement allowing the workstations to evolve separately. Each mammography unit vendor has taken a slightly different approach with different pixel pitch and matrices for their systems, thus, they each produce different sized images. This has created some challenges for the diagnostic workstation to present images of the same size for efficient comparison.

Along with the processing algorithms, each mammogram unit vendor has chosen an optimized window width (WW) and window level (WL) application for their images. As was discussed earlier, LUTs can either be linear or nonlinear for the dynamic range of the image. The workstations, therefore, have the need to be able to apply the correct LUT to any image to produce the optimized image that the vendor intended and the FDA approved. If the wrong LUT table is applied, the image will be degraded either with too much contrast or too flat. This is a point where the buyer must be cautious and knowledgeable to ensure that the workstations that are purchased can perform both linear and nonlinear LUTs so that any FFDM image can be properly displayed. Having FDA clearance to sell digital mammography workstations does not guarantee this functionality.

Because mammography evaluates calcifications of 300 μm on average, detectors are built to have a maximal spatial resolution higher than that and the resultant mammographic images are large. For example, if a detector has a pixel pitch of 50 μm, the matrix can contain more than 20 million pixels. Mammography display monitors typically have only 5 million pixels, and so the mammogram at full resolution will not fit in the field of view for display in most cases. As a result, the workstation has the requirement of intelligently displaying the mammograms with different sampling of the data so that the radiologist can perform the tasks of comparison to priors and close inspection of the current study. Most workstations have the ability to create hanging or display protocols to accomplish this. There are only a few display modes used for all protocols, and they are called fit to viewport, same size, true size, view actual pixels, and magnification.

The radiologist chooses the order of these modes when building a protocol.

Fit to viewport is the mode whereby adjacent pixels' ADUs are averaged together and displayed as 1 ADU to fit the image onto a portion of the monitor. The number of pixels on the diagnostic monitor allocated for display in that step of the protocol and the matrix of the acquisition determines the amount of downsampling (averaging together adjacent pixels) of data for display. Same size is a variation of fit to viewport whereby the workstation takes into account the different matrices from different manufacturers or different paddles (ie, 100 μm vs 70 μm or small detector vs large detector from the same vendor) and scales all the images to look the same size to the radiologist. This allows for much more efficient evaluation of change over time. These modes are used for comparison of current and prior studies and comparison of right and left images. The workstation should readily display the functional pixel pitch of display and what percentage that resolution is compared with both true size and view actual pixels. True size is the mode that displays the true physical size of the breast and is useful when planning for surgery or stereotactic biopsy or when printing hard copy for comparison with screen film mammography. The mode view actual pixels is the mode that displays each acquired pixel on one display pixel. This is the mode that gives full-resolution images and is best for evaluation of calcifications and subtle mass margins. The mammogram is almost always bigger than the monitor in this mode so either manual panning of the image or some predetermined stepwise display of the image is needed to see the entire breast. Zooming the image with optical magnification at the workstation can be done but this is a mathematical up interpolation of data and does not provide more information to the image; it is just making the image larger for ease of viewing and at the same time introduces some noise to the image. Air gap magnification (using a magnification stand exactly like the technique used for screen film mammography) allows a small portion of the breast to be sampled by the detector increasing spatial resolution, because more pixels in the detector are used to sample a smaller area of the breast. For this reason magnification has been shown to be beneficial for evaluating calcifications with digital mammography and should still be used.[27–29]

The solution to all of these issues has come from an organization called Integrating the Healthcare Enterprise (IHE), which has written a digital mammography image profile that outlines exactly what is required of each piece of equipment to ensure correct and consistent display of any mammogram (IHE technical framework www.ihe.net/mammo).[23] To benefit from that functionality the facility must specify in the purchase order that each piece of equipment purchased conforms to this profile. For the profile to work, the equipment that is already present at the facility must also conform and so there is typically some work to be done on the part of the informatics team, in concert with the vendors to ensure that everything conforms and is updated.

PROBLEMS WITH DEDICATED WORKSTATIONS

As a result of all of these special needs, a whole class of stand-alone digital mammography workstations has evolved. Although these workstations perform well with mammograms and can, in some cases, display other images such as ultrasound and magnetic resonance images, they are not typically fully integrated into a facility's picture and archiving communication system (PACS) and thus workflow problems are common. The earliest mammography workstations that offered correct display were produced by the mammography unit vendors and they either had no PACS product or were developed in a subgroup of the company without coordination with their own PACS group.

In part the problem arises because the image sizes are large both from a networking standpoint and a storage standpoint. A single 4-view mammogram is 8 to 54 megabytes (MB), depending on the matrix. Only lossless compression is allowed and so storage and transmission requirements are important. A facility that performs 150,000 mammograms per year can face storage requirements on the order of 4 to 6 terabytes (TB). An early common storage solution was a mini-PACS, which was able to store the digital mammographic images and be directly linked to the stand-alone workstations, but this created an island of information and was suboptimal from a workflow standpoint. Now, most facilities permanently store the digital mammograms on their system-wide PACS, but because there is a frequent lack of linkage to the system-wide PACS, managers (which are intermediary, temporary storage devices) are used to receive the current studies from the acquisition modality and the PACS is queried for the priors. The mammography workstations are then linked to the manager and can display the mammograms. This solution is somewhat constraining in that the managers typically cannot route images to one particular workstation, but instead broadcast all of the cases to each connected workstation. This can cause problems with network speeds because of the excessive data transmission and also creates work list problems for the radiologist at each diagnostic workstation who must then sort through many studies that they do not need to read.

From a network standpoint the mini-PACS and work-around solution is a challenge as well, and becomes more of a challenge as the years pass because many radiologists want to have all of the prior studies available for comparison at the time of interpretation. Therefore, when the manager queries the PACS, more than 1 GB of data per case may be queried. This puts a stain on the bandwidth of busy facilities that are also trying to simultaneously handle the large datasets coming from current computed tomography scanners; not to mention that the manager's memory must be sufficient to house all of the incoming data without slowing down or having cases drop off.

After the cases are interpreted, any annotations that need to be saved must be sent from the diagnostic workstation to the manager and then back to the PACS. To execute all of this storage and transmission most effectively, a team including the radiologist, the informatics group, and the vendors must work together. The solution to these problems lies in cooperation of the vendors who supply the workstations, the PACS, and the information systems (radiology [RIS] or health care [HIS]) so that the mammography workstations can be integrated into the system-wide archive and appear to seamlessly display the mammograms to the radiologists. Much work is still necessary on this front and will only occur with pressure from users to demand it. The beginning of the process is to clearly identify the needs of a facility, the current limitations to workflow that exist, and then to work with the informatics specialists and the vendors to find a solution. The concept of a universal workstation that communicates directly with the PACS and the information system (RIS or HIS) is a good solution in that it would be able to display all modalities well and eliminate all of the problems associated with the mini-PACs described earlier.

SUMMARY

Current day digital mammography acquisition units have already been shown to be equal or better than screen film systems for the detection and classification of breast lesions. The optimal multimodality breast imaging diagnostic workstations and connectivity to existing PACS and information systems is still a work in progress, but with more and more facilities transitioning to digital imaging it is only a matter of time until these hurdles are overcome.

REFERENCES

1. Lewin JM, D'Orsi CJ, Hendrick RE, et al. Clinical comparison of full-field digital mammography and screen-film mammography for detection of breast cancer. AJR Am J Roentgenol 2002;179:671–7.
2. Skaane P, Young K, Skjennald A. Population-based mammography screening: comparison of screen-films and full field digital mammography with soft-copy reading–Oslo I Study. Radiology 2003;229: 877–84.
3. Pisano ED, Gatsonis C, Hendrik E. Diagnostic performance of digital versus film mammography for breast-cancer screening. N Engl J Med 2005; 353:1773–83.
4. DelTurco MR, Mantelli P, Ciatto S, et al. Full-field digital versus screen-film mammography: comparative accuracy in concurrent screening cohorts. AJR Am J Roentgenol 2007;189:860–6.
5. Skaane P, Skjennald A. Screen-film mammography versus full-field digital mammography with soft-copy reading: randomized trial in a population-based screening program – The Oslo II Study. Radiology 2004;232:197–204.
6. Yamada T, Saito M, Ishibashi T, et al. Comparison of screen-film and full-field digital mammography in Japanese population-based screening. Radiat Med 2004;22:408–12.
7. Vinnicombe S, Pinto Pereira S, McCormack VA, et al. Full-field digital versus screen-film mammography: comparison within the UK breast screening program and systematic review of published data. Radiology 2009;251:347–58.
8. Vernacchia FS, Pena ZG. Digital mammography: its impact on recall rates and cancer detection rates in a small community-based radiology practice. AJR Am J Roentgenol 2009;193:582–5.
9. Hambly NM, McNicholas MM, Phelan N, et al. Comparison of digital mammography and screen-film mammography in breast cancer screening: a review in the Irish breast screening program. AJR Am J Roentgenol 2009;193:1010–8.
10. Skaane P. Studies comparing screen-film mammography and full-field digital mammography in breast cancer screening: updated review. Acta Radiol 2009;50:3–14.
11. Yaffe MJ. Detectors for digital mammography. In: Pisano ED, Yaffe MJ, Kuzmiak CM, editors. Digital mammography. Philadelphia: Lippincott, Williams & Wilkins; 2004. p. 15–26.
12. Noel A, Thibault F. Digital detectors for mammography: the technical challenges. Eur Radiol 2004; 14:1990–8.

13. D'Orsi CJ, Newell MS. Digital mammography: clinical implementation and clinical trials. Semin Roentgenol 2007;42:236–42.

14. Yaffe MJ, Mainprize JG, Jong RA. Technical developments in mammography. Health Phys 2008;95:599–611.

15. Yaffe MJ. Physics of digital mammography. In: Pisano ED, Yaffe MJ, Kuzmiak CM, editors. Digital mammography. Philadelphia: Lippincott, Williams & Wilkins; 2004. p. 4–14.

16. Bassett LW, Hendrick RE. Quality determinants of mammography: clinical practice guideline. Darby (PA): Diane Pub Co.; 2004.

17. Samei E, Ranger NT, Mackenzie A, et al. Detector of system? Extending the concept of detective quantum efficiency to characterize the performance of digital radiographic imaging systems. Radiology 2008;249:926–37.

18. Pisano ED, Yaffe MJ. Digital mammogarphy. Radiology 2005;234:353–62.

19. Zanca F, Jacobs J. Evaluation of clinical image processing algorithms used in digital mammography. Med Phys 2009;36:765–75.

20. Chen B, Wang W, Huang J. Comparison of tissue equalization, and premium view post processing methods in full field digital mammography. Eur J Radiol 2009. DOI:10.1016/j.ejrad.2009.05.010.

21. Goldstraw EJ, Castellano I, Ashley S, et al. The effect of premium view post-processing software on digital mammography reporting. Br J Radiol 2010;83(986):122–8.

22. Uematsu T. Detection of masses and calcifications by soft-copy reading: comparison of two post-processing algorithms for full-field digital mammography. Jpn J Radiol 2009;27:168–75.

23. IHE technical framework. Available at: http://www.ihe.net/Technical_Framework/index.cfm#radiology. Accessed August 19, 2010.

24. Draft Guidance for Industry and FDA Staff. Computer-assisted detection devices applied to radiology images and radiology device data – premarket notification [501(k)] submissions. US Food and Drug Administration web site. Available at: http://www.fda.gov/MedicalDevices/DeviceRegulationandGuidance/GuidanceDocuments/ucm187249.htm. Accessed August 19, 2010.

25. Honey ID, Mackenzie A. Artifacts found during quality assurance testing of computed radiography and digital radiography detectors. J Digit Imaging 2009;22:383–92.

26. Ayyala RS, Chorlton MA, Behrman RH, et al. Digital mammographic artifacts on full-field system: what are they and how do I fix them? RadioGraphics 2008;28:1999–2008.

27. Kim MJ, Kim EK, Kwak JY. Characterization of microcalcification: can digital monitor zooming replace magnification mammography in full-field digital mammography? Eur Radiol 2009;19:310–7.

28. Kim MJ, Youk JH, Kang DR. Zooming method ($\times$2.0) of digital mammography vs digital magnification view ($\times$1.8) in full-field digital mammography for the diagnosis of microcalcifications. Br J Radiol 2009. DOI:10.1259/bjr/16967819.

29. Bick U, Dickmann. Digital mammography: what do we and what don't we know? Eur Radiol 2007;17:1931–42.

Digital Mammography: Clinical Image Evaluation

Lawrence W. Bassett, MD[a],*, Anne C. Hoyt, MD[b],
Thomas Oshiro, PhD[c]

KEYWORDS

- Mammography • Digital mammography
- Clinical image evaluation
- Mammography accreditation program

As for screen-film mammography (SFM), obtaining the highest-quality clinical images is an essential goal for digital mammography (DM), either full-field digital mammography (FFDM) or computed radiography mammography (CRM). For the most part, the criteria for a high-quality DM image is similar to that of an SFM examination. However, there are criteria that are especially relevant to DM, which are emphasized in this article.

Learning to recognize specific deficiencies in the clinical images and understanding their possible causes allow the interpreting physician and radiologic technologist to correct image deficiencies as soon as possible. In addition to the recommended daily assessment of clinical images by the interpreting physician and radiologic technologist, an external clinical review of selected clinical images is mandated by the Mammography Quality Standards Act (MQSA)[1,2] at least every 3 years and is performed by specially trained radiologists under the auspices of the Food and Drug Administration's approved accrediting bodies.[3]

THE MAMMOGRAPHY ACCREDITATION PROCESS

The predominant national accrediting body for DM is the American College of Radiology Mammography Accreditation Program (ACRMAP). To become an accredited facility, the site must satisfy minimum requirements for personnel, training, and equipment performance.[4,5] In addition, facilities must submit a 2-view (mediolateral oblique [MLO] and craniocaudal [CC]) screening examination of each breast of a woman with fat density breasts (breast imaging reporting and data system [BI-RADS] type 1 or 2) and of a woman with dense breasts (BI-RADS type 3 or 4) for each mammography unit.[6] If a facility submits mammograms identified as a fatty breast that are identified as dense ($\geq$50% dense) by the reviewer, or mammograms identified as dense that are identified as fatty ($\leq$50% dense), the submitted mammograms are returned to the facility with a request to submit a case that meets the appropriate mammographic density criteria. Because of variations in body habitus or the ability of the patient to cooperate,

[a] Department of Radiological Sciences, David Geffen School of Medicine at UCLA, 200 UCLA Medical Plaza, Room 165-47, Los Angeles, CA 90095, USA
[b] Department of Radiological Sciences, David Geffen School of Medicine at UCLA, 200 UCLA Medical Plaza, Room 165-53, Los Angeles, CA 90095, USA
[c] Department of Radiological Sciences, David Geffen School of Medicine at UCLA, Box 951721, Los Angeles, CA, USA
* Corresponding author.
E-mail address: lbassett@mednet.ucla.edu

Radiol Clin N Am 48 (2010) 903–915
doi:10.1016/j.rcl.2010.06.006
0033-8389/10/$ — see front matter © 2010 Elsevier Inc. All rights reserved.

it is not possible to attain the highest-quality mammograms in all women. Therefore, facilities are requested to submit what they consider to be representative images of their best work. This is an important reason for interpreting physicians to be active in the selection of images that are selected for submission to the accrediting body.

The ACR MAP clinical image evaluation process includes an assessment of these 8 categories: (1) positioning, (2) compression, (3) exposure, (4) contrast, (5) sharpness, (6) noise, (7) artifacts, and (8) labeling. This article reviews each of these image quality categories in detail.

In 1997, a total of 1034 units failed the initial clinical image evaluation submission of analog images to the ACR MAP.[7,8] In these failed initial applications, 6128 categories were cited by reviewers as deficient. These deficiencies included 1250 (20%) deficiencies in positioning, 944 (15%) in exposure, 887 (14%) in compression, 806 (13%) in sharpness, 785 (13%) in contrast, 703 (11%) in labeling, 465 (8%) in artifacts, and 288 (5%) in noise. A significantly higher proportion of failures were attributed to positioning deficiencies for fatty breasts than for dense breasts ($P = .028$). Higher proportions of failures in dense breasts were related to deficiencies in compression ($P<.001$) and exposure ($P<.001$). A follow-up study showed considerable improvement in images submitted in 2003. From 1987 (the inception of the ACR MAP) through 1991, only 70% of the mammography facilities that applied for accreditation for their analog units passed on their first submission. In 2003, 88.3% of the SFM facilities' units passed on their first submission of images, indicating a marked improvement in the quality of mammography since MQSA went into effect and the accreditation program was mandated.

The following text focuses on the 8 categories of the clinical image evaluation process with an emphasis on digital mammography (**Table 1**).

POSITIONING

Breast positioning has improved dramatically over the years. This is because of a better understanding of the anatomy and mobility of the breast and improved capabilities of modern dedicated mammography equipment.[9] The standard screening views are the MLO and CC views. Because these are the only views used for screening mammography, the goal should be to image as much breast tissue as possible on these views.[10]

Before beginning the actual positioning maneuvers, the radiologic technologist performing SFM, CRM, or FFDM (if there is an option) determines which size image receptor is most appropriate for the woman being examined. Both 18 × 24-cm and 24 × 30-cm image receptors are usually available for SFM, CRM, and some FFDM units.

Positioning for the MLO View

The MLO is the view that provides the best opportunity to include most of the breast tissue in a single image (**Fig. 1**A). Because the breast lies primarily on the pectoralis muscle and anterior to the muscle on the MLO view, a generous amount of pectoralis muscle should be included to ensure that far posterior breast tissues are included. The pectoralis muscle should be wide with an anterior convex margin. The muscle should extend to the posterior nipple line (PNL) or below. On the MLO image, the PNL is drawn at an angle approximately perpendicular to the muscle (usually about 45°), extending from the nipple to the pectoralis muscle or to the edge of the film, whichever comes first (see **Fig. 1**B). In addition, the inferior mammary fold should be open and visualized on the image to ensure that the posterior tissues in the lower breast are included. An anterior concave margin occurs when the pectoralis muscle is contracted, resulting in less inclusion of the posterior fibroglandular tissue (**Fig. 2**A). Whenever possible, dense (fibroglandular) tissue should not extend to the posterior edge of the film, as this would suggest that additional tissue was excluded from the image (see **Fig. 2**B).

Skin folds on the image should be avoided because they can obscure a lesion or mimic an abnormality (see **Fig. 2**C). Occasionally, skin folds in the axilla cannot be avoided but these usually do not pose problems in interpretation.

If proper methods have been used during the initiation and application of compression, the breast should not be sagging with the nipple lower than appropriate and the inframammary fold should be open (see **Fig. 2**D).

Positioning for the CC View

The overriding goal for positioning the CC view should be to include all of the posteromedial tissue, as this is the area of the breast most likely to be excluded in the MLO view (**Fig. 3**). If proper methods are used, the radiologic technologist can include almost all the posteromedial fibroglandular tissue without resorting to exaggerated medial positioning of the CC, which may result in unnecessary exclusion of posterolateral tissue. Exaggerated medial positioning may result in unnecessary exclusion of posterolateral tissue (**Fig. 4**A, B). However, although as much lateral tissue as possible should be included, lateral tissue should never be included at the expense

Table 1
The 8 categories for clinical image evaluation

Category	Potential Deficiencies
Positioning	Poor visualization of posterior tissues Sagging breast on MLO Inadequate amount of pectoralis muscle on MLO Inadequate inframammary fold Breast positioned too high on image receptor on MLO Skin folds Posterior nipple line on CC not within 1 cm of MLO Excessive exaggeration on CC view Portion of breast cut off Other body parts projected over breast
Compression	Poor separation of parenchymal densities Nonuniform exposure levels Patient motion
Exposure	Generalized underexposure Generalized overexposure Inadequate penetration of dense areas Excessive penetration of lucent areas
Contrast	Inadequate contrast Excessive contrast
Sharpness	Poor delineation of linear structures Poor delineation of feature margins Poor delineation of microcalcifications
Noise	Visually striking mottle pattern Noise-limited visualization of detail
Artifacts	Image receptor artifacts (ghosting, pixel drop-off) Processing algorithm artifacts (vertical bars, skin tearing) Grid-related artifact Laser printer artifact/scanning lines Cracked compression paddle Hair, deodorant, and so on
Labeling	Failure to properly identify: patient name and additional patient identifier, facility name and location (city, state, and zip), examination date, view and laterality, unit identification or room number (if more than one), technologist identification

of medial tissue. So, this is a challenging trade-off. The radiologist reviewing the images should go by the rule that the nipple should be in the midline on the CC, avoiding exaggeration to the inner or outer breast.

Visualization of the pectoralis muscle on the CC is evidence that sufficient posterior breast tissue has been included. However, the pectoralis muscle is seen in only approximately 30% of properly positioned CC views.[10] The measurement of the PNL is a reliable index as to whether the CC view includes sufficient posterior tissue when the muscle is not visualized. The PNL is drawn from the nipple directly posteriorly to the muscle or to the edge of the image if the muscle is not included. When the muscle is not visualized, a general rule is that

the measurement of the PNL on the CC view should be within 1 cm of its length on the MLO view (see **Fig. 4**C, D).[10] Although the length of the PNL is usually greater on the MLO view, in approximately 10% of correctly positioned cases, the measurement of the PNL is slightly greater on the CC view.

COMPRESSION

Breast compression contributes to digital image quality by immobilizing the breast (reducing motion unsharpness), producing a more uniform, thinner tissue (lower scattered radiation, more even penetration of x-rays, less magnification and geometric blurring, less superposition of tissues), and lower radiation dose.[11] Uniform

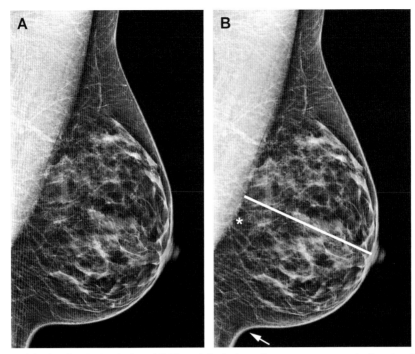

Fig. 1. Proper positioning for the MLO view. (*A*) There is inclusion of a generous amount of pectoralis muscle with a convex anterior margin extending below the posterior nipple line (PNL). (*B*) The PNL is drawn at a 45° angle from the nipple extending to the anterior edge of the pectoralis muscle. There is visualization of retromammary fat (*asterisk*) posterior to the fibroglandular tissues and open inframammary fold (*arrow*).

thickness means that the density of tissues is more likely to correspond to subtle attenuation differences in the tissues rather than to thickness differences. Inadequate compression is manifested by overlapping breast structures, nonuniform tissue exposure, and motion unsharpness (also called blur) (**Fig. 5**). The underlying image receptor device supports the breast on the CC position. Therefore, motion unsharpness caused by patient movement and/or inadequate compression is more commonly seen on the MLO view than on the CC view. (See the section on unsharpness in later discussion.)

CONTRAST

Image contrast can be described as the degree of variation in the different shades of gray on digital images (or variation in optical densities between different areas of the image on a film). The different shades of gray allow the interpreting physician to perceive x-ray attenuation differences in the breast tissues. Image contrast resolution is the term used to describe the ability of a system to differentiate 2 areas that have only slightly different gray levels. Not limited to the fixed optical density characteristics of a specific type of film, the ability to obtain variable contrast is one of the greatest advantages of soft

copy reading with DM. Studies have shown that despite lower spatial resolution, DM systems have at least a 20% improvement in image contrast resolution that compensates for lower spatial resolution.[12]

However, mammography accreditation programs currently require that all images are submitted in a hard copy format. Although it is possible to display digital images in a hard copy format, the advantages of digital technology cannot be fully realized without soft copy display of the mammograms, making electronic display a key and inseparable component of DM. Therefore, when digital images are printed out in a hard copy format, it is important to adjust to the best contrast settings on the laser printer.

Image contrast can be affected by the printer contrast range settings or by manipulating the window-level settings on the soft copy workstation (**Fig. 6**). If the printer contrast range (lookup table) settings or the image window level is too wide, contrast is inadequate on the printed images (see **Fig. 6**B). However, if the printer contrast range settings or the image window level is too narrow, the image contrast is excessive (see **Fig. 6**C).

EXPOSURE

The low peak kilovolt [kV(p)] and high contrast techniques required in mammography result in

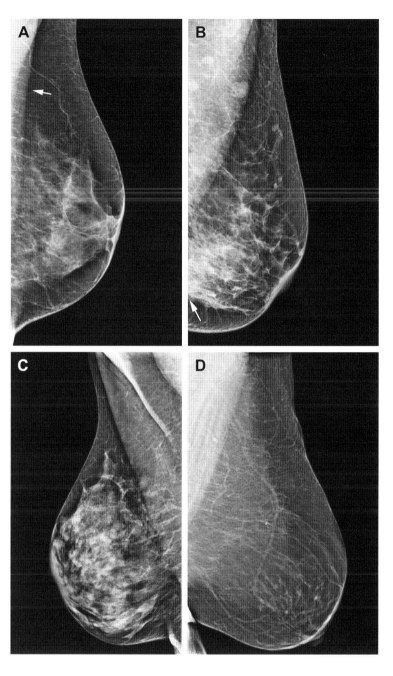

Fig. 2. Deficiencies in positioning for the MLO view. (*A*) The pectoralis muscle extends below the PNL but is not wide enough and has a slightly concave anterior margin (*arrow*), resulting in exclusion of the posterior tissues. (*B*) The fibroglandular tissue extends to the edge of the film (*arrow*), which could result in nonvisualization of a posterior abnormality. Note absence of the inframammary fold. (*C*) Skin folds can potentially obscure a lesion. On this MLO image, there are skin folds at the inframammary fold and the axilla. (*D*) Sagging breast. The radiologic technologist did not hold the breast up and out as compression was applied. Note the low position of the nipple and prominent skin fold at the inframammary area.

a small acceptable exposure latitude.[13] Even small differences in kV(p) or milliampere seconds (mAs) can result in digital mammograms with large variations in gray levels (optical density in SFM). Therefore, kV(p) and mAs must be carefully selected, and automatic exposure control (AEC) performance must be precise over the range of kV(p), breast thickness, and tissue densities encountered in clinical practice. Proper functioning of the phototimer should be evaluated using varying thicknesses of breast-equivalent phantom material during initial calibration of the mammography unit, during the annual survey by the medical physicist, and periodically during the phantom image evaluation by the radiologic technologist.[3] The mammography generator should have sufficient output to adequately image large breasts and dense breasts with reasonably short (<2 seconds) exposure time. The radiologic technologist can monitor exposures for each clinical image based on the length of time of the audible exposure.

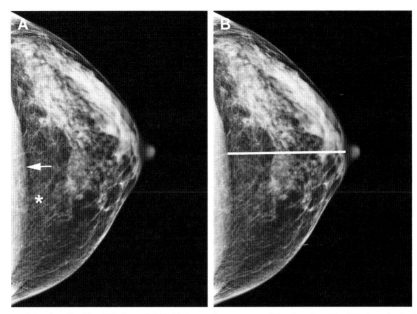

Fig. 3. Proper positioning for the CC view. (*A*) Evidence of proper positioning for the CC view includes location of the nipple in the midline, inclusion of the pectoralis muscle (*arrow*) on the image (not required), and depiction of retromammary fat (*asterisk*) posterior to the medial fibroglandular tissue. Note that some posterior lateral tissue often extends beyond the edge of the film. (*B*) The PNL is drawn directly posterior from the nipple to the muscle or to the posterior edge of the image when the muscle is not visualized.

Proper mammographic exposure should be assessed under correct viewing conditions. For soft copy workstation reading, ambient room light should be approximately equivalent to the workstation monitor's luminance.[14,15] In particular, there should not be any view boxes or other strong light sources directly across the room because they may reflect on the monitor screen. It may be necessary to rearrange a reading room to achieve optimal conditions for interpreting digital mammograms.

Underexposure has been shown to be a more frequent image deficiency than overexposure.[7] Underexposure is manifested by the inability to see image details within dense fibroglandular tissues. Because lesions can be obscured within the underexposed dense tissue, underexposure is a potentially more serious error because it can lead to false-negative results. The pectoral muscle is one of the densest structures seen on the MLO view, and it is important that the muscle be exposed sufficiently to show underlying breast tissues (**Fig. 7**A). Underexposure of the pectoral muscle can result in nonvisualization of underlying breast tissue, lymph nodes, or masses (see **Fig. 7**B). This is more commonly seen in fatty breasts that are easily penetrated, because the AEC system detector that lies under the breast tissue terminates the exposure before the dense pectoralis muscle is fully exposed.

Severe overexposure results in loss of details in the thin or fatty parts of the breast. However, minor overexposure is frequently a recoverable error that can be compensated for with FFDM by adjusting the image at the workstation (analogous to using a high-intensity bright light for SFM). Underexposure is an unrecoverable error that cannot be compensated for by workstation manipulations and requires repeat imaging.

NOISE

Noise is defined as random fluctuations included in the image data when the detector is exposed to an x-ray. Noise is expressed in different ways (eg, variance, standard deviation, noise power spectrum, signal to noise ratio, noise equivalent quanta, detective quantum efficiency), with each quantity providing complementary information.[13] Sometimes referred to as radiographic mottle, noise compromises the ability to discern small details, such as fine calcifications. Quantum mottle is the major source of noise in mammography (**Fig. 8**). It is caused by a statistical fluctuation in the number of x-ray photons absorbed at individual locations in the image receptor.

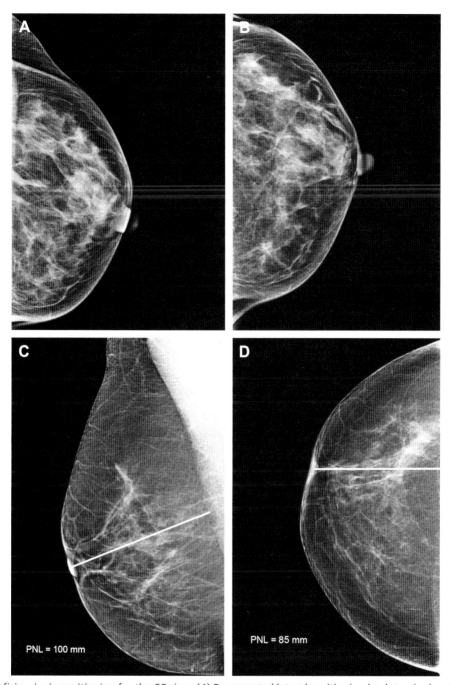

Fig. 4. Deficiencies in positioning for the CC view. (A) Exaggerated lateral positioning leads to nipple not located in the midline and exclusion of posterior medial tissue. There is also a large lateral skin fold. (B) Same patient with proper positioning shows all of the posterior medial tissue. (C, D) Inadequate inclusion of posterior tissue on the CC view. PNL measures 100 mm on the MLO view (C) but only 85 mm on the CC view (D).

Using indirect DM detectors (amorphous silicon), the x-ray photons are first converted to light photons, which then expose the digital image receptor. Using direct DM detectors, the x-ray photons directly expose the digital image receptor (selenium). The fewer the total number of light photons (for indirect digital exposure receptors) or x-ray photons (for direct exposure digital receptors) that produce the image, the greater the amount of quantum mottle that may be observed. Noise is also more likely to be a problem with DM because it has the

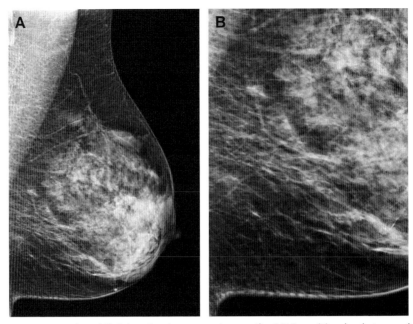

Fig. 5. Inadequate compression. (*A*) Suboptimal compression on the MLO position leads to overlapping breast structures, nonuniform tissue exposure, and motion unsharpness. (*B*) Close-up of the lower breast better depicts these deficiencies, especially blurring of linear structures in the inferior breast.

potential for higher contrast images and higher contrast makes mottle more evident. The increasing public attention to radiation dose presents a real challenge in reducing noise in digital mammograms.[16,17]

SHARPNESS

Sharpness is the ability of the imaging system to define an edge or margin against the surrounding tissue. Unsharpness is manifested by blurring of

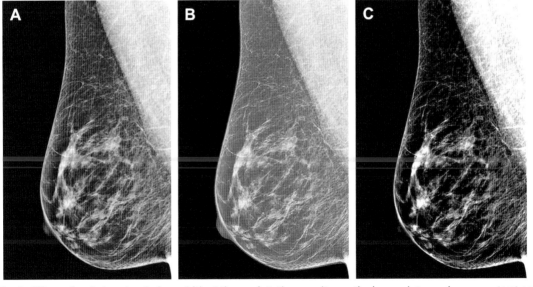

Fig. 6. Effects of variations in window width at the workstation monitor or the laser printer on image contrast on the RMLO view of the same patient. (*A*) Proper window width allows the interpreting physician to perceive subtle x-ray attenuation differences in the breast tissue. (*B*) A window width that is too wide at the soft copy worksta-tion or on the printer settings results in inadequate image contrast. (*C*) A window width that is too narrow causes excessive contrast with loss of image detail, including the skin line.

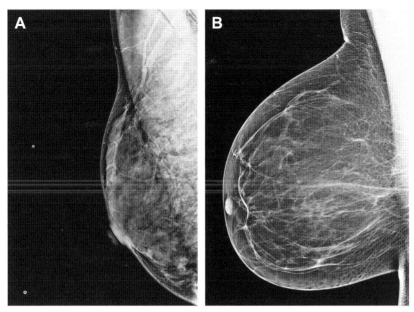

Fig. 7. Proper exposure can be assessed by evaluating the tissue underlying the pectoralis muscle on the MLO view. (*A*) Optimal exposure results in visualization of the pectoralis muscle with any breast tissue, lymph nodes, or masses that project over it. (*B*) An underexposed mammogram resulting in inadequate penetration of the pectoralis muscle resulting in a "white" muscle that may obscure overlying breast tissue, lymph nodes, or masses.

the edges of fine linear structures, tissue borders, and calcifications.

Motion unsharpness in DM is caused by movement of the breast during exposure and is

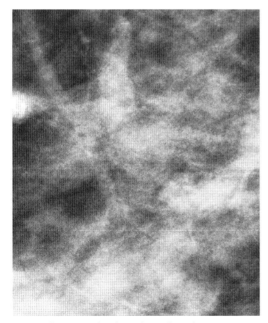

Fig. 8. Close-up of a low-dose digital mammogram demonstrating quantum mottle, the most common source of noise in mammography.

minimized by using a short exposure time and adequate breast compression. Motion unsharpness is most often identified on the lower aspect of the MLO view (see **Fig. 5**B). X-ray tube voltage [kV(p)] may be increased for thick, dense breasts to allow reduction of exposure time.

A larger focal spot size, a longer object-to-film distance (distance from the breast to the image receptor), and a shorter source-to-image distance (distance from the x-ray tube to the image receptor) increases geometric unsharpness. During the last decade, the focal spot sizes of dedicated mammography units have been reduced for contact (the breast placed directly on the image receptor device) and magnification mammography.

Additional unsharpness can be attributed to the spread of signal within the digital image receptor device. Factors including the detector type (direct or indirect capture), pixel size, and postprocessing algorithms can have an effect on the sharpness of the final image.

ARTIFACTS

An artifact can be defined as any density variation on an image that does not reflect true attenuation differences in the subject. FFDM artifacts can result from problems with the x-ray equipment, requiring the attention of the facility's medical physicist and/or contact with the manufacturer.

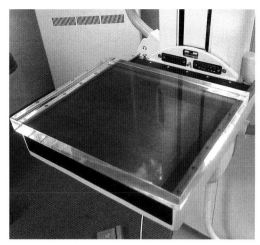

Fig. 9. DM artifacts. Image of a flat-field phantom test setup. When imaged with a homogeneous tissue-equivalent phantom, this test can help identify artifacts within the imaging chain.

Although many artifacts are the same as in SFM mammography (such as gridlines and extraneous objects such as the patient's hair on the image), there are several artifacts that are specific to the digital receptor and digital processing algorithms.[18]

Many digital artifacts can be subtle on clinical images. Therefore, it is important that the facility's quality control program detects and corrects any artifacts. Periodic imaging of a flat field with a homogeneous tissue-equivalent phantom can help identify artifacts within the imaging chain (Fig. 9).

Common artifacts seen on this flat-field test include ghosting and pixel drop-off (bad or failed pixels). A ghosting artifact results from an incomplete erasure of signal from the previous examination (Fig. 10). The ghosting artifact is more frequently identified on the selenium detector than on the amorphous silicon detector. Pixel drop-off can result in a permanent white dot or permanent black dot on the image (Fig. 11A). These failed detector elements can mimic microcalcification on a clinical image (see Fig. 11B). The facility's medical physicist can usually remove ghosting and pixel drop-off artifacts during a detector recalibration.

Although the quality control program can detect many of the artifacts resulting from detector or radiographic system problems, artifacts outside the scope of the regular quality control protocol may also arise. It is important that the interpreting physician be aware of these common artifacts. For

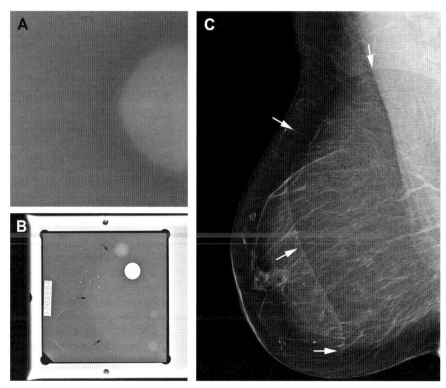

Fig. 10. Ghosting artifacts. (A) This flat-field test demonstrates a ghosting artifact that results from an incomplete erasure of signal from a previous examination. (B) ACR phantom with ghosting artifact (arrows). (C) Clinical image with ghosting artifact (arrows).

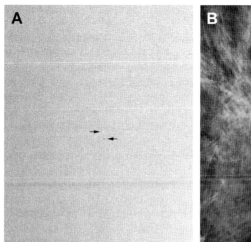
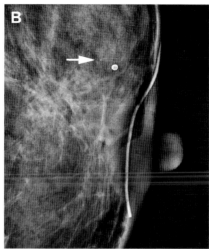

Fig. 11. Pixel drop-off (bad or failed pixel). (A) Flat-field image test showing pixel drop-off as a white-and-black artifact. (B) Magnification view from a postsurgery, preradiotherapy examination of a patient with ductal carcinoma in situ (DCIS). The failed detector element artifact (*arrow*) was misinterpreted as residual DCIS calcification and was recognized as an artifact when it reappeared on additional imaging in the same location and same size despite repositioning of the breast. A recalibration of the detector removed the artifact.

example, DM equipment uses a motor-driven reciprocating grid system. Failure of the motor can occur when imaging in the lateral view because of the additional force needed to drive the grid against gravity. The resulting DM image may have visible fine parallel grid lines (**Fig. 12**).

Because of the limitations in dynamic range of a detector, highly penetrated areas of the detector can be susceptible to truncation or overenhancement when the processing algorithms are applied. One area of the mammographic image susceptible to overpenetration is the skin line. Subsequent processing algorithms can result in the skin-tearing artifact, whereby the skin edge is lost in the background (**Fig. 13**).

Over time, small cracks can develop in the plastic magnification stand or compression paddle resulting in a visible artifact (**Fig. 14**).

LABELING

The interpreting physician is often called on to review mammograms performed at other facilities. A review of mammograms from facilities across the country submitted for clinical image evaluation to ACR MAP in 1993 revealed that nonstandardized labeling practices were common.[19] In addition to nonstandardized formats, labeling often did not contain enough information to adequately identify the patient or the facility where the examination was performed.

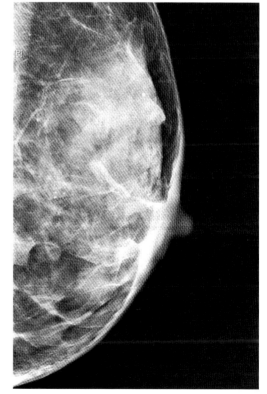

Fig. 12. Grid lines. Fine parallel grid lines are visible on this close-up of a DM medial-lateral view.

For DM, standardized methods for labeling images have been developed by the manufacturers to ensure that the items required for accreditation are included in the digital image. These requirements include unique identifiers for the patient (first and last name and at least 1 other identifier such as medical record number or date of birth), date of examination, the facility where the examination was performed (at least the facility name, city, state, and zip code), the radiologic technologist who performed the examination, and laterality and view for each image (located at the corner of the image closest to the axilla). For facilities with more than one mammography unit, a unit identification or room number is also required.

SUMMARY

Clinical image evaluation is an essential ongoing quality assurance activity that should be performed on a daily basis by every physician who interprets mammograms. The interpreting physician's evaluation of the clinical images complements other quality assurance activities, such as regular phantom image evaluation by the radiologic technologist and medical physicist. Ongoing feedback from the interpreting physician to the radiologic technologist about image deficiencies (and recognition for good-quality images) is important. It should be remembered that the original purpose of the ACR MAP program was to improve the quality of mammography. Learning to recognize the most likely causes of image deficiencies expedites the rapid correction of problems and maintenance of a high-quality breast imaging practice. This article has focused on the clinical imaging evaluation process for DM.

REFERENCES

1. Public Law 102–539. The mammography quality standards act of 1992.
2. Food and Drug Administration. Mammography facilities—requirements for accrediting bodies and quality standards and certification requirements; interim rules. Fed Regist 1993;58:67558.
3. Hendrick RE. Quality assurance in mammography: accreditation, legislation, and compliance with quality assurance standards. Radiol Clin North Am 1992;30:243–55.
4. American College of Radiology. Practice guideline for determinants of image quality in digital mammography. Available at: http://www.acr.org/SecondaryMainMenuCategories/quality_safety/guidelines/breast/image_quality_digital_mammo.aspx. Accessed January 5, 2010.

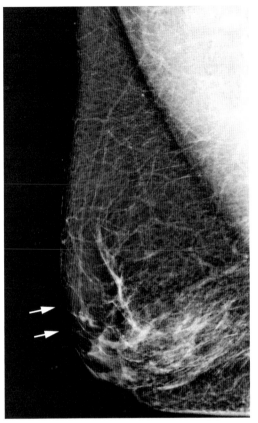

Fig. 13. Skin-tearing artifact. The thinner tissue near the skin line may allow overpenetration of the detector, which when subjected to processing algorithms results in truncation or loss of the normally visible skin line (*arrows*).

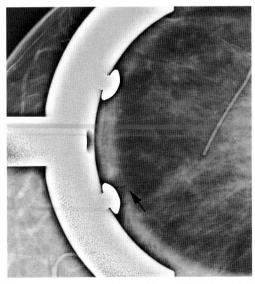

Fig. 14. Spot compression paddle artifact. A crack in the compression paddle may cause a visible artifact (*arrow*). The paddle must be replaced.

5. American College of Radiology. Practice guideline for the performance of screening and diagnostic mammography. Available at: http://www.acr.org/SecondaryMainMenuCategories/quality_safety/guidelines/breast/Screening_Diagnostic.aspx. Accessed January 5, 2010.

6. McLelland R, Hendrick RE, Zinninger MD, et al. The American College of Radiology Mammography Accreditation Program. AJR Am J Roentgenol 1991;157:473–9.

7. Bassett LW, Farria DM, Bansal S, et al. Reasons for failure of a mammography unit at clinical image review in the American College of Radiology Mammography Accreditation Program. Radiology 2000;215:698–702.

8. Destouet JM, Bassett LW, Yaffe MJ, et al. The ACR's Mammography Accreditation Program: 10 years of experience since MQSA. J Am Coll Radiol 2005;2:585–94.

9. Eklund GW, Cardenosa G. The art of mammographic positioning. Radiol Clin North Am 1992;30:21–53.

10. Bassett LW, Hirbawi IA, DeBruhl N, et al. Mammographic positioning: evaluation from the view box. Radiology 1993;188:803–6.

11. Helvie MA, Chan HP, Adler DD, et al. Breast thickness in routine mammograms: Effect on image quality and radiation dose. AJR Am J Roentgenol 1994;163:1371–4.

12. Fischer U, Baum F, Obenauer S, et al. Comparative study in patients with microcalcifications: full-field digital mammography vs screen-film mammography. Eur Radiol 2002;12:2679–83.

13. Curry TS, Dowdey JE, Murry RC. The radiographic image. In: Curry TS, Dowdey JE, Murry RC, editors. Christensen's physics of diagnostic radiology. 4th edition. Philadelphia: Lea & Febiger; 1990. p. 196–218.

14. Alter AJ, Kargas GA, Kargas SA, et al. The influence of ambient and viewbox light upon visual detection of low-contrast targets in a radiograph. Invest Radiol 1982;17:403–6.

15. Siddiqui KM, Chia S, Knight N, et al. Design and ergonomic considerations for the filmless environment. J Am Coll Radiol 2006;3:456–67.

16. Toroi P, Zanca F, Young KC, et al. Experimental investigation on the choice of the tungsten/rhodium anode/filter combination for an amorphous selenium-based digital mammography system. Eur Radiol 2007;17(9):2368–75 [Epub 2007 Feb 1].

17. Tischenko O, Hoeschen C, Dance DR, et al. Evaluation of a novel method of noise reduction using computer-simulated mammograms. Radiat Prot Dosimetry 2005;114(1–3):81–4.

18. Ayyala RS, Chorlton M, Behrman RH, et al. Digital mammographic artifacts on full-field systems: what are they and how do I fix them? Radiographics 2008;28:1999–2008.

19. Bassett LW, Jessop NW, Wilcox PA. Mammography film-labeling practices. Radiology 1993;187:773–5.

Digital Mammography Imaging: Breast Tomosynthesis and Advanced Applications

Mark A. Helvie, MD

KEYWORDS

- Digital breast tomosynthesis • Digital mammography
- Computer-aided detection • Breast cancer
- Breast imaging • Mammography

The Achilles heel of screening mammography is the detection of cancer in women with radiographic dense breasts. Although nearly all cancers will be apparent in fatty breasts, only half will be visible in extremely dense breast.[1] This results, at least in large part, from the masking or camouflaging of noncalcified cancers by surrounding dense tissue. This article discusses several derivative digital technologies being developed to overcome the weakness of conventional mammography (film screen and/or digital mammography [DM]). The emphasis is on digital breast tomosynthesis with secondary discussion of contrast-enhanced DM and combined digital mammographic and ultrasound equipment. All the aforementioned technologies are investigational in the United States at this time and none are approved for clinical use by the US Food and Drug Administration (FDA). The clinical application of these technologies, if any, will be determined by scientific investigation and regulatory approval.

DIGITAL BREAST TOMOSYNTHESIS MAMMOGRAPHY

Digital breast tomosynthesis mammography (DBT) is one technology being developed to improve detection and characterization of breast lesions especially in women with nonfatty breasts. In this technique, multiple projection images are reconstructed allowing visual review of thin breast sections offering the potential to unmask cancers obscured by normal tissue located above and below the lesion. DBT involves the acquisition of multiple projection exposures by a digital detector from a mammographic x-ray source that moves over a limited arc angle.[2–11] These projection image datasets are reconstructed using specific algorithms. The clinical reader is presented with a series of images (slices) through the entire breast that are read at a workstation similar to review of a computed tomography (CT) or magnetic resonance (MR) imaging study. Because each reconstructed slice may be as thin as 0.5 mm, masses and mass margins that may otherwise be superimposed with out-of-plane structures should be more visible in the reconstructed slice. This should allow visualization (detection) and better characterization of noncalcified lesions in particular.

Technique

The advent of DM and computer reconstruction algorithms has allowed derivative technology to be developed including tomosynthesis. In conventional DM, a compressed breast is exposed to

Grant support RO1 091713, R33CA 120234, RO1 CA 095153, MDA 9050210012.
Disclosures: Consultant: General Electric Global Research.
Department of Radiology, University of Michigan Health System, 1500 East Medical Center Drive, SPC 5326, Ann Arbor, MI 48109, USA
E-mail address: mahelvie@umich.edu

Radiol Clin N Am 48 (2010) 917–929
doi:10.1016/j.rcl.2010.06.009

ionizing radiation. Energy that passes through the breast is transformed into an electrical signal by a detector that produces the clinical image. The x-ray tube is stationary, the breast is stationary, and the detector is stationary. The image that is produced in any one projection such as a craniocaudal (CC) or mediolateral oblique (MLO) view is a two-dimensional representation of three-dimensional space. Each pixel is therefore an average of the information obtained through the full thickness of the breast. A three-dimensional depiction of the breast would be advantageous similar to three-dimensional depictions allowed by CT, MR, or ultrasound scanning.

In digital breast tomosynthesis, the x-ray tube is moved through a limited arc angle while the breast is compressed and a series of exposures are obtained (**Fig. 1**). These individual exposures are only a fraction of the total dose used during conventional DM. The total dose used should be within FDA limits and is expected to be near or slightly more than the routine mammographic dose if DBT becomes clinically approved. If there is a 45° arc of movement and an exposure is taken every 3°, there will be 15 individual exposures. These raw projection datasets require reconstruction using algorithms similar to those used in other three-dimensional image sets. The projection datasets are not usually interpreted by the radiologists, but rather the interpretation is based only on the reconstructed tomosynthesis images. Typically, the projection datasets are reconstructed into very thin (eg, 1 mm) slices for radiologist review.

Imaging Technique

Several manufacturers have applied different methods to develop and perform tomosynthesis. There are likely advantages and disadvantages of each technique. However, these differences may produce different clinical results making clinical comparisons between manufacturers difficult. Engineering constraints include total radiation dose, image time, patient motion, detector performance, detector motion, and ability to image the entire breast. There is also the necessity to provide future biopsy capability for those lesions detected only by tomosynthesis.

Manufacturers vary the arc of movement (typically 11–60°), the number of individual exposures (typically 9–25), use of continuous or pulsed exposure, stability or movement of the detector, exposure parameters, total dose, effective size of pixels, x-ray source/filter source, single or binned pixels, and patient position. These theoretic and engineering decisions may lead to different clinical outcomes and different reading recommendations for the different manufacturers. Of particular importance is the assessment of microcalcifications and whether one attempts to accurately depict microcalcifications by DBT. Because of the limited angle of scanning, the images are only quasi three-dimensional. The x-y plane perpendicular to the x-ray beam has the highest resolution. There is less resolution in the parallel plane or z axis. The dataset can be reconstructed for the radiologist to read by displaying different thicknesses. For example, if a 60-cm compressed breast is reconstructed at 1-mm thickness, there will be 60 slices for the physician to review. If the images are reconstructed at 0.5-mm thicknesses, there will be 120 images to be reviewed. If the images are reconstructed at 10-mm thick slabs using maximum intensity projection (MIP) thick slices, there will be 6 images to review.

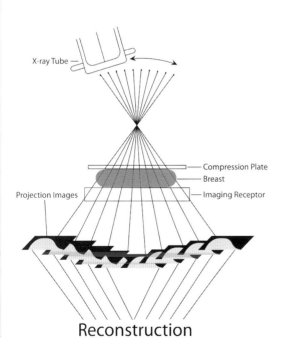

Reconstruction

Fig. 1. Digital breast tomosynthesis. The x-ray tube moves through a narrow arch while the breast is in compression. A series of exposures results in multiple projection image datasets. Each exposure is a fraction of the dose of a conventional mammographic view. Projection image datasets are reconstructed into multiple thin-slice images (eg, 1-mm thickness) for interpretation by the radiologist.

Radiation Dose

A major consideration for DBT manufacturers and regulators is the balance between dose and image quality. Because image quality tends to be directly related to dose, compromises are necessary. All manufacturers have produced equipment with dosing parameters less than the current FDA limit of 300 mrad per exposure. The common conventional mammographic dose per view is 150 to 250 mrad. However, achieving lower doses is optimal. Variations in target filter, breast thickness, and breast density further complicate this analysis. However, if DBT leads to reduction in recall rate or improvement in sensitivity and specificity, a minimally higher dose may be acceptable.

Tomosynthesis Reconstruction Algorithms

Similar to CT and MR, reconstruction algorithms are a critical element for tomosynthesis.[3–8,12–14] It is beyond the scope of this discussion to provide more than a cursory explanation. Unlike historical tomography used for intravenous pylograms in which the projection images were interpreted as is, tomosynthesis reconstructs raw projection image datasets to produce clinical images. Reconstruction techniques include shift-and-add, tuned aperture CT, matrix inversion, filtered back projection, maximum likelihood reconstruction, and simultaneous algebraic reconstruction technique. Certain reconstruction methods may be better for masses and other methods better for calcifications. Details of specific manufacturer algorithms are not always in the public domain.

Potential Benefits of Clinical Breast Imaging with Tomosynthesis

The potential benefits of DBT include improvement in screening sensitivity, improvement in lesion size at detection, improvement in characterization, and decrease in recall rates. DBT may be useful in both the screening and diagnostic evaluation. Neither has been proved in randomized controlled trials.

In theory DBT, with thin section display, should allow superior detection of lesions that historically have been masked by overlying tissue. The primary benefit of DBT would be expected to be for noncalcified mammographic findings such as masses, asymmetries, and distortion (**Figs. 2–5**). In the most basic application, DBT would allow visualization of cancers not apparent by conventional mammography thus improving sensitivity. Although many regard tomosynthesis as a technique for dense breast tissue, it may also have significant applications for those patients with nondense breasts by allowing detection of smaller lesions. This is a variant of improved sensitivity as a decrease in size at time of detection may be associated with improvement in clinical outcome. DBT also offers the possibility that characterization or specificity may be increased by better assessment of detected lesions and reduction in false-positive recalls. This is because the margin of a mass or character of an asymmetry may be better visualized. Malignant lesions may appear more malignant and benign lesions more benign. If these concepts are borne out, DBT may allow for improved sensitivity coupled with improved specificity. Recall rates for asymmetries and possible masses may be lowered if DBT better depicts the morphologic characterization of such findings. Diagnostic evaluation of potential masses and asymmetries found by screening mammography could also be a DBT function. It is unlikely that calcification characterization would improve dramatically.

An understated but important aspect of DBT theory is that the basic technology used is mammography. To date, mammography is the only screening imaging technology that has proved itself in randomized controlled trials to show survival benefit.[15] Improvement in mammographic technology with DBT would therefore be closer to the original mammographic methods than other competing technologies such as MR, ultrasound, or CT with the clinical implication of improved screening.

Proving the superiority of a new technology is more difficult than showing noninferiority. Even if the technology proves useful, there are many clinical considerations that will affect potential use. Given the current cost climate, incremental reimbursement will be challenging. If DBT costs more and takes longer to read, there will be barriers to acceptance. Work-flow issues need careful attention as does technologist and physician training. Obviously, there are many questions to answer before these theories are accepted or refuted.

As no tomosynthetic system is currently clinically approved by the FDA for use in the United States, there are differences of opinion regarding what the best clinical practice acquisition and display methods will be. Of particular interest is whether DBT would replace conventional mammographic views or would be an adjunct to current mammographic views or some combination of the two. The number of DBT views and number of conventional views that would constitute a routine mammogram have not been determined. From a physician's standpoint, 2 extremes can be considered and multiple hybrid reading scenarios can then be postulated. If tomosynthesis is extremely sensitive for masses and calcifications, it may be theoretically possible that a single tomographic view such as the MLO would constitute a routine mammogram. A reader would be presented with a MLO DBT image set for assessment. Masses,

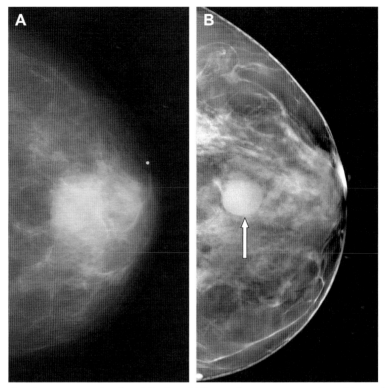

Fig. 2. CC conventional mammography view (*A*) of a middle-aged woman presenting with a palpable mass indicated by a metallic breast biopsy marker. Tomosynthesis 1-mm thick image (*B*) depicts a circumscribed mass (*arrow*). Five such masses were noted by DBT at other levels, all proven to be cysts by ultrasound.

calcifications, distortions, and so forth. would all be detected. At the other extreme of clinical options would be obtaining tomosynthesis images in both the CC and MLO projections and 2 conventional digital images in both the CC and MLO projection (4 views each breast). In this scenario, a physician would read the 2 conventional digital images (CC and MLO) as well as 2 tomosynthetic images. A reader may concentrate on mass detection on the tomosynthesis views and calcifications on the conventional mammograms. In between are hybrid reading scenarios that would have various combinations of these 2 extremes. For example, mammographic study could include a MLO DBT image and conventional CC view. To date, the best or likely method of acquisition has not been scientifically determined. This determination may be manufacturer dependent, technology dependent, and likely will be a compromise among sensitivity, dose, and practice guidelines. Different manufacturers

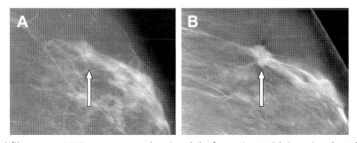

Fig. 3. Conventional film screen MLO mammography view (*A*) of a patient with invasive ductal cancer. The cancer, although vaguely apparent on the conventional mammogram (*arrow*), is much better visualized on the 1-mm thick tomosynthesis image (*B*) (*arrow*). Note the clarity of the spicules and the separation from surrounding tissue.

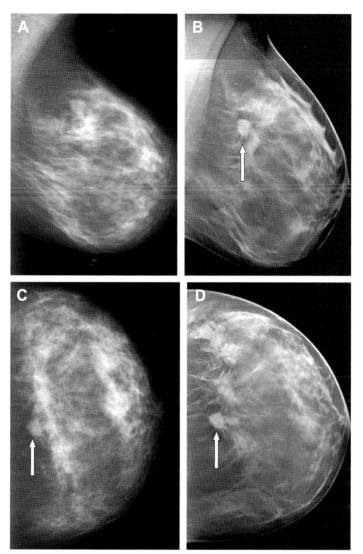

Fig. 4. Mediolateral oblique conventional mammogram (*A*) of a patient with invasive ductal cancer. The cancer was not apparent on the conventional MLO projection but could be vaguely seen on the cranial caudal view (*C*) as a density (*arrow*). 1-mm thick tomosynthesis images in both the MLO (*B*) and CC (*D*) view not only show the cancer (*arrow*) but also the margins.

may seek to solve the same problem with different theories and methods to achieve the same end point.

EARLY CLINICAL TOMOSYNTHESIS EVALUATIONS

We are now able to review several early experimental clinical DBT studies. These DBT studies for masses have generally shown good patient acceptance, physician preference for DBT images, improvement in sensitivity, improvement in characterization, and often longer physician reading times.[16–27] The findings with calcifications have been mixed. The test is neither 100% sensitive nor 100% specific. The real-world performance of DBT may be different than these experimental clinical studies because actual decisions regarding clinical care are not made in these studies. Some of the early studies are reviewed.

Reader Preference Studies

In 2007, Poplack and colleagues[16] evaluated 99 cases with DBT that were recalled for further evaluation from a screening trial. Only 14% of the recalls were for calcifications. One of 2 readers was asked to determine his/her preference regarding image quality. For 51% of cases,

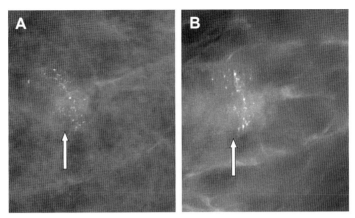

Fig. 5. Conventional CC digital mammogram (*A*) and tomosynthesis 11-mm thick MIP image (*B*) of microcalcifications proven to represent ductal carcinoma in situ. Both conventional and DBT images show calcifications well (*arrows*). The MIP image does not necessarily show microcalcifications above or below the 11-mm thick slice.

readers determined the DBT image quality was equal, 37% were considered superior, and 11% were considered inferior. Calcification assessment was problematic. Of those cases deemed of inferior image quality, 72% were for calcifications. In this select population, the investigators concluded that the recall rate could have been diminished by 40% if tomosynthesis images had been obtained at time of screening examination. This decrease in recall rate, however, is likely an overstatement of clinical practice as they did not study the potential increase in recall rate if tomosynthesis had been initially applied to a larger group of patients.

Good and colleagues[17] assessed 9 physicians' opinion on image quality with DBT. They evaluated 30 mixed diagnostic cases consisting of two-thirds masses and one-third calcifications. The readers determined that DBT image quality was somewhat better (44%) or significantly better (23%) in 67% of cases. Thirty-one percent were comparable and only 1.9% of DBT images were worse than conventional images. These results were similar to Poplack and colleagues'[16] results. This study also measured reading time, which was longer for DBT than conventional reading, with a mean time for conventional reading of 1.6 minutes and 2.7 minutes for DBT, a difference of 69%.

Andersson and colleagues,[18] using several expert readers and 40 cases that were considered extremely subtle or occult, assessed visibility of cancers by DBT. In this series, only 12% of cases were calcifications. The readers rated DBT image quality higher in 55%, equal in 32%, and inferior in 2%. Ten percent of cases were false-negative by both DBT and DM. The differences in perceived image quality were significant to a statistical value of $P = .01$.

Clinical Trials of DBT

Helvie and colleagues,[19] using 4 readers and a diagnostic set of mass cases scheduled for biopsy, determined that more masses were detected by DBT (49.5) than conventional mammography (36.5), an increase of 35.6%, which was significant for each reader. Only 7 malignant cases were included in the initial study. However, DBT detected 100% of cancers by all readers, whereas only 71% were detected by conventional mammography, an incremental cancer detection increase of 40%. Lo and colleagues,[20] in a similar study of diagnostic cases and lesion detection, also noted a 40% incremental detection rate for DBT (91% vs 65%) although no difference in cancer detection was noted in 4 cases of cancer.

Rafferty and colleagues[21] analyzed 310 DBT and DM cases using receiver operating curve (ROC) methods and 15 readers. They compared 3 reading methods: DM alone, DM and MLO DBT, and DM compared with DM and both CC DBT and MLO DBT. This reading method was different in that DBT was used as an adjunct to conventional DM. They found significant improvement in ROC area under the curve (AUC) values when DBT views were combined with DM compared with DM alone. For fatty breasts, the AUC was 0.880 for DM alone, 0.898 for DM and MLO DBT, and 0.915 for DM plus CC DBT with MLO DBT. The incremental advantage of using DBT with DM for dense breasts using the same study methods were proportionally greater, AUC of 0.786, 0.832, and 0.877 respectively. Still, the best DBT AUC was highest for women with fatty breasts (0.915) compared with dense breasts (0.877) suggesting that although DBT may improve test performance for cancer in women with dense breasts proportionally more than fatty breasts, maximum performance is still for women with fatty breasts.

Moore and colleagues[22] compared the recall data on 1957 patients screened with MLO DBT and standard 2-view DM. In this study, 10 readers read the conventional digital mammograms and 2 readers read the DBT studies. The standard DM screening mammography recall rate was 7.5% and the single-view DBT recall rate was 4.3%. The decline in recall rate by 43% is similar to the decline noted by Poplack and colleagues[16] and Rafferty and colleagues.[21] These studies suggest the potential for DBT to improve recall rates while maintaining sensitivity, at least in experimental reading situations.

Gur and colleagues[23] reported a retrospective reader study comparing DM with DBT alone and combined DM and DBT using an enriched population of 125 cases that included 35 known cancers. Of 90 benign study cases, 49% had either benign findings or had been recalled from screening. In an organized reader study, 8 radiologists reviewed images in several reading situations including 2-view (CC, MLO) DM alone, 2-view (CC, MLO) DBT images alone, and combined DM and DBT images of a single breast. The investigators noted a nonsignificant improvement in sensitivity when reading DBT alone (93%) was compared with DM alone (88%). The combination of DM and DBT did not improve sensitivity compared with DBT alone. Specificity was greatest with DBT combined with DM, compared with DBT alone, or with DM alone (0.72 vs 0.64 vs 0.60). There was a corresponding 10% relative decrease in unnecessary recall rate for benign findings by DBT versus DM alone. There was a significant 30% reduction in recall rate for cancer-free cases if DBT was used as an adjunct in combination with DM compared with DM alone. In this experimental situation, the mean time to read DBT was greater than DM (2.05 minutes vs 1.22 minutes) for a single breast. DBT plus DM reading time was even longer at 2.39 minutes. Although encouraging, the investigators cautioned that further evaluation in a more realistic clinical situation was warranted.

Not all DBT studies have yielded positive results. Teertstra and colleagues[24] in the Netherlands compared 513 diagnostic digital mammograms with tomosynthesis. The diagnostic patients included abnormal screen examinations (26%), women with palpable findings (44%), and those seeking a second opinion (30%). There were 344 cases that had histologic proof of diagnosis with 112 newly detected cancers. A single observer assessed the DBT examination alone 1 to 3 months after the clinical study, but 1 of 7 different observers reported the initial clinically performed DM study at the time of the clinic visit. Using a positive threshold of Breast Imaging Reporting and Data System (BIRADS) category 0, 3, 4, and 5, the investigators reported similar sensitivity of 92.9% for both DBT and DM. Specificity was 86.1% with DM and 84.4% for DBT, a nonsignificant difference. There were 8 cancers that were false-negative to DBT. These results suggested no improvement for diagnostic DBT. However, if the more commonly used positive threshold for cancer was category 0, 4, or 5, then the sensitivity of DBT was greater than DM (80% vs 73%) with specificity of 96% and 97%. This was caused by/because of the large number of cancers (21%) classified as probably benign by mammography in the study. These assessments for category 3, probably benign, may vary from practice in the United States. The investigators noted all clusters of malignant calcifications detected by DM were also detected at breast DBT.

Characterization of Masses

One of the touted advantages of DBT has been for characterization and margin assessment of masses. Helvie and colleagues[25] reported results of 4 readers who assessed the margins of masses scheduled for biopsy. When masses were visible by both DBT and conventional mammography, readers were able to visualize 77% of the perimeter of a mass with DBT versus 53% of the perimeter of a mass by conventional mammography. The increase in incremental visible margin was significant for all readers. A weakness of this study was that the conventional mammograms consisted of a mixed population of film screen and digital studies. In another study of 382 DBT views of biopsy-proved masses, BIRADS margin characterization of benign masses versus malignant masses showed that circumscribed masses were much more common with benign masses than cancer (70 vs 5%).[26] Conversely, spiculated or indistinct margins were much more common with cancer than benign masses (81% vs 11%). Thus, most benign masses appeared circumscribed and most malignant masses were spiculated. Using a threshold of cancer probability of 2% for category 3, in this experimental situation, it was estimated that 39% of masses recommended for biopsy would have been classified as BIRADS 1, 2 or 3, theoretically decreasing the biopsy rate. The real-world clinical performance would likely be less.

Anderson and colleagues[18] explored the theoretic incremental characterization assessment change when reviewing DBT with a single-view DM mammography versus a 2-view conventional mammography for subtle breast cancers. They noted a 25% incremental upgrade rate (from category 1, 2, or 3 to category 4 or 5) when DBT was compared with a single-view conventional DM image. That is, lesions that were considered benign by conventional imaging were deemed more suspicious by DBT and a biopsy recommendation was made. This upgrade rate decreased to 20% when the DBT image was compared with a 2-view DM. This study suggests a small incremental yield even for subtle cancers when a 2-view (single DBT and single DM) study is compared with a 3-view study (single DBT plus CC DM and MLO DM).

Microcalcifications by DBT

There is limited literature regarding clinical microcalcification assessment by DBT for detection and characterization. The engineering, physics, and reconstruction of different manufacturers' equipment may lead to different results and completely different conclusions even though all are tomosynthesis. X-ray source, motion, pixel size, and reconstruction algorithms are of particular concern. Although the in-plane resolution of DBT is good, out-of-plane resolution is poor. Because calcifications may be dispersed in three-dimensional space, viewing thin DBT images may make perception of calcification clusters difficult as only 1 or 2 may be seen on a slice. To overcome this issue, manufacturers have developed MIP images consisting of thick slices such as 1 to 2 cm for reviewing calcifications (see **Fig. 5**). In a feasibility study, we showed that for cases that were subjected to biopsy based on conventional imaging, calcifications were visible by DBT in either CC or MLO view in 100% (93 of 93) of cases.[27] However, the per view visualization was less. By view, 96% of benign lesions and 97% of malignant lesions were apparent by DBT. This study merely assessed if calcifications were visible by DBT, not reader preference or performance between DBT and conventional mammograms. Poplack and colleagues[16] DBT study of image quality showed a disproportionate number of calcification cases to be inferior. When image quality was considered inferior, 72% of lesions were calcifications. Yet in the study population, only 14% of cases were for calcifications. Teertstra and colleagues[24] showed all malignant calcification cases that were visualized by DM were also visualized by DBT. Much more work is necessary before conclusions can be drawn regarding microcalcifications and DBT.

COMPUTER-AIDED DETECTION TOMOSYNTHESIS

Because of the marked increase in number of images for physician review, with potential increased time necessary for interpretation, DBT may impose clinical work-flow challenges. It can be postulated that secondary to increased workload and the increased number of images to review, physician oversight of findings could increase. Computer-aided detection (CAD) may be important for clinical DBT and have a more significant clinical role than with conventional DM mammography in improving work performance. It is possible that CAD will also perform better with tomosynthesis images compared with DM images because of better margin visibility of masses. Several researchers have developed CAD systems for DBT. Chan and colleagues[28,29] reported on CAD for masses with DBT. Mass detection sensitivity of 90% has been achieved at 2.0 false-positive cases per breast volume. At 80% sensitivity, 1.2 false-positives per case has been achieved. Singh and colleagues[30] also has developed a CAD program for mass detection. Their reported optimal performance was 85% sensitivity for masses at 2.4 false-positives per breast. Reiser and colleagues[31,32] developed mass and calcification detection programs for DBT. In a small series of calcifications, performance sensitivity of 86% was achieved at 1.3 false-positives per volume. This performance was noted to be better than CAD performance for DM systems. The development of these CAD systems was based on limited enriched DBT datasets but show encouraging results. Like DM, CAD will be a supplemental adjunct to human observation and characterizations and act as a second, not primary reader.

IMPORTANT CONSIDERATIONS FOR ASSESSMENT OF NEW TECHNOLOGY SUCH AS DBT

Although preliminary experimental clinical studies have generally been favorable for tomosynthesis, more rigorous scientific investigation is underway to establish the true nature of tomosynthesis and potential application for clinical breast imaging. There are several biases to be considered when reviewing preliminary clinical investigations. Experimental clinical trials do not exactly replicate real-world clinical realities. Readers may have heightened awareness for cancer detection given enriched cancer populations, which may overstate sensitivity and specificity compared with normal lower cancer incidence encountered in clinical practice. Another important but overlooked positive bias relates to the initial performance versus subsequent test performance on a screened population. Prevalent detection bias occurs when a new screening technology is applied to a population that has not been previously exposed to that technology. In general, cancer detection rates and outcomes are higher at prevalent detection than subsequent annual incident screening. The magnitude of this bias is often underappreciated. For conventional mammography, the prevalent detection rate is 6 to 10/1000 and the annual incident detection rate is 2 to 4/1000.[33] A study of MR imaging of high-risk women showed the prevalent detection of MR imaging of 13.2 per 1000, which decreased to 5.3 per 1000 at incident detection.[34] In the same study, mammography prevalence detection was 16.5 per 1000, which decreased to 2.1 per 1000 at incident screening. Therefore, when analyzing new technology, one must be aware of potential positive bias induced by the prevalent (first) testing situation. In almost all reported cases, DBT has been tested as a prevalent test. Simply increasing the number of views for a radiologist to interpret may by itself increase sensitivity even without the addition of new a technology, which may have an effect when assessing trials using DBT as an adjunct to mammography.

Extensive physician training will be necessary if DBT proves efficacious in clinical trials. Radiologist mammographic interpretation and performance variability remains a major weak link in the assessment of mammographic images. Technologist training with a new modality will also be important for proper image acquisition. Training regarding appropriate reading time, methods, and thresholds for recall and biopsy will all be necessary. In particular, determining which structures are normal and which require intervention will be an ongoing educational process. It is possible that further refinements of what constitutes a BIRADS category 3, probably benign lesion, and what constitutes a category 2 benign lesion will be necessary. Completely circumscribed masses such as cysts may be able to be classified as category 2 by DBT. Conversely, some lesions such as fibroadenomas that may currently be classified as category 3 because of circumscribed margins by DM may show more margin variability by DBT, which could change their classification to category 4A. Lesions that are considered suspicious but only visualized on DBT will require manufacturers to develop biopsy capability, which will further increase the training need for physicians using DBT.

OTHER NEW DM SYSTEMS
Contrast-Enhanced DM

Combining high-resolution DM with the functional attributes obtained with contrast enhancement offers another potential derivative application for DM. The advantage of contrast-enhanced digital mammography (CEDM) would be to obtain functional contrast information attributed to malignant neovascularity directly linked to high-quality anatomic information. Breast MR imaging has used this principle for years. The potential advantages postulated for using CEDM would be the widespread installation of mammography units, superior resolution, patient acceptance of mammography, and potential lower cost. The disadvantage of such a technique for screening is the necessity for an intravenous contrast administration, adverse consequences of contrast, increased cost, increased time, and patient acceptance compared with standard DM. Competing against CEDM is a body of work using contrast-enhanced MR imaging. Potential applications could be similar to MR imaging including screening, diagnostic, staging, and treatment monitoring. Currently, screening for MR has been stratified based on high risk for breast cancer. If CEDM proves efficacious, its application may follow a pattern of high-risk or special situation application.

There are 2 main methods described for CEDM: serial examinations over time and dual energy imaging.[35–41] Both use iodinated contrast material and modified DM units for imaging. Higher kilovolts, often 45 to 49 kV, are used to take advantage of the K-edge of iodine. Serial imaging can be obtained for a single projection only. Although this may have application for diagnostic or staging reasons, it would be less applicable to screening situations. For this reason, dual energy methods have been developed to allow imaging of both breasts with a single contrast administration. Early work has shown technical and clinical feasibility. The actual number of patients studied to date has been limited so the application if any for future potential clinical use is uncertain.

Serial CEDM

Serial or temporal CEDM is similar to contrast-enhanced breast MR imaging. The patient's breast is placed in compression in a single view such as the MLO. Before contrast injection, a noncontrast image is obtained. Next, following contrast administration, a series of images are obtained. Each image is a fractional dose of conventional mammography. There is insufficient visible enhancement to allow primary interpretation, and for this reason the enhanced images are subtracted from the baseline image leaving areas of enhancement visible. Using this methodology, enhancement curves can be obtained. Weaknesses of this type of study include the ability to only image the breast in a single projection at a time significantly limiting application to a routine screening situation. Technically, motion may cause misregistration errors limiting sensitivity, visualization of enhancing lesions, and overall confidence in interpretation.

Dual Energy CEDM

A conceptually different approach uses dual energy technology. The technology makes use of different iodine K-edge x-ray absorption at low and high energies. Dual energy mammography requires a modified mammographic machine that is capable of producing both normal mammographic images and images obtained at higher energy (45–50 kV) acquired in rapid succession after contrast administration. The patient is injected with contrast and placed in compression. Two paired exposures are obtained, one at low kilovolts and the other at high kilovolts. A subtraction image is produced that highlights areas of iodine concentration or enhancement. The mammographic image at low energy can be used as a routine grayscale mammographic interpretation. With efficient technologists, 4 views (2 views of each breast) can be obtained during a single administration of contrast. This technique does not allow for kinetic assessment of enhancement curves.

Early studies have shown the clinical feasibility of CEDM with test sensitivity ranging from 80% to 91%. Jong and colleagues[37] reported enhancement by serial CEDM in 8 of 10 (80%) cancers in a 22-patient study. Lewin and colleagues,[38] using dual energy CEDM, showed strong enhancement in 11/13 (85%) malignancies and moderate or weak enhancement in the remaining 2 cases. A similar 80% sensitivity was noted by Dromain and colleagues[35] for 20 malignant cases undergoing single CC view serial CEDM. Chen and colleagues[41] combined CEDM with DBT in a feasibility study with 13 patients in which 10 of 11 (91%) patients with malignancies had abnormal enhancement visible by CEDM. Most recently, a multicenter 5-reader retrospective study of 85 lesions (68 cancers) compared DM alone with DM plus CEDM.[40] The investigators demonstrated sensitivity improvement for readers from 0.81 to 0.86 with the addition of CEDM and the area under the ROC curve was greater for all readers although significant for only 2 readers.

Although CEDM seems technically feasible in small series, the clinical usefulness has yet to be established. Both types of CEDM compete against a large body of breast MR knowledge and clinical experience. It is possible that CEDM techniques would be less expensive that current MR imaging examinations, and possibly generate similar information. However, some of the issues limiting breast MR would apply to CEDM including the necessity of intravenous contrast administration, which is a barrier to routine screening of a general population compared with routine DM, breast ultrasound, or potentially DBT. Patient motion is a problem with repetitive time sampling leading to misregistration and potential diagnostic problems. There are many patients who are unable to tolerate MR scanning so this technology could be used for such individuals. Unlike MR, compression is applied for CEDM to limit motion. However, excessive compression may inhibit blood circulation within the breast, which could limit enhancement.

COMBINING DM WITH OTHER IMAGING TECHNOLOGY

Digital imaging allows the potential to coregister different technologies to produce fused images. Screening breast ultrasound detects mammographically occult cancers in women with dense breasts. The ACRIN 6666 trial showed a 4.2/1000 improvement in cancer detection with the addition of physician-performed hand-held ultrasound screening of high-risk women with dense breasts.[42] However, there are potential limitations of whole-breast ultrasound screening by physician because of the time necessary to perform the examination and resources available. In Berg and colleagues'[42] study, the mean scanning time was approximately 20 minutes. Automated ultrasound scanning methods have appeal. Methods to combine simultaneous mammography and automated ultrasound would have the theoretic advantage of the improved sensitivity of ultrasound with an automated approach and the ability to simultaneously correlate the sonographic findings with the mammographic findings. Screening and diagnostic scanning could occur simultaneously.

Equipment and methods have been developed that allow automated DM (with or without tomosynthesis) and automated ultrasound at the same patient sitting.[43–45] Using prototypes, the patient's breast is compressed as with a typical mammographic image. A conventional mammographic image is obtained. Subsequently, while still under compression, the breast is scanned mechanically by ultrasound.

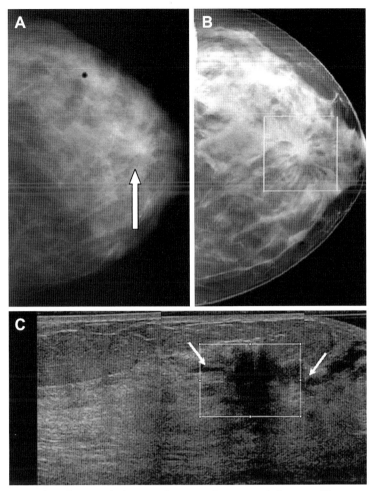

Fig. 6. Images from a combined DBT and ultrasound system. The DBT and ultrasound image were obtained automatically during a single compression. Conventional film screen (CC) mammogram (*A*), DBT 1-mm thick image (*B*), and the corresponding automated ultrasound image (*C*) of a patient with invasive cancer. The cancer is subtle on conventional mammogram (*arrow*) and apparent on the DBT (*within box*), and very apparent on ultrasound image (*within box, arrows*).

The mammograms and ultrasound images can be reviewed independently. In addition, a direct three-dimensional registration is possible, which allows correlation of a lesion found by one technology with the other technology (**Fig. 6**). For example, a circumscribed mass detected by mammography could be correlated with a simple cyst found at sonographic scanning and no recall would be necessary. Conversely, if a sonographic suspicious finding is detected and the mammogram is normal, the improved sensitivity of ultrasound screening could be realized. There are other potential combined systems under early investigation including combining DM with nuclear medicine functional imaging or optical scanning.

SUMMARY

Advanced digital mammographic technology such as digital breast tomosnythesis is an exciting new development for breast cancer screening and diagnostic applications. Favorable preliminary experimental clinical trial results, especially for masses, must be confirmed with larger more representative clinical trials. The assessment of microcalcifications awaits further study. Major advantages of DBT as a new imaging technology include the linkage to the scientific basis for screening mammography, the existent extensive installed mammographic base, familiarity with existing digital equipment, and decades-old medical and radiologic experience with mammography.

Patient acceptance would be expected to be good. If successful, and borne out by rigorous clinical trials, this technology has the potential to change conventional mammographic screening and diagnostic imaging with possible improvements in cancer detection, decreased call backs, and fewer false-positive biopsies.

ACKNOWLEDGMENTS

Thanks to Nancy Gage and Sarah Abate for assistance in manuscript preparation. Thanks to patient volunteers and the Breast Imaging Team at the University of Michigan for their dedicated efforts in patient care and breast cancer research.

REFERENCES

1. Roubidoux MA, Bailey JE, Wray LA, et al. Invasive cancers detected after breast cancer screening yielded a negative result: relationship of mammographic density to tumor prognostic factors. Radiology 2004;230:42–8.
2. Niklason LT, Christian BT, Niklason LE, et al. Digital tomosynthesis in breast imaging. Radiology 1997;205:399–406.
3. Niklason LE, Kopans DB, Hamberg LM. Digital breast imaging: tomosynthesis and digital subtraction mammography. Breast Dis 1998;10:151–64.
4. Wu T, Moore RH, Rafferty EA, et al. A comparison of reconstruction algorithms for breast tomosynthesis. Med Phys 2004;31:2636–47.
5. Wu T, Moore RH, Kopans DB. Voting strategy for artifact reduction in digital breast tomosynthesis. Med Phys 2006;33:2461–71.
6. Zhang Y, Chan H-P, Sahiner B, et al. A comparative study of limited-angle cone-beam reconstruction methods for breast tomosynthesis. Med Phys 2006;33:3781–95.
7. Claus BEH, Eberhard JW, Schmitz A, et al. Generalized filtered back-projection reconstruction in breast tomosynthesis. In: Astley SM, Brady M, Zwiggelaar R, editors. Lecture notes in computer science – digital mammography. Manchester (UK): Springer-Verlag; 2006. p. 167–74.
8. Hsiao IT, Khurd P, Rangarajan A, et al. An overview of fast convergent ordered-subsets reconstruction methods for emission tomography based on the incremental EM algorithm. Nucl Instrum Methods Phys Res A 2006;569(2):429–33.
9. Eberhard JW, Albagli D, Schmitz A. Mammography tomosynthesis system for high performance 3D imaging. In: Astley SM, Brady M, Zwiggelaar R, editors. 8th international workshop on digital mammography. Lecture notes in computer science – digital mammography. Manchester (UK): Springer-Verlag; 2006. p. 137–43.
10. Schulz-Wendtland R, Wenkel E, Lell M, et al. Experimental phantom lesion detectability study using a digital breast tomosynthesis prototype system. Rofo 2006;178:1219–23.
11. Gong X, Glick SJ, Liu B, et al. A computer simulation study comparing lesion detection accuracy with digital mammography, breast tomosynthesis, and cone-beam CT breast imaging. Med Phys 2006;33:1041–52.
12. Diekmann F, Meyer H, Diekmann S, et al. Thick slices from tomosynthesis data sets: phantom study for the evaluation of different algorithms. J Digit Imaging 2009;22:519–26.
13. Dobbins J, Godfrey D. Digital x-ray tomosynthesis: current state of the art and clinical potential. Phys Med Biol 2003;48:R65–106.
14. Suryanarayanan S, Karellas A, Vedantham S, et al. Evaluation of linear and nonlinear tomosynthetic reconstruction methods in digital mammography. Acad Radiol 2001;8:219–24.
15. Smith RA, Duffy SW, Gabe R, et al. The randomized trials of breast cancer screening: what have we learned? Radiol Clin North Am 2004;42:793–806.
16. Poplack SP, Tosteson TD, Kogel CA, et al. Digital breast tomosynthesis: initial experience in 98 women with abnormal digital screening mammography. Am J Roentgenol 2007;189:616–23.
17. Good WF, Abrams GS, Catullo VJ, et al. Digital breast tomosynthesis: a pilot observer study. Am J Roentgenol 2008;190:865–9.
18. Andersson I, Ikeda D, Zackrisson S, et al. Breast tomosynthesis and digital mammography: a comparison of breast cancer visibility and BIRADS classification in a population of cancers with subtle mammographic findings. Eur Radiol 2008;18:2817–25.
19. Helvie MA, Roubidoux MA, Hadjiiski L, et al. Tomosynthesis mammography versus conventional mammography: comparison of breast masses detection and characterization. In: Radiological Society of North America 93rd Scientific Assembly and Annual Meeting. Chicago (IL), November 24–30, 2007.
20. Lo JY, Durham NC, Baker JA. Breast tomosynthesis: assessing patient compression, comfort, and preference. In: Radiologic Society of North America 92nd Scientific Assembly and Annual Meeting. Chicago (IL), November 25–December 1, 2006.
21. Rafferty EA, Smith AP, Niklason LT. Assessing radiologist performance in dense versus fatty breasts using combined full-field digital mammography and breast tomosynthesis compared to full-field digital mammography alone. In: Radiologic Society of North America 95th Scientific Assembly and Annual Meeting. Chicago (IL), November 28–December 4, 2009.
22. Moore RH, Boston MA, Kopans DB, et al. Initial callback rates for conventional and digital breast tomosynthesis mammography comparison in the screening setting. In: Radiologic Society of North

America 92nd Scientific Assembly and Annual Meeting. Chicago (IL), November 24–30, 2007.

23. Gur D, Abrams GS, Chough DM, et al. Digital breast tomosynthesis: observer performance study. AJR Am J Roentgenol 2009;193:586–91.

24. Teertstra H, Loo C, van den Bosch M, et al. Breast tomosynthesis in clinical practice: initial results. Eur Radiol 2010;20(1):16–24.

25. Helvie MA, Roubidoux M, Zhang Y, et al. Tomosynthesis mammography versus conventional mammography: lesion detection and reader preference - initial experience. Chicago: Radiological Society of North America; 2006.

26. Helvie MA, Hadjiiski L, Goodsitt MM, et al. Characterization of benign and malignant breast masses by digital breast tomosynthesis mammography. In: Radiological Society of North America 94th Scientific Assembly and Annual Meeting. Chicago (IL), November 29–December 5, 2008.

27. Helvie MA, Chan HP, Hadjiiski L, et al. Digital breast tomosynthesis mammography: successful assessment of benign and malignant microcalcifications. In: Radiologic Society of North America 95th Scientific Assembly and Annual Meeting. Chicago (IL), November 28–December 4, 2009.

28. Chan HP, Wei J, Zhang Y, et al. Computer-aided detection of masses in digital tomosynthesis mammography: comparison of three approaches. Med Phys 2008;35:4087–95.

29. Chan HP, Wei J, Sahiner B, et al. Computer-aided detection system for breast masses on digital tomosynthesis mammograms: preliminary experience. Radiology 2005;237:1075–80.

30. Singh S, Tourassi GD, Baker JA, et al. Automated breast mass detection in 3D reconstructed tomosynthesis volumes: a featureless approach. Med Phys 2008;35:3626–36.

31. Reiser I, Nishikawa RM, Edwards AV, et al. Automated detection of microcalcification clusters for digital breast tomosynthesis using projection data only: a preliminary study. Med Phys 2008;35:1486–93.

32. Reiser I, Nishikawa RM, Giger ML, et al. Computerized mass detection for digital breast tomosynthesis directly from the projection images. Med Phys 2006; 33:482–91.

33. US Department of Health and Human Services. Quality determinants of mammography. Clinical practice guideline. Rockville (MD): Public Health Service; 1994.

34. Kriege M, Brekelmans C, Boetes C, et al. Differences between first and subsequent rounds of the MRISC breast cancer screening program for women with a familial or genetic predisposition. Cancer 2006;106:2318–26.

35. Dromain C, Balleyguier C, Muller S, et al. Evaluation of tumor angiogenesis of breast carcinoma using contrast-enhanced digital mammography. AJR Am J Roentgenol 2006;187:W528–537.

36. Diekmann F, Diekmann S, Jeunehomme F, et al. Digital mammography using iodine-based contrast media: initial clinical experience with dynamic contrast medium enhancement. Invest Radiol 2005;40:397–404.

37. Jong R, Yaffe M, Skarpathiotakis M, et al. Contrast-enhanced digital mammography: initial clinical experience. Radiology 2003;228:842–50.

38. Lewin JM, Isaacs PK, Vance V, et al. Dual-energy contrast-enhanced digital subtraction mammography: feasibility1. Radiology 2003;229:261–8.

39. Diekmann F, Bick U. Tomosynthesis and contrast-enhanced digital mammography: recent advances in digital mammography. Eur Radiol 2007;17:3086–92.

40. Dromain C, Balleyguier C, Adler G, et al. Contrast-enhanced digital mammography. Eur J Radiol 2009;69:34–42.

41. Chen SC, Carton AK, Albert M, et al. Initial clinical experience with contrast-enhanced digital breast tomosynthesis. Acad Radiol 2007;14:229–38.

42. Berg WA, Blume JD, Cormack JB, et al. Combined screening with ultrasound and mammography vs mammography alone in women at elevated risk of breast cancer. JAMA 2008;299:2151–63.

43. Booi RC, Krucker JF, Goodsitt MM, et al. Evaluating thin compression paddles for mammographically compatible ultrasound. Ultrasound Med Biol 2007; 33:472–82.

44. Kapur A, Carson PL, Eberhard J, et al. Combination of digital mammography with semi-automated 3D breast ultrasound. Technol Cancer Res Treat 2004; 3:325–34.

45. Sinha SP, Goodsitt MM, Roubidoux MA, et al. Automated ultrasound scanning on a dual-modality breast imaging system: coverage and motion issues and solutions. J Ultrasound Med 2007;26:645–55.

Cystic Breast Masses and the ACRIN 6666 Experience

Wendie A. Berg, MD, PhD[a,b,*], Alan G. Sechtin, MD[b],
Helga Marques, MS[c], Zheng Zhang, PhD[c]

KEYWORDS

- Ultrasound • Sonography • Breast • Cyst
- Complex cystic • Breast cancer

Masses due to cystic lesions of the breast are extremely common findings on mammography, ultrasonography, and magnetic resonance (MR) imaging. Although many of these lesions can be dismissed as benign simple cysts, requiring intervention only for symptomatic relief, complex cystic and solid masses require biopsy. Perhaps the most challenging are complicated cysts, that is, cysts with internal debris. When the debris is mobile or a fluid-debris level is seen, complicated cysts can be dismissed as benign. Breast Imaging Reporting and Data System (BI-RADS)[1] 2, findings. When the debris is homogeneous and hypoechoic, it is often difficult to distinguish a complicated cyst from a solid mass. As an isolated finding, homogeneous complicated cysts can be classified as probably benign, BI-RADS 3, with intervention only considered if there is interval development or enlargement, if abscess is suspected, or if suspicious features develop. When multiple and bilateral complicated and simple cysts are present (ie, at least 3 cysts, with at least 1 in each breast), a benign, BI-RADS 2, assessment is usually appropriate. Clustered microcysts are common benign findings in pre- and perimenopausal women, although short-interval surveillance may be appropriate for many such lesions in postmenopausal women,

particularly if the lesion is new or rather small or deep (ie, diagnostic uncertainty). Intradermal cysts, such as epidermal inclusion cysts and sebaceous cysts, are benign findings, which are not included in this review.

Increasing use of whole breast screening ultrasonography reveals many, otherwise occult, cystic lesions of the breast; a thorough understanding of their imaging findings and management is important. In addition to reviewing the literature on such lesions, the authors present results from the American College of Radiology Imaging Network (ACRIN) 6666 protocol of screening breast ultrasonography.[2] In the ACRIN protocol, women at high risk for breast cancer were screened annually with mammography and independent, physician-performed, freehand sonography for 3 years.[3] The reference standard for a given lesion in the ACRIN protocol includes not only biopsy within the first year of follow-up or at least 11-month follow-up imaging but also any biopsy results for procedures performed through a minimum of 33 months of follow-up. A summary of studies reviewed after systematic literature search (PubMed, National Library of Medicine, on January 2, 2010) and associated reference standards are presented in Table 1.

Meticulous technique is critical in evaluating cystic lesions, and technical issues with breast

Supported by Avon Foundation and NCI U01 CA79778, U01 CA80098.

Financial disclosures: WAB received elastography software from Siemens, Inc, a laptop computer and software from MediPattern, Inc, and has been a consultant to SuperSonic Imagine.

[a] 301 Merrie Hunt Drive, Lutherville, MD 21093, USA

[b] American Radiology Services Inc, Johns Hopkins Green Spring, 10755 Falls Road, Suite 440, Lutherville, MD 21093, USA

[c] Center for Statistical Sciences, Brown University, 121 South Main Street, G-S121-7, Providence, RI 02912, USA

* Corresponding author. American Radiology Services Inc, Johns Hopkins Green Spring, 10755 Falls Road, Suite 440, Lutherville, MD 21093.

E-mail address: wendieberg@gmail.com

Radiol Clin N Am 48 (2010) 931–987

doi:10.1016/j.rcl.2010.06.007

Table 1
Summary of studies evaluating cystic breast lesions

Study, Year	Description of Population	Reference Standard
Omori et al,[46] 1993	6000 consecutive sonograms, 70 cases of mixed cystic and solid lesions	Surgical excision of 56 reported cases
Kolb et al,[23] 1998	3626 screening sonograms in women with at least minimal scattered fibroglandular density; normal mammography and clinical breast examination	Aspiration (n = 30) or follow-up (n = 126) for lesions described
Venta et al,[24] 1999	4562 consecutive diagnostic sonograms, 252 women with 308 complex[a] cysts	141 lesions were attempted for aspiration, but 24 failed and had biopsy; 2 bloody, atypical cytology, biopsy benign
Buchberger et al,[20] 2003	6113 asymptomatic women with at least minimal scattered fibroglandular density, and 687 women with palpable or mammographic masses; 133 complex[a] cysts identified	All 133 lesions aspirated; 7 could not be aspirated and had core biopsy
Berg et al,[19] 2003	2072 image-guided biopsies, 150 cystic lesions identified	All lesions biopsied; follow-up after biopsy in 126
Berg,[35] 2005	1900 consecutive sonograms with 79 clustered microcysts; 4 palpable	13 biopsied lesions overlap with prior series,[19] 66 lesions followed
Chang et al,[21] 2007	212 patients with symptomatic cystic lesions among 57,437 sonograms	175 lesions with pathologic proof reported
Daly et al,[22] 2008	186 patients consecutively presenting for aspiration of 243 complicated cysts, including 15 clustered microcysts (ie, 228 were complicated cysts)	Pathologic proof for all lesions: 243 lesions aspirated, 33 did not yield fluid; 32 biopsied and 1 resolved; benign lesions followed for a mean of 21.9 mo
Tea et al,[47] 2009	Retrospective review of records reporting complex cyst; 151 lesions in 131 patients. Nonstandard terminology used: impossible to compare with prior literature for most subgroups	Excision of all lesions
ACRIN 6666	2809 women at elevated risk of breast cancer enrolled for 3 rounds of annual screening ultrasonography, blinded to mammography	11-month follow-up or biopsy available for 2659 women year 1; 2493 women, year 2; 2321 women, year 3; total 2662 unique participants

[a] The term complex is used, but the description is that of complicated cysts: mass resembles a cyst except that internal echoes are present or posterior enhancement is absent; mass has circumscribed margins with no perceptible intracystic mass or solid component.

ultrasonography are discussed in this article. Use of high-frequency, broadband, linear array transducers, with center frequency of at least 10 MHz, is required for adequate breast ultrasonography.

SIMPLE CYSTS

Simple cysts are epithelium-lined, fluid-filled, round or oval structures that are thought to occur secondary to obstructed ducts. The epithelium can be bland or apocrine type. The latter is a tall, cuboidal, secretory epithelium and can make the inner wall of the cyst appear fuzzy on high-resolution ultrasonography. Cysts can be isolated or diffuse and can occur in any quadrant. Ectopic breast tissue (tail of Spence) can extend into the axillary tail regions, but breast tissue and therefore cysts and other breast lesions are not usually found within the axillae proper.

Cysts are the most common type of breast mass, with peak incidence between ages 35 and 50 years. Simple cysts represented 25% of consecutive breast masses in the series by Hilton and colleagues.[4] In the ACRIN 6666 protocol, cysts were seen in 998 (37.5%) of 2659 women in the first round of screening ultrasonography and in 1255 (47.1%) of 2662 participants over the 3 years. Of the participants with simple cysts, nearly half (48%) had cysts in both breasts. Being hormonally sensitive, cysts can fluctuate in size and number with the menstrual cycle, being most prominent in the premenstrual phase. In postmenopausal women, cysts are more common in women on hormone replacement therapy[5,6] and were reported in 6% of such women in 1 series.[6] Based on the ACRIN 6666 experience, it seems that postmenopausal cysts are much more common. In the first year of ACRIN 6666 trial, 406 (29.8%) of 1362 postmenopausal women were found to have cysts, decreasing to 298 (24.7%) of 1208 by year 3. Cysts were seen at some time during the 3-year study in 537 (39.4%) of 1363 postmenopausal women compared with 516 (65.1%) of 793 premenopausal women (P<.0001) (Table 2). Among 1363 postmenopausal women in the ACRIN 6666 trial, 73 (5.4%) were using estrogen replacement therapy. Over the 3-year study, cysts were seen in 48 (66%) of 73 women using estrogen compared with 489 (37.9%) of 1290 who were not (P<.0001) (see Table 2).

The natural history of cysts is to develop and regress. In a series following 68 newly appearing benign cysts, Brenner and colleagues[7] reported that 47% had completely regressed within 1 year and 69% within 5 years. In any given year, up to 12% of the cysts had increased in size.[7]

Imaging Findings

Mammographically, cysts present as solitary or multiple, often bilateral, low-density, circumscribed, round, oval, or occasionally mildly lobulated masses (Figs. 1–4), which vary in size from several millimeters to 5 to 6 cm. The margins are frequently obscured by surrounding parenchyma. When at least 75% of the margin of the mass is seen as circumscribed and the rest is not worse than obscured, the mass is still considered circumscribed.[8] Cysts can have thin calcified walls and can contain calcium. Calcium in cysts, ie, milk of calcium, appears amorphous, round, or smudgy on the craniocaudal (CC) view and changes in appearance to layer on a true lateral (mediolateral or lateromedial) view like leaves in the bottom of a tea cup (Fig. 5). With the exception of macrocysts containing milk of calcium, cysts cannot be distinguished from solid masses mammographically.

When multiple and bilateral (with at least 3 cysts in total and at least 1 in each breast), partially circumscribed, partially obscured (PCPO) masses can be dismissed as benign findings, BI-RADS 2,[9] with the usual etiologies being cysts (see Figs. 3

Table 2
Prevalence of simple cysts among 2662 unique participants in ACRIN 6666

	Number of Participants	Number with Cysts (%)
Premenopausal	793	516 (65.1)
Postmenopausal	1363	537 (39.4)
No HRT[a]	1290	489 (37.9)
HRT	73	48 (66)[b]
Surgical Menopause	484	193 (39.9)
Unknown Menopausal status	22	9 (41)
Total	2662	1255 (47.1)

[a] HRT, any estrogen-containing hormone replacement therapy.
[b] Simple cysts were more common in postmenopausal women taking HRT rather than not taking HRT (P<.0001).

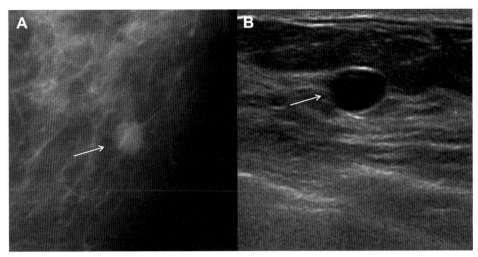

Fig. 1. A 74-year-old woman was noted to have a new mass on screening mammography and no history of hormone use. (A) Spot magnification craniocaudal (CC) view shows partially circumscribed, partially obscured 7-mm mass (*arrow*). (B) Targeted ultrasonography shows anechoic circumscribed mass (*arrow*) with minimal posterior enhancement, that is, a simple cyst, corresponding to the mammographic abnormality, a benign finding. (*Courtesy of* Wendie A. Berg, MD, PhD, Lutherville, MD.)

and **4**), complicated cysts, and fibroadenomata. With multiple bilateral PCPO masses, ultrasonography is appropriate when there is a dominant or palpable mass (see **Fig. 4**; **Figs. 6** and **7**) or if 1 or more masses have suspicious features (**Fig. 8**). Ultrasonography can also be performed electively for supplemental screening when there is concern that a suspicious mass could be obscured by the PCPO masses and/or dense parenchyma.

Sonography should be performed using high-frequency transducers, with a center frequency of at least 10 MHz and peak frequency of at least 12 MHz. With high-frequency transducers, cysts as small as 2 to 3 mm in size can be identified and characterized, although characterization of cysts was variable until a size of at least 8 mm was reached in an observer study.[10] With gentle compression, a cyst frequently flattens, unlike most solid lesions.

If the mass is deeper than 3 cm from the skin, the transducer's frequency may need to be decreased for adequate penetration. A sonographically simple cyst with the classic

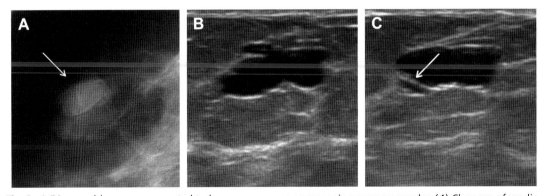

Fig. 2. A 54-year-old woman was noted to have a new mass on screening mammography. (A) Close-up of mediolateral oblique (MLO) mammogram shows lobulated, circumscribed mass (*arrow*). (B, C) Targeted ultrasonography shows lobulated simple cyst corresponding to the mammographic abnormality, a benign finding. Apparent thin septation in image (C) (*arrow*) is due to lobulation of the cyst. (*Courtesy of* Wendie A. Berg, MD, PhD, Lutherville, MD.)

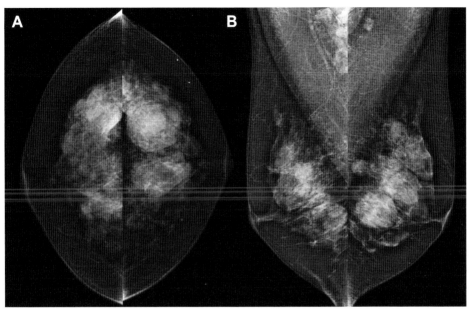

Fig. 3. A 43-year-old woman was noted to have a changing pattern of multiple bilateral partially circumscribed, partially obscured (PCPO) masses on screening (A) CC and (B) MLO mammograms, most compatible with cysts, which were confirmed on screening ultrasonography (not shown). (*Courtesy of* Wendie A. Berg, MD, PhD, Lutherville, MD.)

appearance (avascular, anechoic, oval or round mass with imperceptible wall and posterior enhancement) can be dismissed as a benign finding, although posterior enhancement may not always be apparent.[4] Spatial compounding improves margin detection and decreases speckle and noise, although posterior features are less conspicuous (Fig. 7D, E).

Reverberation artifacts (Fig. 9) typically parallel the anterior wall of a cyst: on its way back to the transducer, the beam is reflected again off the anterior wall of the cyst to insonate deeper tissues again and thus takes longer to return to the transducer, and the imaged structure appears deeper than it really is. Tissue harmonic imaging can be used to reduce artifactual internal echoes.

Thin (<0.5 mm) septations can be present in lobulated simple cysts (Figs. 2C, 10 and 11) or can appear to be present when several cysts abut each other (Fig. 12). Cysts can communicate with ducts (Figs. 13 and 14).

Elastography provides a measure of the stiffness of a lesion and is an option available on most standard ultrasonographic equipment. Cysts are typically soft and many malignancies are hard. Compression elastography is an evolving technology, and different methods and algorithms are used by different manufacturers. Devices manufactured by Toshiba and Hitachi require gentle

pressure to be applied with the transducer and released; cysts can have a trilaminar appearance on such an equipment (Fig. 15).[11] With equipments from Siemens and Philips, normal patient respiratory motion is sufficient to generate an elastogram, although superficial or very deep lesions cannot be readily imaged, and there must be at least several centimeters of breast thickness. Softer lesions appear bright (Siemens and Philips) or green (Toshiba and Hitachi) and smaller on elastography than on B-mode ultrasonography, whereas stiffer lesions will appear darker (Siemens and Philips) or blue (Toshiba and Hitachi) and larger on elastography. With Siemens and Philips, a target or bull's-eye appearance can be seen on elastography of cysts (Fig. 16)[12,13] and cystic areas within complex masses (Fig. 17), and such appearance is due to subtle motion of the fluid (Richard Barr, MD, PhD, personal communication, 2010). With shear-wave elastography, low-frequency shear waves are propagated in tissue and elasticity of the tissue is quantitatively and reproducibly assessed (Claude Cohen-Bacrie, PhD, personal communication, 2010). Cysts can appear black internally on shear-wave elastography because shear waves do not propagate in nonviscous liquid (Fig. 18); fat and soft masses appear blue, and stiff lesions appear red on SuperSonic equipment (SuperSonic Imagine, Aix-en-Provence, France). Manufacturers are encouraged

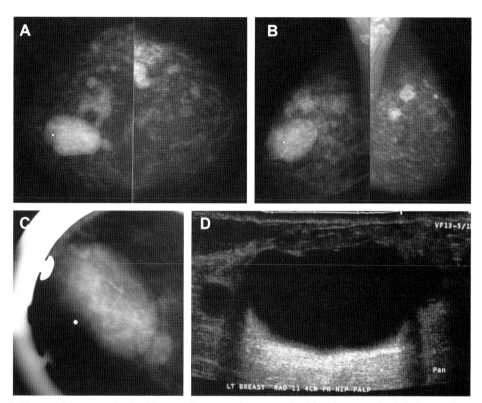

Fig. 4. A 43-year-old woman had a history of cysts and presented with a lump in the left breast. (*A*) Bilateral CC and (*B*) MLO mammograms show minimal scattered fibroglandular density and multiple bilateral PCPO masses consistent with the history of cysts. Ultrasonography is appropriate at least to evaluate the dominant, palpable mass (marked with a radiopaque marker). (*C*) Spot compression view was performed, but, in this case, it is not necessary before (*D*) targeted ultrasonography, which confirmed a benign simple cyst. Aspiration is typically only performed for symptomatic relief or diagnostic uncertainty. (*Courtesy of* Wendie A. Berg, MD, PhD, Lutherville, MD.)

to adopt a consistent approach to color code stiffness.

With MR imaging, there is no contrast enhancement of simple cysts. The signal intensity of simple cysts parallels that of water (ie, hypointense on T1 and hyperintense on T2 or short T1 inversion recovery [STIR]).

Differential Diagnosis

Meticulous sonographic technique must be used, with the focal zone at the level of the mass and appropriate gain and gray scale. With too narrow a dynamic range, hypoechoic solid lesions can appear anechoic and mimic cysts (see **Fig. 7**). Metastatic adenopathy (**Fig. 19**), high-grade infiltrating ductal carcinoma (IDC) not otherwise specified (NOS), and mucinous and medullary carcinomas (2 special types of IDC) can present

as nearly anechoic masses with posterior enhancement.[14,15] Metastatic nodes are usually located in the axilla and may show vascularity on color or power Doppler; cysts do not show internal vascularity. Margin characterization is important: most cystic-appearing IDC or other malignancies show at least a focally indistinct margin or thickened wall and may show internal vascularity (**Figs. 20** and **21**). Images of all lesions, including cysts, should be documented without calipers (and electively with calipers also) in 2 perpendicular planes, so that the margins can be fully assessed by the interpreting physician (see **Fig. 7**).

Management

A palpable mass in a patient younger than 30 years should be evaluated initially with ultrasonography,[16] and mammography is typically performed

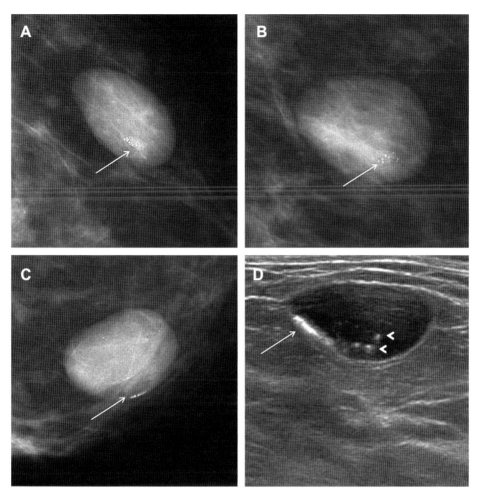

Fig. 5. On screening mammography, a 65-year-old woman was noted to have a circumscribed oval mass containing calcifications that were punctate and amorphous and changed appearance between (*A*) CC and (*B*) MLO views (*arrows*). (*C*) True lateral view was obtained, showing the calcifications to layer in the inferior aspect of the mass (*arrow*), compatible with milk of calcium within a cyst. Layering calcifications were also evident on (*D*) ultrasonography (*arrow*), although not all the echogenic calcifications layer (*arrowheads*). (*Courtesy of Wendie A. Berg, MD, PhD, Lutherville, MD.*)

only if sonographic and/or clinical features are suspicious for malignancy. If the patient is 30 years or older, typically mammography is performed first, followed by ultrasonography.

Simple cysts are primarily asymptomatic, although they can be palpable as soft mobile masses when they are large. Relaxed cysts, which are oval (flat), are usually asymptomatic. Tense, round cysts may require aspiration for symptomatic relief. A clearly benign cyst recommended for aspiration because of symptoms is still appropriately coded BI-RADS 2, benign[1] and is not included as a positive imaging finding for auditing purposes (Edward A. Sickles, MD, personal communication, 2009).

The fluid of simple cysts can be clear or cloudy and yellow or greenish black. Cysts that communicate with ducts can produce nipple discharge. Greenish-black nipple discharge is typical of fibrocystic change communicating with the nipple and does not require further evaluation. Clear or milky nipple discharge only with stimulation is usually physiologic and does not require further evaluation.[17] Spontaneous clear nipple discharge can be caused by papillomas or cysts or rarely by cancer (with 6% malignancy rate in one series[18])

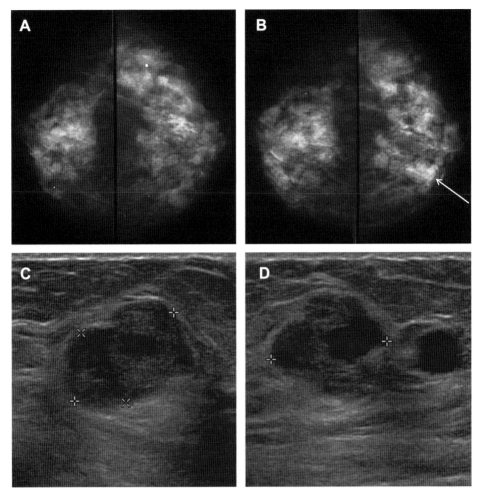

Fig. 6. A 64-year-old woman has a changing pattern of bilateral PCPO masses on (A) initial CC views and (B) CC views obtained 3 years later. One slightly larger mass (*arrow*) was recalled for additional evaluation on the latter examination. (*C*) Radial and (*D*) antiradial ultrasonography targeted to the recalled mass showed a complex cystic and solid mass (*denoted by calipers*), as well as an adjacent simple cyst. Ultrasound-guided core biopsy and excision showed benign phyllodes tumor. Multiple simple cysts were also present in both breasts. (*Courtesy of* Wendie A. Berg, MD, PhD, Lutherville, MD.)

and merits further evaluation with mammography and ultrasonography and rarely MR imaging or galactography. Bloody nipple discharge is typically caused by benign or malignant papillary lesions, with a 24% rate of malignancy in one series.[18]

COMPLICATED CYSTS: CYSTS WITH DEBRIS

Complicated cysts are masses that otherwise meet the criteria for simple cysts except that they are not anechoic, that is, they appear at least partially hypoechoic internally (**Fig. 22**). The internal echoes represent proteins from cell turnover, hemorrhage, or pus, and such proteins can be collectively termed debris.

Demographically, there is no difference between simple and complicated cysts with peak incidence for both at 35 to 50 years of age. In the ACRIN trial, participants with and without cysts, complicated cysts, and other cystic lesions had the same demographics as the overall patient population of ACRIN 6666, with a median age of 49 to 54 years (range, 26–87 years).

Complicated cysts are frequently asymptomatic and often accompany simple cysts and can be painful and/or palpable when they are tense, inflamed, infected, or rapidly enlarging. Infected cysts are often associated with overlying erythema. Rarely, nipple discharge can occur if there is communication with a duct. Over time,

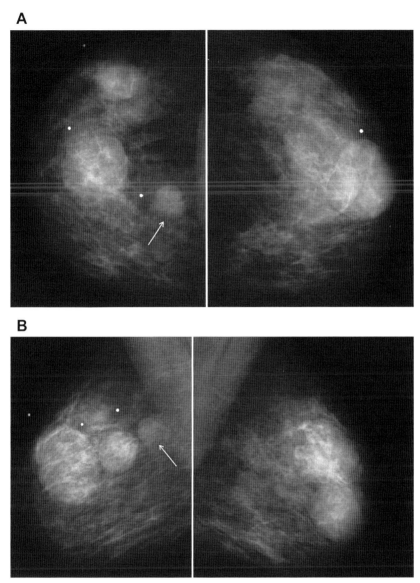

Fig. 7. A 45-year-old woman had a history of cysts and now had bilateral tender palpable masses marked by radi-opaque markers on (A) CC and (B) MLO mammograms. (C) Multiple static ultrasonographic images of the palpable lumps were interpreted as bilateral cysts. One lump was aspirated (upper inner right breast [marked by arrows in A and B]), yielding malignant cytology. (D) Repeat ultrasonography of the known malignant mass in the right breast at 2-o'clock position shows it to be indistinctly marginated and lobulated both without and (E) with spatial compounding. Any lesion documented on ultrasonography should have images recorded without calipers to facilitate margin assessment. Images of the tumor from the initial ultrasonography in part C (the *bottom left* image) had too narrow a dynamic range (effectively too few shades of gray); hence, the solid mass appeared anechoic. (F) Sagittal image from 3-dimensional fat-suppressed spoiled gradient echo (SPGR) MR imaging 1.5 minutes after 0.1 mmol/kg of gadolinium-based contrast injection shows an irregular enhancing mass (*arrow*) corresponding to the known grade III invasive ductal carcinoma. (*Courtesy of* Wendie A. Berg, MD, PhD, Lutherville, MD.)

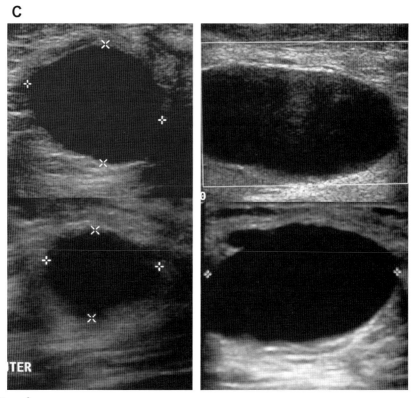

Fig. 7. (*continued*)

both simple cysts and cysts with debris can wax and wane in size and many will resolve spontaneously in weeks to years.

Across 6 prior series,[19–24] only 2 (0.23%) of 868 lesions that were thought to be complicated cysts on sonography proved to be malignant (**Table 3**). One malignancy was a 3-mm ductal carcinoma in situ (DCIS) within a papilloma[24] and the other was a 4-mm grade II IDC NOS.[22] Of the 243 lesions that were prospectively classified as complicated cysts (including 15 clustered microcysts) in the series by Daly and colleagues,[22] 210 (86.4%) yielded fluid at diagnosis, 8 resolved or nearly resolved (3.2%) on puncture, and 7 (2.9%) had enough material for cytologic examination, 1 of which was atypical and showed myxoid fibroadenoma at excision. Of the 33 suspected complicated cysts not yielding fluid, a total of 19 were biopsied, of which 1 was malignant.[22] Importantly, in the series by Buchberger and colleagues,[20] 7 (5.2%) of 133 complicated cysts did not yield fluid on attempted aspiration, with no malignancies; 24 (17%) of 141 did not yield fluid on attempted aspiration in the series by Venta and colleagues[24] (including the 1 malignancy); and 33 (14%) of 243

did not yield fluid on attempted aspiration in the series by Daly and colleagues[22] (including the 1 malignancy). Thus, over these 3 series,[20,22,24] 64 (12%) of 517 lesions that were thought to be complicated cysts proved solid, with 2 (3.1%) of such 64 solid lesions proving malignant.

In the ACRIN 6666 protocol, complicated cysts in the setting of bilateral simple cysts could be dismissed as benign findings (BI-RADS 2).[3] A solitary probable complicated cyst seen only on initial ultrasonography was classified as probably benign (BI-RADS 3).[3] Aspiration was generally recommended only for isolated new probable complicated cysts or those with other suspicious features (BI-RADS 4).[3] In year 1, of 296 complicated cysts, 132 (44.6%) were given BI-RADS 2 assessment; 135 (45.6%), BI-RADS 3; and 28 (9.5%), BI-RADS 4A (with 1 unknown). By year 3, of 224 complicated cysts, 176 (78.6%) were given BI-RADS 2 assessment; only 37 (17%), BI-RADS 3; and only 9 (4.0%), BI-RADS 4A. New complicated cysts in the setting of multiple simple cysts were dismissed as benign unless there were other suspicious features. Using this approach, only 1 malignancy was followed (**Fig. 23**), and 1 other

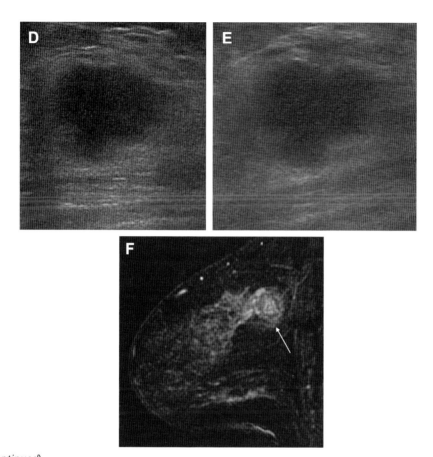

Fig. 7. *(continued)*

malignancy was identified as a new complicated cyst on ultrasonography with biopsy recommended (**Fig. 24**). One other participant had bilateral complicated cysts during the first screening and was recommended for a 6-month follow-up, at which time a new mass was noted on ultrasonography and found to be malignant. Complicated cysts were seen in 376 (14.1%) ACRIN participants. Of those 376 participants with complicated cysts, 301 (80%) also had at least 1 simple cyst and 84 (22%) had multiple bilateral complicated cysts. Of the 7473 ultrasonographic studies in the 3 years of the ACRIN 6666 trial, 644 (8.6%) examinations showed at least 1 complicated cyst, with 475 such lesions identified (counting multiple bilateral similar complicated cysts as 1 lesion). Of the 475 lesions, 2 (0.42%) possible cysts with debris proved malignant (see **Figs. 23** and **24, Table 4**) and 2 were high-risk lesions (1 an atypical papilloma and 1 a ruptured cyst in year 1, which was excised in year 2 showing

lobular carcinoma in situ). The malignancies were each found in breasts with concurrent ipsilateral cancer: for one, the lesion mistaken for a complicated cyst was a 6-mm invasive lobular carcinoma (see **Fig. 23**) ipsilateral to grade I IDC+DCIS, node negative; for the other, the lesion was IDC+DCIS ipsilateral to a second grade II IDC+DCIS, with nodal metastases (see **Fig. 24**).

Imaging Findings

Mammographically, both simple and complicated cysts are manifest as solitary or multiple, bilateral, PCPO, round or oval masses, and both simple and complicated cysts can show milk of calcium or, rarely, rim calcification. As with simple cysts, a pattern of fluctuation, with some regressing and others developing, is common. This pattern does not require further imaging (ie, ultrasonography) unless there is a new dominant or palpable

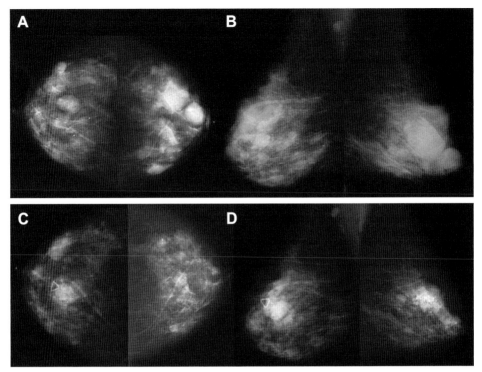

Fig. 8. A 57-year-old woman had multiple bilateral PCPO masses on (*A*) CC and (*B*) MLO screening mammograms, compatible with cysts or other benign nodules. (*C*) CC and (*D*) MLO mammograms of the same woman, obtained 3 years later, show changing pattern of bilateral cysts as well as interval development of an indistinctly margin-ated dense mass at the site of a new palpable mass (*marked by triangular markers*). The mass is seen better on (*E*) spot compression CC and (*F*) close-up MLO views. (*G*) Transverse and (*H*) sagittal ultrasonographic images show an irregular complex cystic and solid mass with a surrounding echogenic halo, highly suggestive of malignancy. Ultrasound-guided biopsy and excision showed grade III infiltrating ductal carcinoma not otherwise specified, ER+, her2/neu−, with negative sentinel nodes. (*Courtesy of* Wendie A. Berg, MD, PhD, Lutherville, MD.)

lesion, although ultrasonography can be per-formed electively.

Most simple and complicated cysts are identi-fied on sonography that is performed for evalua-tion of a clinical or mammographic abnormality or for screening. An oval, or less often round, mass with imperceptible walls, internal echoes, and posterior acoustic enhancement is classic. When a fluid-debris level is observed with no suspicious features (**Fig. 25**) or when the internal echoes are mobile on real-time evaluation (**Fig. 26**), the appearance is pathognomonic,[1] although such appearances are relatively uncommon. In the ACRIN 6666 protocol, of the 376 participants with complicated cysts, 28 (7.4%) were reported to have fluid-debris levels and 23 (6.1%) had mobile internal echoes. Power Doppler can impart energy, which can allow motion of the debris to be visible. Rarely,

a fluid-debris level can be present because of hemorrhage from an intracystic mass (**Figs. 27** and **28**). In such cases, turning the patient from supine to supine oblique position will prompt a change in appearance of debris and can allow visualization of any underlying mass (see **Fig. 28; Fig. 29**). If the debris is thick, up to 5 minutes may be needed between initial and repeat imaging.

Complicated cysts with homogeneous low-level echoes can be difficult to distinguish from solid masses, and, indeed, as described earlier, 64 (12%) of 517 lesions prospectively classified as complicated cysts proved solid across three series.[20,22,24] Complicated cysts are usually accompanied by simple cysts (as in 80% of AC-RIN 6666 participants previously described). Internal vascularity is not present in cysts and should prompt biopsy (**Fig. 30**). Harmonics can

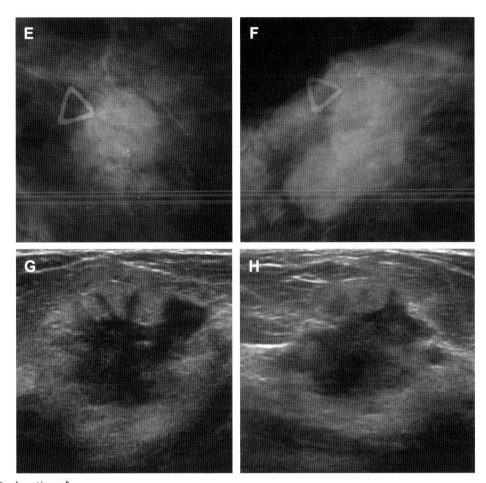

Fig. 8. (*continued*)

reduce false internal echoes. Spatial compounding improves margin evaluation and decreases speckle and noise at the expense of posterior feature characterization.

Elastography can sometimes help distinguish a benign complicated cyst (**Fig. 31**) from a suspicious solid mass (**Figs. 32** and **33**), although further validation of this approach is needed.

T1-weighted MR imaging demonstrates an oval, round, or gently lobulated mass with its signal dependent on the internal contents. Hemorrhagic and proteinaceous cysts appear hyperintense on T1 and hypointense on T2 or STIR. A fluid-fluid or fluid-debris level may be seen (**Fig. 34**).

Differential Diagnosis

Small simple cysts can appear hypoechoic, with 21% of cysts measuring 4 mm or smaller in size described as solid masses in one series, as were 13% of cysts measuring 4.1 to 6 mm and 8% of cysts measuring 6.1 to 8 mm; all simple cysts larger than 8 mm were appropriately classified.[10] Reverberation artifacts (see **Fig. 9**) can mimic debris.

Fibroadenomata are typically circumscribed oval masses, which are slightly hypoechoic or iso-echoic to fat, with or without posterior enhancement (see **Fig. 32**). Internal echogenic septations may be evident within fibroadenomata and

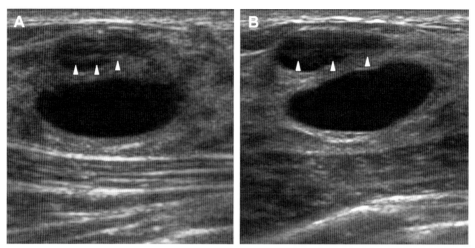

Fig. 9. A 30-year-old woman presented for evaluation of palpable masses. The masses were shown to be cysts on (A) radial and (B) antiradial ultrasonographic images. The more superficial cyst shows reverberation artifacts paralleling the anterior wall of the cyst (*arrowheads*). (*Courtesy of* Wendie A. Berg, MD, PhD, Lutherville, MD.)

lactating adenomas (**Fig. 35**), and there can be vascularity adjacent to or even within such solid masses. Popcorn calcifications are best seen on mammography and are pathognomonic of fibroadenomata.

Sonographically, oil cysts can be anechoic or can have low-level echoes or fluid-debris levels (discussed later). They may or may not show posterior enhancement and can even shadow. Mammographically, oil cysts are lucent and can

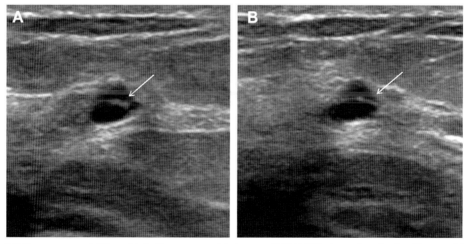

Fig. 10. (A) Transverse and (B) sagittal ultrasonographic images (L12-5 MHz transducer) of a 47-year-old woman with incidental cyst containing a thin (<0.5 mm) septation (*arrows*) on ACRIN 6666 screening ultrasonography, which was stable for 3 years. This is a benign finding. (*Courtesy of* Wendie A. Berg, MD, PhD, Lutherville, MD.)

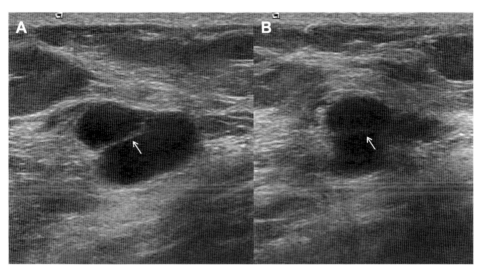

Fig. 11. A benign cyst showing thin internal septation (*arrows*) on (*A*) radial and (*B*) antiradial ultrasonographic images in a 46-year-old woman. Often such cysts will be shown to communicate with each other if aspiration is attempted. (*Courtesy of* Wendie A. Berg, MD, PhD, Lutherville, MD.)

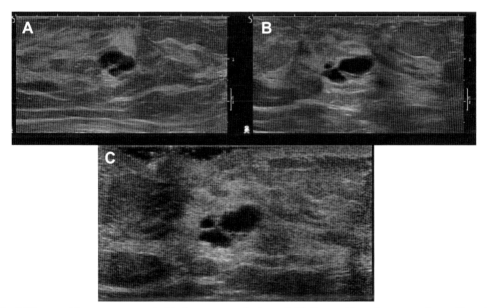

Fig. 12. A 35-year-old woman was noted to have a mass that was initially questioned as a complex cystic and solid mass on (*A*) transverse sonography (L15-4 MHz transducer). On (*B*) sagittal and (*C*) radial images, the mass was shown to correspond to a group of adjacent small cysts. This is a benign finding. (*Courtesy of* Dr Linda Hovanessian Larsen, Keck University School of Medicine, University of Southern California, Los Angeles, CA, via SuperSonic Imagine.)

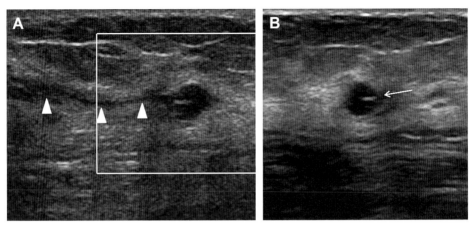

Fig. 13. In the ACRIN 6666 protocol, on baseline screening a 54-year-old woman by (*A*) radial and (*B*) antiradial ultrasonography, a small cyst was incidentally identified, which communicates with a duct (*arrowheads*). The cyst contains a single thin septation (*arrow*). This is a benign finding. (*Courtesy of* Wendie A. Berg, MD, PhD, Lutherville, MD.)

develop rim/dystrophic calcification, the latter contributing to posterior shadowing on ultrasonography. There may be other evidence of fat necrosis (discussed later).

Galactoceles are associated with pregnancy or breastfeeding. Finding an echogenic fat plug (**Fig. 36**) or fluid-debris level with nondependent hypoechoic fat can suggest the diagnosis of galactocele (**Fig. 37**). Internal vascularity implies a solid mass and should prompt biopsy (**Fig. 38**).

Abscesses are most often found near the nipple, with bacteria entering through cracks in the skin (**Fig. 39**). Abscesses usually produce clinically evident pain and often erythema and are more

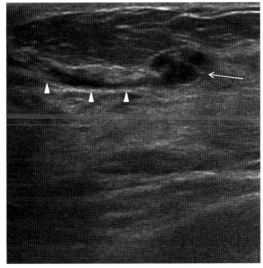

Fig. 14. Radial ultrasonographic image shows incidental group of small cysts (*arrow*) communicating with a duct (*arrowheads*) in a 51-year-old woman who underwent screening ultrasonography due to a strong family history of breast cancer and dense breasts. (*Courtesy of* Wendie A. Berg, MD, PhD, Lutherville, MD.)

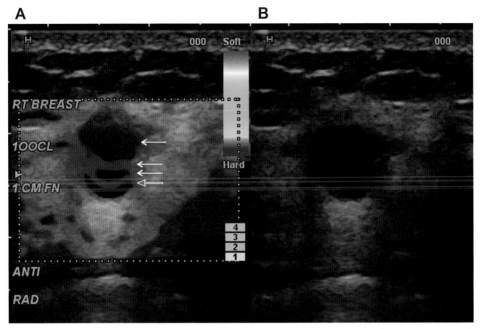

Fig. 15. A 39-year-old woman was followed up for cysts and complicated cysts. On (*A*) elastography with Hitachi equipment (or also Toshiba), cysts can have a layered and usually trilaminar appearance (*arrows*), appearing stiffer (blue on these devices) anteriorly and softer (red on these devices) posteriorly. Sometimes there is an apparent fourth layer (*open arrow*) in the region of posterior enhancement, analogous to the bright area on Siemens and Philips equipment. This is a simple cyst on (*B*) B-mode ultrasonography image. (*Courtesy of* Dr Christopher Comstock, Memorial Sloan Kettering Cancer Center, New York, NY.)

frequent with breastfeeding, trauma, or surgery. Most abscesses will have a thick and/or irregular wall (ie, complex cystic lesion), although 6 (33%) of 18 abscesses appeared to be complicated cysts in one series.[19] In the series of symptomatic cystic lesions reported by Chang and colleagues,[21] of the 35 complicated cysts with homogeneous low-level echoes, 21 (60%) were abscesses, 9 (26%) fibrocystic changes, 4 (11%) cysts had debris, and 1 (3%) was a mucocele-like tumor excised, (benign). With abscesses, there is usually increased echogenicity in the surrounding parenchyma because of associated edema. Increased vascularity may be evident adjacent to abscesses on color or power Doppler.

As mentioned earlier, malignancies are rarely mistaken for complicated cysts. Intraductal papillary DCIS rarely can bleed and obscure the mass and produce a fluid-debris level (see **Figs. 27** and **28**). High-grade IDC, NOS, can present as a round or oval hypoechoic mass with posterior acoustic enhancement (see **Fig. 30**).[15] Although most of the margin can appear circumscribed with IDC NOS, usually at least a portion of the margin is indistinct or angular and/or there will be evidence of a complex cystic and solid mass (discussed

later) with thickened wall, thick septations, or intracystic mass.

Management

Mammographic or sonographic bilateral fluctuating cysts, both simple and complicated, may be dismissed as benign, BI-RADS 2, with routine mammographic (and, optionally sonographic) screening performed.

Asymptomatic complicated cysts with fluid-debris levels or mobile internal echoes are benign, BI-RADS 2, with no follow-up needed.

An isolated noncalcified mass, which may be a fibroadenoma or complicated cyst on ultrasonography, noted on baseline examination or incidentally noted on ultrasonography can be considered probably benign, BI-RADS 3, with 6-, 12-, and 24-month surveillance. Gradual enlargement, defined as a 20% or less increase in diameter in 6 months, is acceptable for fibroadenomata[25] and certainly also for complicated cysts. Although typically biopsy is performed for palpable masses compatible with fibroadenomata, surveillance seems to be a reasonable alternative, with 1 malignancy (1.5-mm DCIS) among 375 palpable masses in

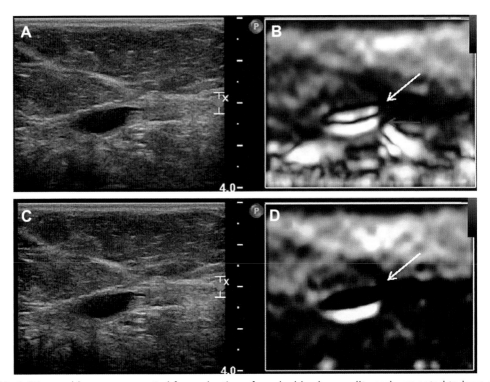

Fig. 16. A 35-year-old woman presented for evaluation of a palpable abnormality and was noted to have a cyst on (A) and (C) conventional ultrasonography (L17-5 MHz transducer, Philips Ultrasound, Bothell, WA, USA). (B) On EI (elastography imaging) setting 2, a target or bull's-eye appearance is seen (*white arrow*) in which the cyst is a void with a central bright area because of the motion of cyst fluid. Also, a bright area is noted just deep to the cyst (*red arrow*). (D) On EI setting 1, the cyst a black void (*arrow*) with posterior bright area. (*Courtesy of* Richard G. Barr, MD, PhD, Radiology Consultants, Youngstown, OH.)

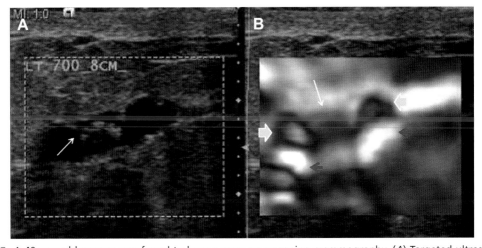

Fig. 17. A 40-year-old woman was found to have a mass on screening mammography. (A) Targeted ultrasonography showed an intraductal mass (*arrow*), which was hypervascular on power Doppler (not shown). (B) Elasticity image shows bull's-eye appearance to the fluid (*solid arrows*) on either side of the solid, gray, stiffer, biopsy-proven papilloma (*white arrow*). Posterior bright areas (*red arrows*) are also noted deep to the cystic portions. (*Courtesy of* Richard G. Barr, MD, PhD, Radiology Consultants, Youngstown, OH.)

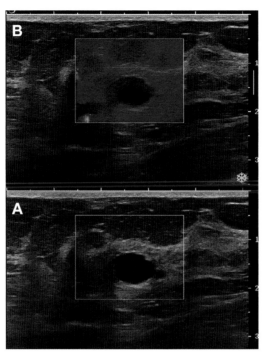

Fig. 18. Simple cyst on (A) gray-scale (L15-4 MHz transducer) and (B) shear-wave elastography. Cysts typically appear mostly black or dark blue (ie, soft) on this type of elastography. (*Courtesy of* Dr Philippe Henrot, Nancy, France, via SuperSonic Imagine.)

one series (0.3% malignancy rate[26]) and no malignancies among 157 such masses in another series.[27]

A BI-RADS 4 assessment, with recommendation for aspiration and possible biopsy if the mass proves to be solid, is appropriate in the following situations:

1. Palpable, tender, possible abscess
2. Diagnostic uncertainty (ie, possibly solid) and mass is new, or enlarging (more than 20% increase in diameter in 6 months)
3. Other suspicious features are present, such as suspicious calcifications, indistinct margin on mammography, distortion, or mass is actually a complex cystic lesion (ie, intracystic mass, thick wall of ≥0.5 mm, thick septations of ≥0.5 mm, mixed cystic and solid lesion).

Aspiration is performed with an 18- to 20-gauge needle. Use of ultrasonographic guidance facilitates aspiration to resolution. An equal volume of room air can be instilled at the conclusion of the procedure to decrease the risk of recurrence.[28,29] Typical cyst fluid is clear or cloudy and yellow or greenish black. Unless the fluid is bloody (especially old blood) or pus, it can be discarded. When bloody, the fluid should be sent for cytologic examination and the cyst should be marked with a clip placed under sonographic guidance, although the risk of malignancy in this situation is exceedingly low. Indeed, among 6782 aspirates sent for cytologic examination in the series by Ciatto and colleagues,[30] no malignancies were identified, although there were 5 papillomas among the 2% of aspirates which were bloody. Sending typical cyst fluid for cytologic examination may result in false-positive results and unnecessary further treatment. In the series by Smith and colleagues,[31] 660 aspirates were sent for cytologic examination and 33 (5%) produced an atypical result with no malignancies on surgery or follow-up and 86 (13%) were acellular and nondiagnostic but none were malignant. Similarly, Hindle and colleagues[32] reported all 689 nonbloody aspirates in their series produced only acellular, benign, or nondiagnostic cytology.

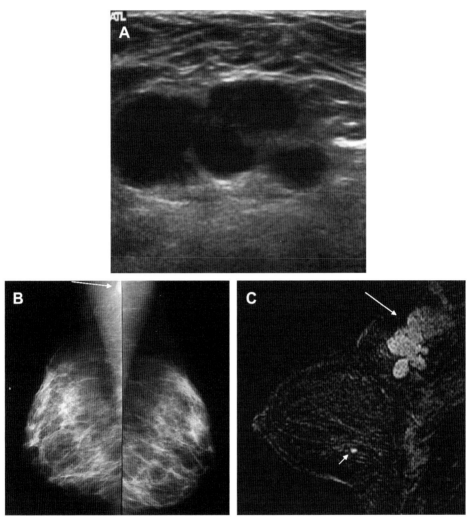

Fig. 19. This 42-year-old woman had a palpable axillary mass, incorrectly attributed to cysts on (*A*) transverse sonography. (*B*) MLO mammograms show portion of a dense mass corresponding to the palpable axillary mass (*arrow*). Ultrasound-guided core biopsy showed metastatic grade III invasive ductal carcinoma. (*C*) Sagittal subtraction image from contrast-enhanced spoiled gradient echo (SPGR) MR imaging shows bulky, enhancing, axillary adenopathy (*long arrow*). Tiny enhancing breast lesion (*short arrow*) proved benign, and the primary was never identified. The patient underwent excision of the nodes, chemotherapy, and radiation therapy to the breast and was disease free 5 years later. (*Courtesy of* Wendie A. Berg, MD, PhD, Lutherville, MD.)

OIL CYSTS

An oil cyst is a round or oval, liquid, fat-containing, encapsulated lesion. The cause is usually trauma, although the trauma can be so minor as to be unnoticed by the patient. Oil cysts can often occur after surgery and irradiation. Oil cysts are most commonly seen in superficial subcutaneous and subareolar tissues, which are the most mobile and most vulnerable regions to trauma. Ischemia can result in cell death and fat necrosis, particularly at the periphery (upper outer quadrant) of transverse rectus abdominis myocutaneous flap reconstructions, where the blood supply is most tenuous.

Oil cysts are a special type of fat necrosis, which occurs when fat cells are damaged and release their lipid content into surrounding parenchyma. The lipids are broken down into fatty acids, which then are surrounded by a fibrous capsule. The capsule calcifies over

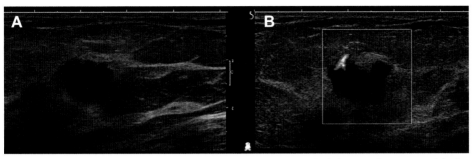

Fig. 20. A 60-year-old woman was noted to have a nearly anechoic but slightly irregular mass on (A) ultrasonography. Internal vascularity was demonstrated on (B) power Doppler. Biopsy showed medullary carcinoma, a special type of invasive ductal carcinoma. (*Courtesy of* Dr Catherine Balu-Maestro, Centre Antoine Lacassagne, Nice, France, via SuperSonic Imagine.)

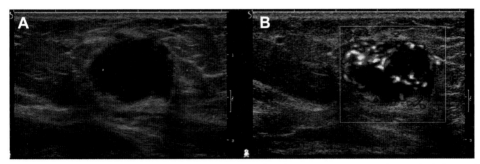

Fig. 21. A 64-year-old woman underwent (A) ultrasonography, demonstrating a nearly anechoic irregular mass with posterior enhancement. (B) On power Doppler, marked internal vascularity was demonstrated, confirming the solid nature of this spindle cell sarcoma. (*Courtesy of* Dr David Cosgrove, Charing Cross Hospital, London, UK, via SuperSonic Imagine.)

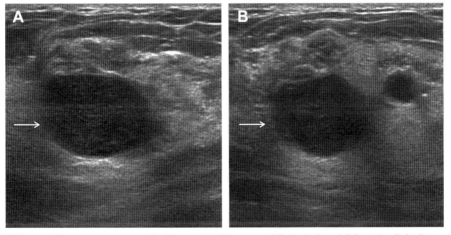

Fig. 22. A 41-year-old woman presented with a palpable mass. (A) Radial and (B) antiradial ultrasonographic images (L12-5 MHz) showed oval circumscribed mass (*arrows*) with homogeneous low-level echoes and posterior enhancement, which is typical of a complicated cyst with debris. This mass was aspirated to resolution at patient request, yielding a cloudy yellow fluid that is typical of benign cyst content and therefore it was discarded. An adjacent simple cyst was incidentally noted. (*Courtesy of* Wendie A. Berg, MD, PhD, Lutherville, MD.)

Table 3
Summary of outcomes of lesions described sonographically as complicated cysts

Study, Year	Number	Number Aspirated or Biopsied (%)	Number Malignant (%)	Details of Malignancies	Details of Benign	Follow-up Details
Kolb et al,[23] 1998	126	30 aspirated	0	NA	Not distinctly reported	96 followed
Venta et al,[24] 1999	308	123	1 (0.32)	3-mm DCIS in a papilloma (6-mm mass)	11 FA, 10 FCC, 5 cyst walls, 3 fibroses, 1 hamartoma, 1 lymph node	161 followed, 24 no follow-up
Buchberger, et al[20] 1999	133	133 aspirated, 7 also core biopsied	0	NA	Not distinctly reported	
Berg et al,[19] 2003	38	38	0	NA	19 cysts, 6 abscesses, 5 FCC, 2 fat necroses, 1 papilloma	26 resolved, 1 enlarging papilloma excised, 1 each recurrent cyst and fat necrosis excised; 1 recurrent galactocele
Chang et al,[21] 2007	35	26 aspirated, 7 core biopsied, 2 excised	0	NA	21 abscesses, 9 FCC, 4 cysts, 1 mucocelelike tumor	
Daly et al,[22] 2008	228	Aspiration attempted on all, no fluid in 33[a]	1 (0.44)	4-mm grade II IDC NOS, did not yield fluid (6-mm mass)	4 abscesses, 2 FA, 1 ALH, rest were cysts and FCC	
Total	868		2 (0.23)			

Abbreviations: ALH, atypical lobular hyperplasia; DCIS, ductal carcinoma in situ; FA, fibroadenoma; FCC, fibrocystic change; NA, not applicable, no entries.
[a] Includes women with lesions prospectively classified as either clustered microcysts or complicated cysts; mean size 13 mm.

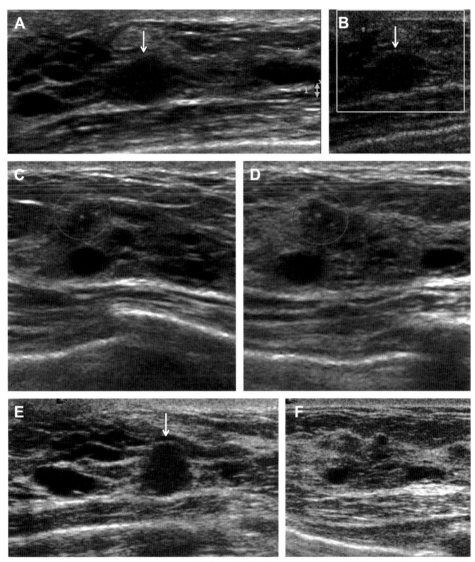

Fig. 23. A 52-year-old ACRIN 6666 participant had multiple findings on her third annual screening ultrasonography, including multiple cysts. On (A) radial and (B) antiradial ultrasonography with power Doppler, a mass seen at 2-o'clock position in the left breast was thought to be a complicated cyst and was recommended for a 6-month follow-up. On (C) radial and (D) antiradial ultrasonographic images of the right breast, at the 12-o'clock position, a few calcifications were noted (red circles), which were dismissed as fibrocystic changes adjacent to several small cysts. No calcifications were seen mammographically. At follow-up after 7 months, (E) radial ultrasonography showed that the left breast mass had enlarged (arrow), prompting ultrasound-guided biopsy. This mass proved to be a 6-mm node-negative invasive lobular carcinoma. (F) Radial ultrasonography of the 12-o'clock position in the left breast appeared unremarkable. Follow-up (G) transverse and (H) sagittal ultrasonography on the right side showed an enlarging isoechoic mass with calcifications (red ovals). This mass proved to be a 6-mm grade I IDC+DCIS and node negative. Seen only on (I) CC and not on (J) MLO mammograms, a subtle area of distortion was noted in the 12-o'clock position of the left breast (short solid arrow), which proved to be a 5-mm tubular carcinoma (grade I IDC, special type) with associated DCIS. (Courtesy of Wendie A. Berg, MD, PhD, Lutherville, MD.)

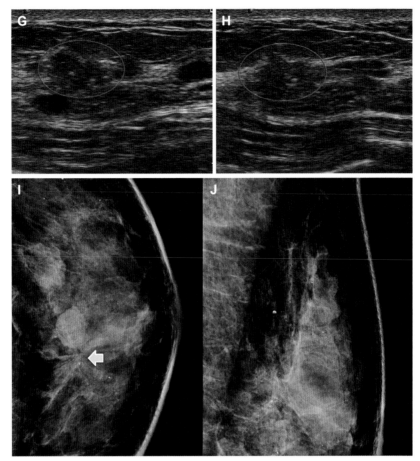

Fig. 23. (*continued*)

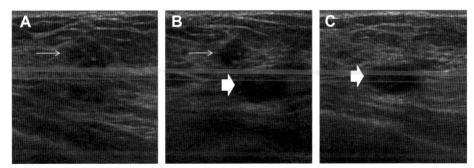

Fig. 24. A 59-year-old ACRIN 6666 participant had prior left breast conservation therapy for cancer. On the third annual screening ultrasonography, 2 masses were noted in the outer right breast on (*A*) oblique, (*B*) antiradial, and (*C*) radial images. The first mass was nearly isoechoic, microlobulated, and contained echogenic calcifications (*arrows*) and was recommended for biopsy. Just deep to this mass was an oval mass with probable fluid-debris level which was thought to be a complicated cyst (*short solid arrows*). The first mass was proved to be a 12-mm grade II IDC with DCIS. The deeper mass was also excised and also proved to be grade II IDC with DCIS. Sentinel node showed metastatic disease. (*Courtesy of* Wendie A. Berg, MD, PhD, Lutherville, MD.)

Table 4
Prevalence and outcomes of cystic lesions in ACRIN 6666 among 2662 unique participants over 3 annual screening ultrasonographic examinations

Description[a]	Number of Participants (%)	Number of Unique Lesions[b]	Number of such Lesions Biopsied (%)	Number of such Lesions Aspirated (%)	Number Malignant (%)	Details of Pathology
Complicated Cysts[c]	376 (14.1)	475	34 (7.2)[d]	40 (8.4)	2 (0.42)	1 ILC, 1 IDC-DCIS, 1 atypical papilloma, 1 ADH, 1 LCIS, 7 FA, 12 ruptured cysts, 1 granuloma/chronic inflammation, 4 FCC, 1 FIBR, 2 SA, 1 lymph node, 1 duct ectasia
Clustered Microcysts[e]	104 (3.9)	123	5 (4.1)	3 (2.4)	1 (0.8)[e]	1 ILC,[e] 1 AM, 1 FCC, 1 ruptured duct, 1 SA
Complex Cystic and Solid Lesions[f]	42 (1.6)	45	20 (48)[e]	6 (13)	0	1 ADH, 4 papillomas, 4 FA, 2 ruptured cysts, 2 FCC, 2 AM, 2 FIBR, 1 duct ectasia, 1 SA, 1 was granulomatous
Hypoechoic Solid with Tiny Cystic Areas[g]	32 (1.2)	35	17 (49)	4 (11)	0[e]	6 FA, 4 FCC, 1 AM, 2 SA, 1 FNx, 1 duct ectasia, 1 BBT, 1 PASH

Abbreviations: ADH, atypical ductal hyperplasia; AM, apocrine metaplasia; BBT, benign breast tissue; FA, fibroadenoma; FCC, fibrocystic change; FIBR, fibrosis; FNx, fat necrosis; ILC, invasive lobular carcinoma; LCIS, lobular carcinoma in situ; PASH, pseudoangiomatous stromal hyperplasia; SA, sclerosing adenosis.

[a] Lesions are listed by their initial description; participants are listed more than once, if they had several types of cystic lesions.

[b] Multiple bilateral complicated cysts were seen in 84 participants and are considered one such lesion each as were multiple bilateral clustered microcysts in 4 participants.

[c] Seven lesions initially described as complicated cysts changed description on follow-up; none of which were malignant: 3 changed to complex, 1 to hypoechoic with cysts, and 3 to clustered microcysts.

[d] Twelve complicated cysts also underwent initial attempt at cyst aspiration, as did 4 complex cystic and solid lesions, not listed among aspirations.

[e] Four lesions initially classified as clustered microcysts changed description on follow-up: 1 became hypoechoic solid with tiny cystic areas and was biopsied, showing ILC; 2 became complex with no biopsy; and 1 became complicated.

[f] One lesion initially classified as complex was later classified as clustered microcysts.

[g] One lesion initially classified as hypoechoic solid with tiny cystic areas was later considered complicated and one was later considered complex.

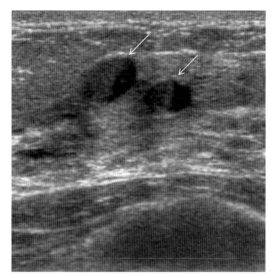

Fig. 25. On screening ultrasonography, a 54-year-old ACRIN 6666 participant was noted to have 2 small adjacent cysts with fluid-debris levels (*arrows*). These are complicated cysts with debris, benign findings, and such lesions do not require any follow-up. (*Courtesy of* Wendie A. Berg, MD, PhD, Lutherville, MD.)

time, with calcifications typically seen 2 years after the original trauma.

Clinical presentation is related to underlying cause and ranges from asymptomatic on screening to tender or nontender palpable masses. No treatment is needed as there is no association with malignancy. Oil cysts occur at any age in men and women, being much more frequent in women.

Imaging Findings

Oil cysts are easily recognized on mammography as round or oval, circumscribed, lucent masses with

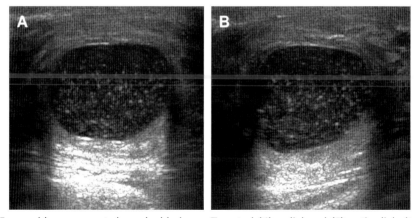

Fig. 26. A 45-year-old woman noted a palpable lump. Targeted (*A*) radial and (*B*) antiradial ultrasonography show a complicated cyst containing echogenic cholesterol crystals, which were mobile on real-time evaluation. Aspiration can be performed electively for symptomatic relief, but this is a benign finding. (*Courtesy of* Wendie A. Berg, MD, PhD, Lutherville, MD.)

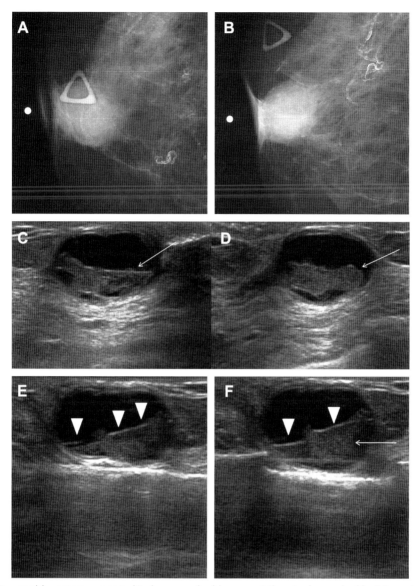

Fig. 27. A 68-year-old woman was noted to have a palpable mass at the nipple, marked by triangular markers on (A) spot compression CC and (B) MLO mammograms that show the palpable abnormality to correspond to a dense indistinctly marginated mass with overlying skin retraction. (C) Radial and (D) antiradial ultrasonography show intracystic mass (arrows). Additional oblique ultrasonographic images (E, F) show fluid-debris level (arrowheads) formed due to hemorrhage from the intracystic mass (arrow). A 14-gauge core biopsy showed atypical papilloma. Excision showed 8 mm of DCIS involving a papilloma, with 3-mm microinvasive colloid carcinoma. (Courtesy of Wendie A. Berg, MD, PhD, Lutherville, MD.)

a thin capsule. Over time, usually beginning after 1.5 to 2 years,[33] the capsule can calcify due to saponification of the fatty acids. Eggshell or rim calcification of a lucent mass is pathognomonic of an oil cyst (Fig. 40), and dystrophic calcifications are simply more densely calcified oil cysts/fat necrosis.

The sonographic appearance of oil cysts is variable and depends on the composition of the lesion (Figs. 41 and 42). The mass is typically round or oval and anechoic if simple liquid fat is present (see Fig. 42). With increasing complexity and calcification, internal septations and echogenic bands can

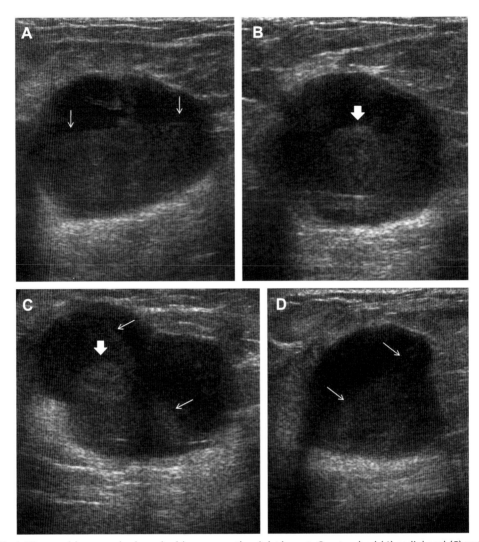

Fig. 28. A 52-year-old woman had a palpable mass on the right breast. On standard (A) radial and (B) antiradial ultrasonographic images, the mass was cystic with a fluid-debris level (*arrows*). There was also a question of an intracystic mass (*short solid arrow*). The patient was then positioned (C) in the right-side decubitus and then (D) the left-side decubitus positions. The fluid-debris level shifted accordingly (*arrows*), and the intracystic mass persisted (*short solid arrow*). Ultrasound-guided aspiration was performed, yielding bloody fluid. Core biopsy of the residual mass showed papillary DCIS (which had bled, causing the fluid-debris level). (*Courtesy of* Wendie A. Berg, MD, PhD, Lutherville, MD.)

be seen, as can thickened walls, echogenic mural masses (see **Fig. 41**C, D), and fluid-debris levels (see **Fig. 41**E, F) with the fat echogenic and nondependent as in galactoceles. Posterior enhancement can be seen, but posterior shadowing is common with oil cysts (see **Fig. 42**) and is sometimes caused by peripheral calcification. No flow is seen with color or power Doppler. Acutely, other stigmata of fat

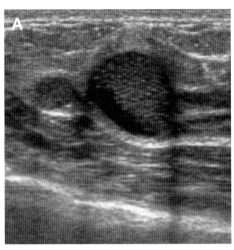
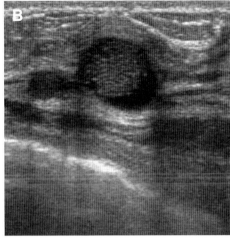

Fig. 29. On screening ACRIN 6666 ultrasonography, a 54-year-old woman was noted to have a circumscribed oval mass with posterior enhancement in the outer right breast on (*A*) supine position. Internal echoes were noted, and it was uncertain whether the echoes represented debris or an intracystic mass. (*B*) The patient was then positioned in left lateral decubitus (LLD) position and reimaged after 3 minutes, showing a shift in the contents, which is consistent with debris. This is a benign complicated cyst with no evidence of an intracystic mass. (*Courtesy of* Wendie A. Berg, MD, PhD, Lutherville, MD.)

necrosis can be seen, such as edema in the surrounding parenchyma and mixed anechoic and hyperechoic collections from trauma or surgery.

MR imaging demonstrates a well-defined, hyperintense, round to oval mass on T1-weighted images, which has decreased signal on T2W images. With contrast, a thin enhancing rim can occasionally be seen.

Differential Diagnosis

Imaging findings of oil cysts are pathognomonic on mammography and MR imaging. Sonographic findings can be correlated with the mammogram by placing a radiopaque marker under ultrasonography and repeating the mammogram if needed.

Management

Oil cysts are benign findings, BI-RADS 2.

CLUSTERED MICROCYSTS

Clustered microcysts represent the terminal duct lobular unit, or a portion of it, where there has been cystic dilatation of individual acini (**Fig. 43**).[1,34] Clustered microcysts are a part of the spectrum of benign cystic change of the breast and can be lined with bland or apocrine metaplastic epithelium (see **Fig. 43**; **Figs. 44**

and **45**). Stigmata of fibrocystic changes, with simple cysts, fibrosis, and adenosis, are also often present.

Clustered microcysts are most common in perimenopausal women aged 39 to 50 years (median 48 years)[35] and were found in 5.8% of consecutive breast ultrasonographic examinations in one series.[35] Typically, these are found as an incidental finding on mammography, ultrasonography, or both. One-half of clustered microcysts are stable at 1-year follow-up, and at 2 years, approximately 20% resolve, approximately 20% decrease in size, and approximately 10% increase in size, after which they are stable or they resolve.[35]

Across 4 prior series, no malignancies were found among 112 lesions described as clustered microcysts (**Table 5**). On the initial screening ultrasonographic examination in the ACRIN 6666 trial, 64 (2.4%) of 2659 women were reported to have clustered microcysts, although this may be underreported as some may have been included among simple cysts. Over the 3-year ACRIN 6666 experience, of 123 unique lesions described as clustered microcysts, 1 (0.8%) proved malignant (a 4-mm node-negative invasive lobular carcinoma). The malignant lesion appeared solid with distortion during the second screening and may not have even been the same lesion (**Fig. 46**). Over three years of ACRIN 6666, clustered microcysts were found in 104 (3.9%) of 2662 participants.

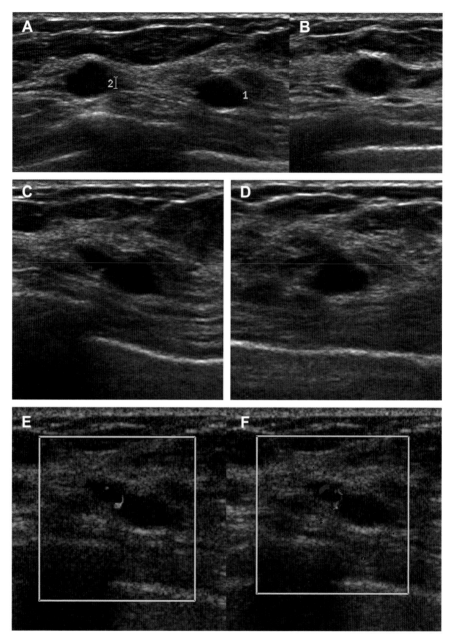

Fig. 30. A 59-year-old woman with dense breasts was referred for biopsy of indeterminate calcifications in the right breast. Screening ultrasonography was performed, demonstrating 2 adjacent, mostly circumscribed, hypo-echoic masses with posterior enhancement suggestive of complicated cysts (labeled 1 and 2) on (A) radial and (B) antiradial sonograms of mass 1. (C) Radial and (D) antiradial images of mass 2. Radial power Doppler images (E, F) of mass 2 show internal vascularity, which is not found with cysts. As such, biopsy was performed of both masses, showing multifocal grade III invasive ductal carcinoma. The original calcifications referred for biopsy proved to be high nuclear grade DCIS. (*Courtesy of* Wendie A. Berg, MD, PhD, Lutherville, MD.)

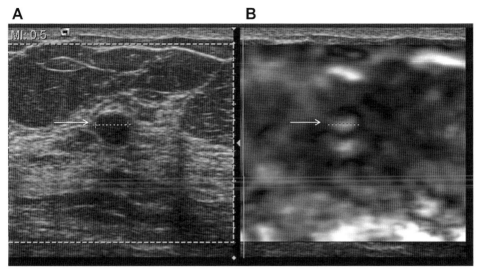

Fig. 31. A 52-year-old woman underwent screening ultrasonography that showed an incidental circumscribed oval mass with uniform low-level echoes on (*A*) gray-scale image (*arrow*) compatible with either complicated cyst or solid mass. (*B*) Elastogram (Antarres, Siemens-Acuson, Mountain View, CA, USA) shows the lesion to have a bull's-eye appearance, being centrally white and peripherally dark (*arrow*), that is typical of a cyst (in this case, a complicated cyst with debris). The lesion measured the same diameter on both images (*dotted lines*). Stiff lesions, including many cancers, tend to appear larger on elastography. (*Courtesy of* Wendie A. Berg, MD, PhD, Lutherville, MD.)

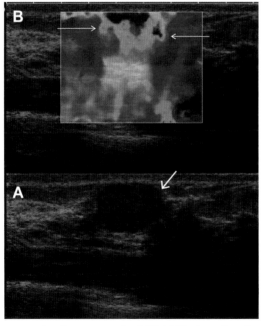

Fig. 32. (*A*) On conventional gray-scale ultrasonography (L15-4 MHz transducer), a mass (*arrow*) is noted which appears mostly circumscribed with posterior enhancement and could be mistaken for a complicated cyst. (*B*) Shear-wave elastography, in which low-frequency shear waves are induced in the tissue, shows the lesion to be hard (as evidenced by the orange and red overlay, *arrows*) compared with the softer (*blue*) surrounding tissue, suggesting malignancy. This proved to be a fibroadenoma. (*Courtesy of* Dr Valerie Juhan, MD, Hospital La Timone, Marseille, France, via Super Sonic Imagine, Aix, Provence, France; with permission.)

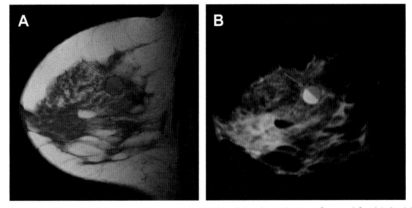

Fig. 33. A 48-year-old woman with an oval mass on (A) radial (L15-4 MHz transducer) ultrasonography. The margins are mostly circumscribed, and there is a question of a fluid-debris level (*arrow*), suggesting a complicated cyst. (B) On a shear-wave elastogram, the lesion appears irregular (*short solid arrow*) and portions are stiff (*red*). Biopsy showed grade III IDC. (*Courtesy of* Dr Valerie Juhan, Hospital La Timone, Marseille, France, via SuperSonic Imagine.)

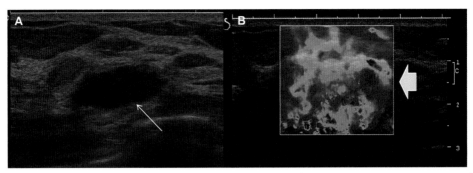

Fig. 34. On sagittal (A) T1- and (B) inversion-recovery weighted MR imaging performed for high-risk screening in a 47-year-old woman with a personal history of contralateral cancer, a smooth round mass with fluid-fluid level is seen (*arrows*), which is typical of a benign complicated cyst with debris. The more posterior component has a higher protein content than the anterior fluid. (*Courtesy of* Wendie A. Berg, MD, PhD, Lutherville, MD.)

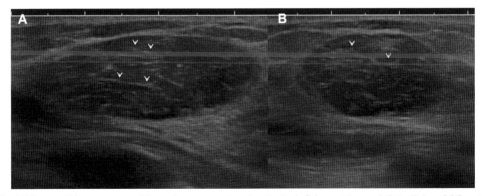

Fig. 35. A 30-year-old woman was 24 weeks pregnant and noted a left breast lump. (A) Radial and (B) antiradial ultrasonographic images show a circumscribed oval mass isoechoic to fat with internal echogenic septations (*arrowheads*). Biopsy showed lactating adenoma. (*Courtesy of* Dr Ellen Mendelson, Feinberg School of Medicine, Northwestern University, Chicago, IL, via SuperSonic Imagine.)

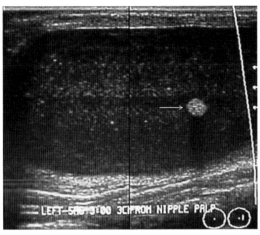

Fig. 36. A 18-year-old pregnant woman noted a palpable mass in her left breast. On targeted ultrasonography, a circumscribed mass with low-level internal echoes and posterior enhancement was noted, as well as a focal echogenic area representing a fat plug (*arrow*) in this galactocele, which was aspirated to resolution. (*Courtesy of* Wendie A. Berg, MD, PhD, Lutherville, MD.)

Imaging Findings

Mammographically, clustered microcysts manifest as a microlobulated or oval mass with circumscribed or partially obscured margins of equal or low density when compared with the surrounding parenchyma (**Fig. 47**). Milk of calcium can be seen (**Fig. 48**).

Sonographically, a circumscribed, microlobulated or oval mass is seen, composed of multiple small adjacent cysts separated by thin (<0.5 mm) septa (see **Figs. 43–48; Fig. 49**). The septations represent the equivalent of 2 acini walls lying back to back (ie, epithelial and myoepithelial layers of each acinus). Mean size is 8 mm with a range from 5 to 30 mm, with individual microcysts ranging from 1 to 7 mm.[35] Posterior enhancement can be seen. When lined by apocrine metaplastic epithelia, the internal septi may be fuzzy (see **Figs. 43** and **44**), although the outer margin

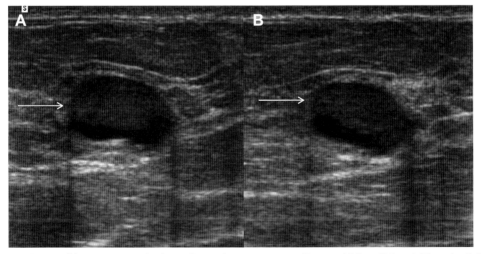

Fig. 37. A 36-year-old woman noted a lump 6 months post partum. Targeted (*A*) radial and (*B*) antiradial ultrasonography demonstrate nondependent fat-containing echogenic debris (*arrows*) with fluid-debris level, typical of benign galactocele. (*Courtesy of* Wendie A. Berg, MD, PhD, Lutherville, MD.)

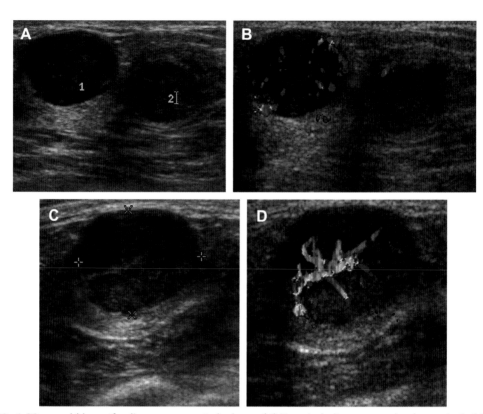

Fig. 38. A 36-year-old breastfeeding woman noted a lump. (*A*) Targeted ultrasonography demonstrated 2 adjacent hypoechoic masses (labeled 1 and 2). Mass 1 appears mostly circumscribed but has internal vascularity on (*B*) color Doppler. The suspicious nature of these findings was not initially recognized, and the patient was recommended for a 3-month follow-up ultrasonography. (*C*) On follow-up ultrasonography, both masses had enlarged, and (*D*) mass 1 was shown to be even more vascular on color Doppler. Ultrasound-guided core biopsy showed grade III IDC from both masses. (*Courtesy of* Wendie A. Berg, MD, PhD, Lutherville, MD.)

appears circumscribed. When associated with milk of calcium, dependent echogenic material can be seen (see **Fig. 48**). Individual microcysts can be complicated with fluid-debris levels or low-level echoes (see **Fig. 44**). The latter may be difficult to differentiate from a solid component. Associated simple and complicated cysts can be present. Spatial compounding may better depict the internal septa. Harmonics may help to prove individual microcysts are truly anechoic. With color Doppler, no flow is present.

On T1-weighted MR images, clustered microcysts appear as oval or microlobulated masses that are iso- or hypointense to the parenchyma. The fluid components within clustered microcysts appear bright on T2W images (**Fig. 50**). Apocrine metaplastic change can enhance, although the cystic components do not.

Differential Diagnosis

Clustered microcysts are typically caused by fibrocystic change and can have milk of calcium. Individual acini can have apocrine metaplasia. Multiple, adjacent, tiny, simple cysts can mimic clustered microcysts.

Apparent solid components in individual microcysts are most often debris, that is, complicated microcysts (see **Fig. 44**). Papillary apocrine metaplasia is a high-risk lesion and is more likely to have solid components. Of greater concern, complex cystic and solid masses, when small, can mimic benign clustered microcysts (**Figs. 51** and **52**), but complex masses are suspicious for malignancy as discussed later.

Small microlobulated, predominantly solid, masses such as fibroadenomata, papillomas,

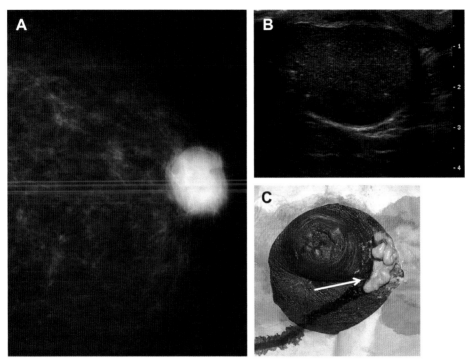

Fig. 39. A 43-year-old woman had a history of recurrent subareolar abscesses in the left breast. (A) CC mammogram shows a dense oval mass in the subareolar region. (B) Transverse ultrasonography shows a circumscribed oval mass with posterior enhancement at the site of a mammographic and palpable tender mass. Sonographically this mass has the appearance of a complicated cyst with debris. (C) On incision for ultrasound-guided aspiration, pus spontaneously drained from the mass (arrow). (Courtesy of Wendie A. Berg, MD, PhD, Lutherville, MD.)

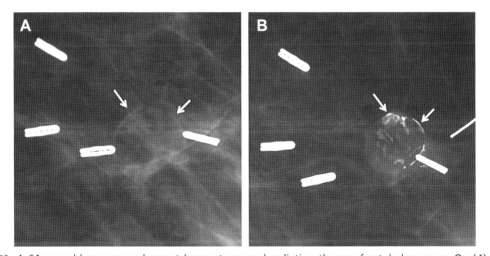

Fig. 40. A 64-year-old woman underwent lumpectomy and radiation therapy for tubular cancer. On (A) MLO mammography 18 months after surgery, a circumscribed lucent mass is noted at the lumpectomy site, which is compatible with an oil cyst (arrows). On (B) follow-up MLO mammography 6 months later, the oil cyst is slightly smaller and has developed peripheral rim calcification (arrows). (Courtesy of Wendie A. Berg, MD, PhD, Lutherville, MD.)

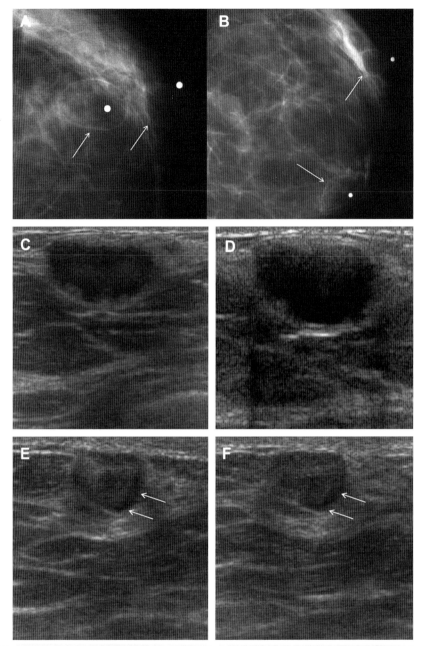

Fig. 41. A 37-year-old woman is 18 months postreduction mammoplasty and noted 2 palpable lumps (marked with radiopaque markers). On close-up (A) CC and (B) MLO mammograms, the masses are shown to be circumscribed and lucent, typical of benign oil cysts (*arrows*). Ultrasonography was nonetheless performed because of other abnormalities. (C) Transverse and sagittal ultrasonographic images of the mass in the 6-o'clock position show a nearly anechoic mass with thick nodular wall and no posterior features. Without the mammogram, the sonographic appearance would be indeterminate. (E) Radial and (F) antiradial ultrasonographic images of the oil cyst at 12-o'clock position show it to be mostly (but not completely) circumscribed, nearly isoechoic to surrounding fat, and to contain a thin eccentric rim of fluid (*arrows*). (*Courtesy of* Wendie A. Berg, MD, PhD, Lutherville, MD.)

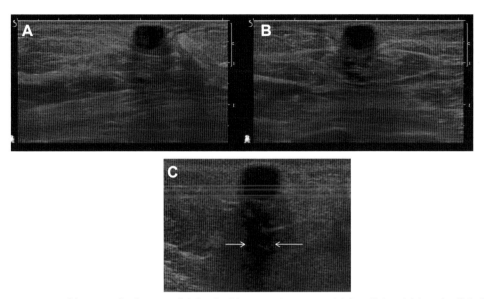

Fig. 42. A 72-year-old woman had a superficial palpable mass. On targeted (*A*) radial and (*B*) antiradial ultraso-nography, the mass appeared circumscribed but produced minimal low-level echoes. Posterior shadowing (*arrows*) was evident in (*C*) fundamental ultrasonographic image without spatial compounding. These features are fundamentally indeterminant on ultrasonography but can be seen with oil cysts, as in this case, which was aspirated, showing red oily fluid. (*Courtesy of* Dr Valerie Juhan, Hospital La Timone, Marseille, France, via Super-Sonic Imagine.)

phyllodes tumor (**Fig. 53**), DCIS, IDC, infiltrating lobular carcinomas, lactating adenomas, and tubular adenomas, rarely can be difficult to distin-guish from clustered microcysts.

Management

When the typical sonographic appearance is seen, clustered microcysts can be dismissed as benign, BI-RADS 2. When small or deep and difficult to

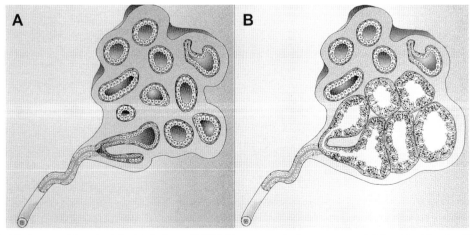

Fig. 43. (*A*) A normal terminal duct lobular unit (TDLU) composed of numerous acini lined by bland epithelium. (*B*) A group of acini are cystically dilated with tall cuboidal epithelium: ie, apocrine metaplasia. When imaged with ultrasonography, the TDLU in *B* is seen as clustered microcysts. (*Reprinted from* Warner JK, Kumar D, Berg WA. Apocrine metaplasia: mammographic and sonographic appearances. AJR Am J Roentgenol 1998;170:1375–9; with permission.)

Apocrine Metaplasia

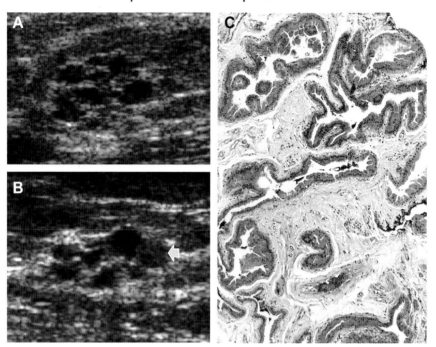

Fig. 44. (A) Radial and (B) antiradial ultrasonographic (10 MHz linear array transducer) images of an incidental mass on baseline screening mammography in a 95-year-old woman show typical appearance of clustered microcysts, one of which appears to contain debris (arrow). (C) Low-power (10× magnification) view of hematoxylin-eosin staining of 14-gauge core biopsy shows distended acini with tall, cuboidal, apocrine metaplastic epithelium. (Reprinted from Warner JK, Kumar D, Berg WA. Apocrine metaplasia: mammographic and sonographic appearances. AJR Am J Roentgenol 1998;170:1375–9; with permission.)

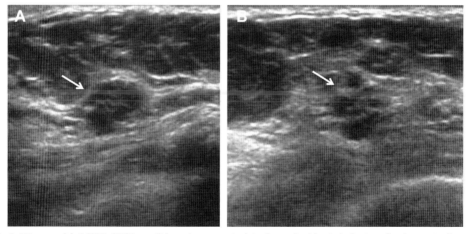

Fig. 45. A 70-year-old ACRIN 6666 participant was noted to have incidental clustered microcysts (arrows) on screening (A) radial and (B) antiradial ultrasonographic images. Ultrasound-guided core biopsy was performed because of diagnostic uncertainty and it showed fibrocystic changes, apocrine metaplasia, cyst wall inflammation, and periductal fibrosis. (Courtesy of Wendie A. Berg, MD, PhD, Lutherville, MD.)

Table 5
Summary of outcomes of lesions described sonographically as clustered microcysts

Study, Year	Number	Number of Lesions Biopsied	Follow-up Details	Number Malignant	Results of Biopsies
Berg,[19] 2003	16	16	After biopsy, 9 resolved, 2 decreased, 2 stable, 2 NA, 1 rebiopsied was benign	0	7 AM, 6 FCC, 2 cysts, 1 FA
Berg,[35] 2005	79, only 66 new[a]	13[a]	≥2-y follow-up on 66 lesions: 35 (53%) stable, 15 (23%) resolved, 12 (18%) decreased, 4 (6%) initially increased then were stable or decreased	0	5 AM, 5 FCC, 2 cysts, 1 FA[a]
Chang et al,[21] 2007	15	10 aspirated, 4 core biopsied, 1 excised	Follow-up of some lesions, details not clear	0	15 cysts or FCC
Daly et al,[22] 2008	15	218 aspirated, 32 biopsied[b]	All followed, details not specified	0	See Table 1
Total	112[a]			0	

Abbreviations: AM, apocrine metaplasia; FA, fibroadenoma; FCC, fibrocystic changes; NA, not available.
[a] All 13 biopsied lesions in the study by Berg, 2005[35] overlap with the 16 lesions reported in the study by Berg et al, 2003[19] and are thereby excluded from the total of 79 lesions in the study by Berg, 2005,[35] that is, only the 66 lesions which were followed (not biopsied) in the study by Berg, 2005[35] are new and therefore listed in the overall total.
[b] Includes women with lesions prospectively classified as either clustered microcysts or complicated cysts; mean size 13 mm.

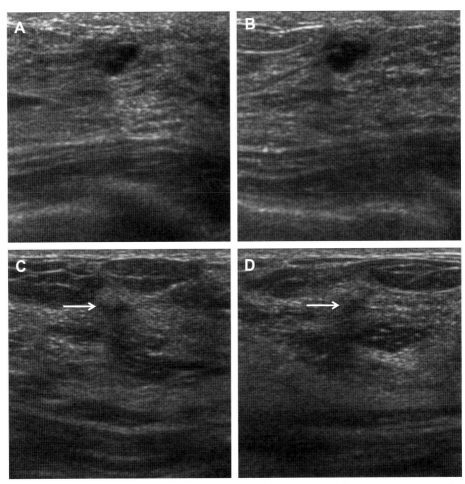

Fig. 46. A 42-year-old ACRIN 6666 participant was noted to have a mass attributed to clustered microcysts on screening ultrasonography (*A*, radial and *B*, antiradial images). At screening ultrasonography 12 months later, ultrasonography of the same area demonstrated a subtle irregular isoechoic mass (*arrows*) on (*C*) radial and (*D*) antiradial images. It seems that the original clustered microcysts resolved and a new lesion has formed. Biopsy showed a 4-mm invasive lobular carcinoma. (*Courtesy of* Wendie A. Berg, MD, PhD, Lutherville, MD.)

adequately characterize, a probably benign assessment, BI-RADS 3, with 6-, 12-, and 24-month follow-up may be appropriate, using the imaging modality on which the lesion is best seen. Greater caution is appropriate with new clustered microcysts in a postmenopausal woman, particularly in the absence of hormone replacement therapy; with a typical appearance, a BI-RADS 3 assessment can be used in this setting. If the margins are not circumscribed, or if there are other suspicious features, a BI-RADS 4 assessment and biopsy may be appropriate.

Debris within microcysts can mimic a solid component. Provided there is no dominant solid component, and margins appear circumscribed, surveillance is reasonable. Biopsy should be performed (with BI-RADS 4 assessment) if the overall appearance is that of a complex cystic and solid mass (see **Fig. 51**), rapid growth has occurred (see **Figs. 51** and **52**), or any suspicious findings are present clinically or on any imaging (see **Fig. 53**).

COMPLEX CYSTIC AND SOLID MASSES

Complex cystic and solid masses are those with solid components such as a thick wall ($\geq$0.5 mm), thick septations ($\geq$0.5 mm), an intracystic mass,

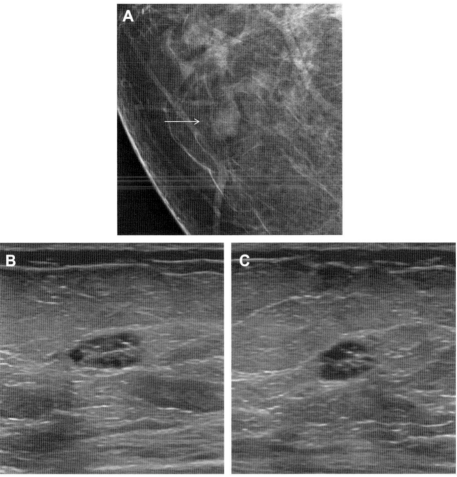

Fig. 47. A 59-year-old woman who used hormone replacement therapy had a PCPO low-density mass (*arrow*) in the inner right breast, as seen on (*A*) spot compression mammographic image. (*B*) Radial and (*C*) antiradial targeted ultrasonography (13 MHz linear array transducer) demonstrates an oval circumscribed mass composed of microscopic cysts, that is, clustered microcysts. The mass has been stable for 4 years. (*Courtesy of* Wendie A. Berg, MD, PhD, Lutherville, MD.)

or solid masses with cystic areas. Such masses are uncommon but are suspicious for malignancy, BI-RADS 4, and merit biopsy. When malignant, the cystic portion can be due to areas of necrosis within a high-grade malignancy. As mentioned earlier, invasive cancers can mimic cysts or complicated cysts (see **Figs. 7** and **30**), although often slightly indistinct or angular margins or thickened walls are present (see **Figs. 20** and **21**; **Fig. 54**).[15] High-grade cancers are typically rapidly enlarging and often palpable. With the high prevalence of benign cystic lesions, it can be especially difficult to recognize the few malignancies with such presentation, when they are nonpalpable incidental findings on imaging. Papillary DCIS can present as an intraductal or intracystic mass (see **Figs. 27** and **28**); it is difficult on imaging to exclude focal invasion.

Across prior series, 97 (36%) of 270 complex cystic and solid lesions proved malignant (**Table 6**). In the ACRIN 6666 protocol, 19 (0.7%) of 2659 participants had such lesions on the initial screening, as did 42 (1.6%) of 2662 participants over the 3-year protocol, with 45 such lesions

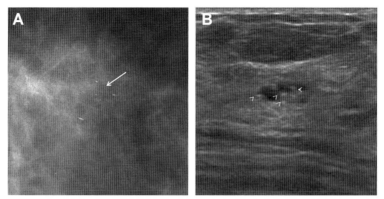

Fig. 48. A 62-year-old woman was noted to have loosely grouped punctate calcifications on (*A*) mediolateral magnification mammogram (*arrow*). The calcifications were shown to be within clustered microcysts on (*B*) targeted ultrasonography (*arrowheads*). (*Courtesy of* Wendie A. Berg, MD, PhD, Lutherville, MD.)

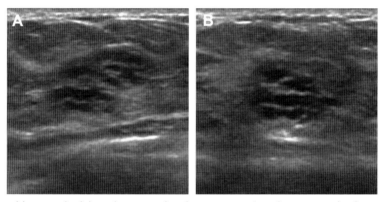

Fig. 49. A 49-year-old woman had dense breasts and underwent screening ultrasonography demonstrating multiple bilateral simple and complicated cysts as well as this lesion of clustered microcysts on (*A*) transverse and (*B*) sagittal ultrasonographic images. Within 2 years, this mass had resolved on ultrasonography, and other clustered microcysts developed elsewhere over subsequent screening ultrasonographic examinations. (*Courtesy of* Wendie A. Berg, MD, PhD, Lutherville, MD.)

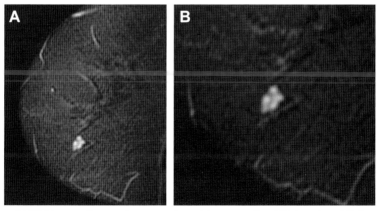

Fig. 50. A 54-year-old BRCA mutation carrier was referred for screening MR imaging. (*A*) On sagittal inversion recovery (STIR) MR imaging, hyperintense fluid-filled clustered microcysts with hypointense thin internal septations were incidentally noted. (*B*) Close-up. No enhancement was noted after contrast injection. (*Courtesy of* Wendie A. Berg, MD, PhD, Lutherville, MD.)

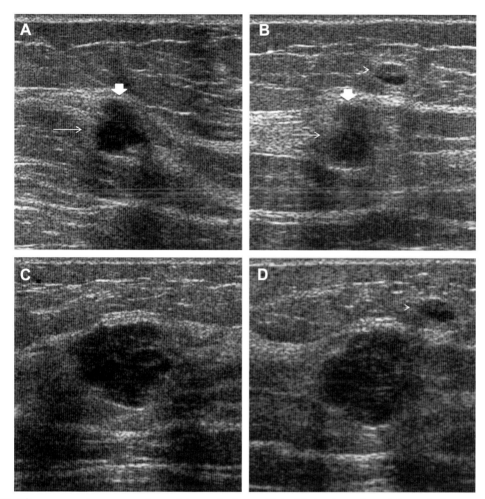

Fig. 51. Ultrasonography was performed to evaluate multiple bilateral small nodules noted on screening mammography in a 58-year-old woman. Multiple cysts were noted. One nodule (A, radial and B, antiradial ultrasonography, *thin arrows*) was thought to be clustered microcysts but was recommended for a 6-month follow-up ultrasonography. An incidental adjacent complicated cyst with fluid-debris level was noted (*arrowhead*). At 6-month follow-up (C, radial and D, antiradial ultrasonography), the mass had enlarged. Biopsy was performed showing a 2-cm grade III IDC. The adjacent complicated cyst was stable (*arrowhead*). In retrospect, the mass is indistinctly marginated with probable solid component on the initial ultrasonographic images (A, B, short fat arrows). (*Courtesy of* Wendie A. Berg, MD, PhD, Lutherville, MD.)

initially so classified, and no malignancies (see **Table 4**). These lesions were retrospectively reviewed. Only 20 (44%) of the 45 lesions were actually complex cystic lesions: 7 intracystic masses, 5 thick-walled cystic lesions, 3 mixed cystic and solid masses, 3 hypoechoic masses with tiny cystic areas, 1 intraductal mass, and 1 postsurgical collection. The other 25 were not complex cystic lesions: 10 complicated cysts (including 4 with fluid-debris levels), 4 clustered microcysts, 4 simple cysts with a single thin septation (see **Figs. 10** and **13**), 3 groups of simple cysts with intervening normal tissue, 2 simple cysts, and 1 each microlobulated anechoic mass and indistinctly marginated anechoic mass.

Of the 2662 participants, 35 (1.2%) had masses described as hypoechoic with few tiny cystic areas (ie, predominantly solid with cystic components), and none of the 35 such lesions initially so classified proved malignant, although 1 lesion initially

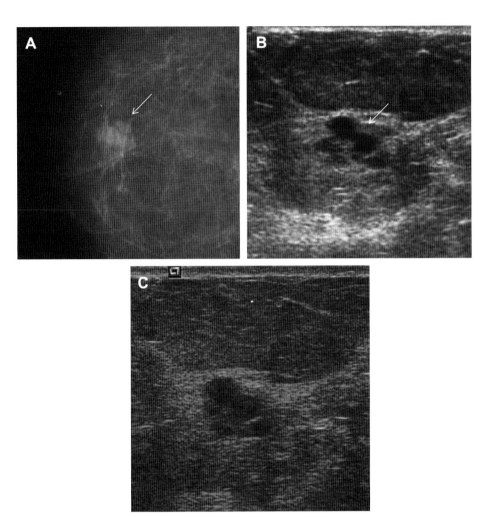

Fig. 52. A 78-year-old woman was noted to have a new mass on screening mammography, as seen on (*A*) CC mammogram (*arrow*). (*B*) Targeted ultrasonography demonstrated what appeared to be clustered microcysts (*arrow*). The patient was not on hormonal therapy. Short-interval follow-up was recommended. At (*C*) 6-month follow-up ultrasonography, the mass seemed to have thick septations and indistinct margins. Biopsy was recommended, showing grade III IDC with associated high nuclear grade DCIS. (*Courtesy of* Wendie A. Berg, MD, PhD, Lutherville, MD.)

appearing as clustered microcysts was later described as hypoechoic with few tiny cystic areas and proved malignant (see **Fig. 46**).

Imaging Findings

Mammographically, such lesions may have additional suspicious features such as indistinct margins, higher density than surrounding parenchyma, and associated suspicious calcifications.

Amorphous calcifications can be seen in papillary lesions.

Complex cystic and solid masses are defined by their sonographic appearance. Lesions included in this category may have any or all of the following: thick wall ($\geq$0.5 mm), thick internal septations, intracystic mass, and both solid and cystic components. Typically, posterior enhancement is seen because of the cystic portion of the mass. Rarely, intracystic hemorrhage can produce a fluid-debris

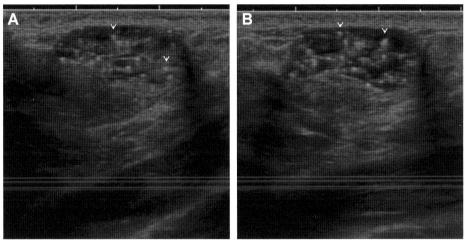

Fig. 53. A 31-year-old woman had a mass in the right breast. On (*A*) radial and (*B*) antiradial ultrasonography, the mass appeared complex, cystic, and solid with many tiny cystic areas and numerous echogenic microcalcifications (*arrowheads*). Excision showed benign phyllodes tumor. (*Courtesy of* Dr Valérie Juhan, La Timone University Hospital, Marseille, France, via SuperSonic Imagine.)

level and obscure the underlying malignancy or papilloma (see **Figs. 27** and **28**). It can be difficult to distinguish intracystic from intraductal masses, although the latter are typically more tubular (see **Fig. 17**). As stated, malignant complex cystic and solid masses may show angular, indistinct, or microlobulated margins (see **Figs. 7, 20, 21, 51,** and **54**) or thick walls (**Fig. 55**). Low-grade malignancies are more likely to have spiculated margins than high-grade cancers[15]; similarly, necrosis is uncommon with low-grade malignancies. As such, malignant complex cystic and solid lesions are most often either high-grade invasive cancers or intracystic papillary DCIS. Scars and postoperative collections should be seen to connect to the overlying skin incision (**Figs. 56** and **57**).

Most suspicious lesions in this category show enhancement of the solid portions of the lesion on MR imaging, with the cystic portion following fluid signal characteristics. Slow, persistent enhancement of a smooth wall around, what is otherwise, a cyst suggests a ruptured cyst (**Fig. 58**), whereas malignancy often shows rapid, intense, plateau, or washout enhancement and the wall tends to be nodular, indistinct, and/or

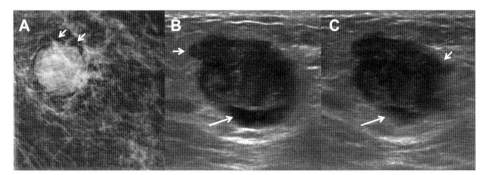

Fig. 54. A 74-year-old woman noted a lump in her left breast. (*A*) Spot compression mammogram demonstrated a mostly circumscribed dense mass. A portion of the margin appears lobulated (*short arrows*). Targeted (*B*) radial and (*C*) antiradial ultrasonography demonstrated a complex mostly solid mass with eccentric cystic area (*arrows*). The margins are focally angular (*short arrows*). Ultrasound-guided biopsy showed grade III IDC. (*Courtesy of* Wendie A. Berg, MD, PhD, Lutherville, MD.)

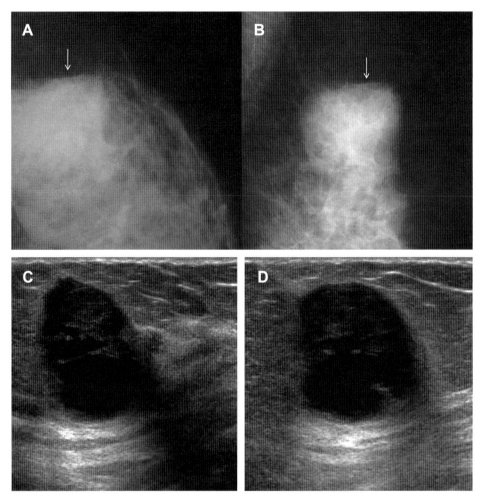

Fig. 55. A 43-year-old woman felt a lump, which corresponded to a dense, slightly indistinctly marginated mass on spot compression (A) XCCL and (B) MLO mammograms (arrows). Targeted (C) sagittal and (D) transverse ultrasonography (L17-5 MHz transducer) showed a complex cystic and solid mass. The mass was found to have internal vascularity on (E) sagittal and (F) transverse power Doppler ultrasonographic images. Repeat (G) radial and (H) transverse ultrasonography at the time of biopsy 2 weeks later (L12-5 MHz transducer) showed the mass to have thick walls. Ultrasound-guided 14-gauge core biopsy showed grade III IDC. (*Courtesy of* Wendie A. Berg, MD, PhD, Lutherville, MD.)

irregular (**Fig. 59**). Hematomas have a characteristic signal on MR imaging (**Fig. 60**).

Differential Diagnosis

Thick-walled cystic lesions with or without thick internal septations

Benign causes of thick-walled cystic lesions include ruptured/inflamed cysts (see **Fig. 58**; **Figs. 61** and **62**) and fibrocystic change, especially with apocrine metaplasia. Abscesses, fat necrosis, and seromas and hematomas can present as thick-walled cystic lesions but they usually show surrounding edema and history and clinical findings are usually exculpatory.

The concern with a thick-walled cystic lesion is that it could represent a rapidly growing invasive carcinoma, which is most often a poorly differentiated (grade III) IDC NOS (see **Fig. 55**). Medullary carcinoma can also have this appearance.[19]

Intracystic masses

Tumefactive debris in benign complicated cysts can mimic an intracystic mass (see **Figs. 61** and **62**) and usually requires aspiration for diagnosis. Papillary lesions, including benign and atypical papillomas and papillary DCIS with or without invasion, are the most common cause of intracystic masses (see **Figs. 27** and **28**; **Figs. 63** and **64**),

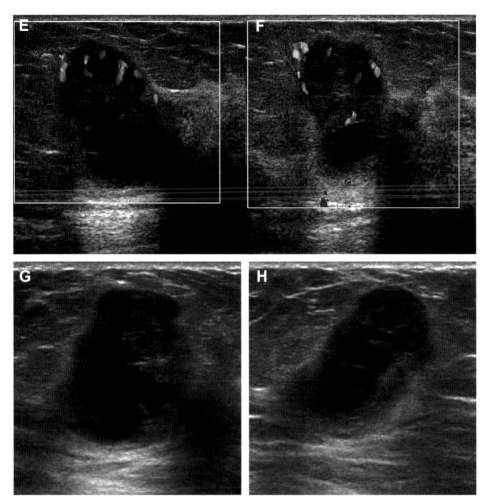

Fig. 55. (*continued*)

with an age range of 40s to 50s for papillomas and a mean age of 63 to 67 years for papillary carcinomas. Intracystic papillary carcinoma (papillary DCIS) is uncommon, representing 0.6% to 0.8% of all breast cancers.[19,36] Doppler imaging may demonstrate a vascular stalk in benign and malignant papillary lesions. Presentation depends on cause and ranges from an asymptomatic to palpable, tender or nontender mass, with or without spontaneous clear and/or bloody nipple discharge. From 22% to 34% of papillary carcinomas produce nipple discharge. Mucinous (colloid) carcinoma rarely presents as a nearly anechoic mass or an intracystic mass (**Fig. 65**).

Mixed cystic and solid lesions

Complex fibroadenomata are those that have superimposed fibrocystic change in the glandular elements (**Fig. 66**). Cystic foci were reported in 3% of fibroadenomata in one series.[19] Lactational change can also produce cystic areas within fibroadenomata (also known as lactating adenoma). Phyllodes tumors often have cystic spaces (see **Figs. 6** and **53**), as reported in 7 (23%) of 30 such tumors in the series by Liberman and colleagues,[37] and may be more common with malignant phyllodes tumors (see **Fig. 59**). Intracystic masses can be primarily solid with eccentric cystic areas: papillary lesions can

Table 6
Summary of outcomes of sonographically complex cystic lesions[a]

Type of Lesion Author, Year	Number	Number Malignant (%)	Details of Malignancies	Details of Benignity
Intracystic Masses				
Omori et al,[46] 1993	21	10 (42)	Not detailed	6 FCC, 3 papillomas, 2 abscesses
Berg et al,[19] 2003	18	4 (22)	2 DCIS, 1 IDC, 1 IDC+DCIS	5 papillomas, 3 FCC, 2 abscesses, 1 each galactocele, cyst, AM, and ruptured cyst
Tea et al,[47] 2009[b]	19	4 (21)	Not detailed[b]	
Total of this subgroup	58	18 (31)		
Thick Walls with or without Thick Septations				
Berg et al,[19] 2003	23	7 (30)	6 IDC, 1 IDC+DCIS	7 abscesses, 4 papillomas, 3 FCC, 3 cysts, 2 mucocelelike tumors, 1 fibroadenoma
Chang et al,[21] 2007[c]	27	7 (26)	5 high-grade IDC (1 medullary), 2 papillary carcinomas	
Tea et al,[47] 2009[b]	36[b]	11 (31)[b]	Not specifically detailed[b]	
Total of this subgroup	86	25 (29)		
Complex Cystic and Solid Masses				
Omori et al,[46] 1993	35	14 (40)	Not detailed	12 FCC, 3 FA, 2 papillomas, 2 abscesses, 1 ruptured epidermal inclusion cyst, 1 hemangioma
Berg et al,[19] 2003	38	7 (18)	2 IDC, 2 IDC+DCIS, 1 each DCIS, ILC, and IDC+ILC+DCIS	14 FCC, 11 FA, 2 AM, 1 each cyst, abscess, fat necrosis, and lactating adenoma
Chang et al,[21] 2007	53	33 (62)	19 IDC, 5 malignant phyllodes, 4 metaplastic carcinoma, 2 DCIS, 2 mucinous carcinoma, 1 papillary carcinoma	8 FA, 7 FCC, 2 abscesses, 2 papillomas, 1 phyllodes tumor
Total of this subgroup	126	54 (43)		
Overall Total	**270**	**97 (36)**		

Abbreviations: AM, apocrine metaplasia; FA, fibroadenoma; FCC, fibrocystic change; ILC, invasive lobular carcinoma.

[a] All such lesions were biopsied in the reported series.

[b] In the report by Tea et al,[47] masses with an intracystic solid mass may overlap with the group with wall thickness and/or septation. For wall thickness, 11 (31%) of 36 lesions were malignant compared with 7 (9.7%) of 72 lesions with septation not otherwise detailed and with some overlap of these categories not detailed: only wall-thickness group is included herein. Overall, 21 malignancies were identified among 151 complex cystic and solid masses, of which 8 (38%) were invasive, including 6 IDC, 1 ILC, and 1 invasive papillary carcinoma.

[c] Includes lesions with mural masses (ie, intracystic masses).

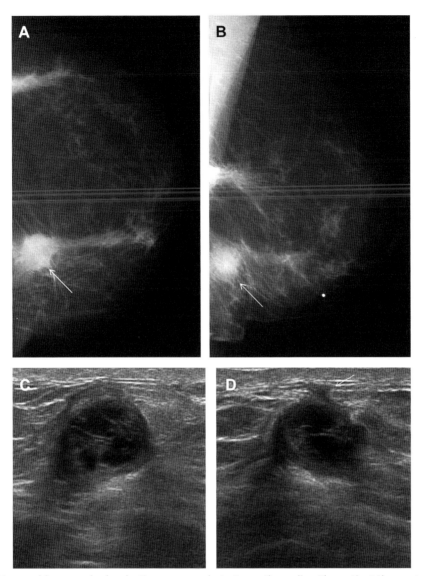

Fig. 56. A 55-year-old woman had reduction mammoplasty 3 months earlier. The patient then noted a lump in the lower inner left breast. The lump corresponded to a dense irregular mass on (A) CC and (B) MLO mammograms (arrows). (C) Radial and (D) antiradial targeted ultrasonography demonstrate a thick-walled complex cystic mass with thick internal septations, compatible with postoperative seroma or hematoma. Track to overlying skin incision was evident (arrow). The mass decreased on a 6-month follow-up. (Courtesy of Wendie A. Berg, MD, PhD, Lutherville, MD.)

appear mostly solid (Fig. 67) or entirely solid and can have calcifications, which are usually punctate or amorphous. High-grade invasive ductal carcinoma is the most common malignancy to appear predominantly solid with eccentric cystic areas, although mucinous and medullary carcinomas can have this appearance, as can metaplastic carcinomas and sarcomas (see Fig. 59) and rarely metastases such as from melanoma.

Management

Given the substantial risk of malignancy with complex cystic and solid lesions, biopsy is appropriate, with BI-RADS 4 assessment. Various approaches have been taken to biopsy such masses, including direct excision. Aspiration alone is unlikely to be diagnostic, and, as for complicated cysts, atypia can be found, prolonging the

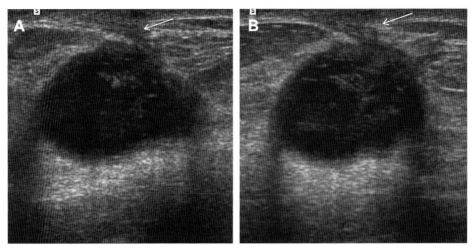

Fig. 57. A 51-year-old woman had lumpectomy for cancer 2 years earlier. The thick-walled collection with thick internal septations seen on (*A*) radial and (*B*) antiradial ultrasonographic images is consistent with postoperative seroma or hematoma. With careful technique, the track to the overlying skin incision can be demonstrated (*arrows*), thus helping to confirm this impression. (*Courtesy of* Wendie A. Berg, MD, PhD, Lutherville, MD.)

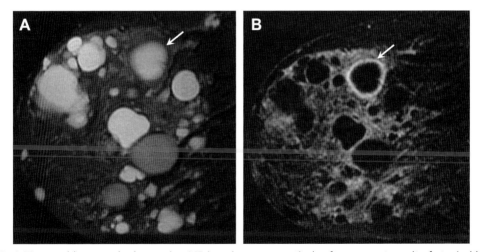

Fig. 58. A 52-year-old woman had screening MR imaging preoperatively after a recent result of atypical lobular hyperplasia on core biopsy. On (*A*) sagittal STIR image, multiple cysts are demonstrated, some of which are proteinaceous with decreased signal intensity. One cyst in the upper central breast (*arrow*) showed a slow persistent smooth thin (<2 mm) rim of enhancement on (*B*) sagittal fat-suppressed spoiled gradient echo T1-weighted image obtained 2 minutes after intravenous injection of 0.1 mmol/kg gadolinium-based contrast (*arrow*). This appearance is typical of a ruptured or inflamed cyst and does not require intervention. (*Courtesy of* Wendie A. Berg, MD, PhD, Lutherville, MD.)

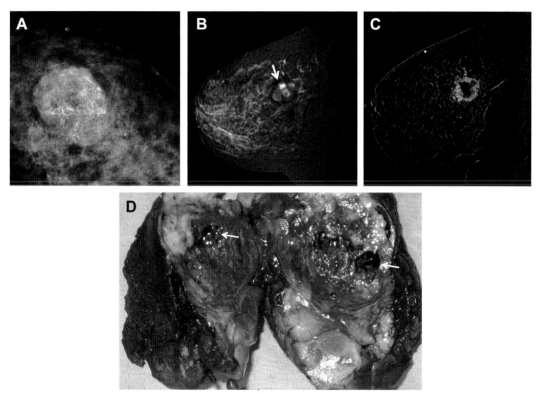

Fig. 59. A 52-year-old woman noted a lump in her left breast. On (A) spot magnification CC mammography, the mass was found to be dense, with unusual amorphous coalescent calcifications and indistinct margins. On (B) sagittal STIR MR images, the lump appeared as a partially cystic mass (arrow) which was peripherally hypointense, probably due to the calcification. On (C) 3-dimensional fat-suppressed spoiled gradient echo MR imaging 1.5 minute after injecting 0.1 mmol/kg of gadolinium-based contrast, the mass showed nodular, thick, rim enhancement with washout kinetics. Ultrasound-guided core biopsy and excision showed metaplastic sarcoma with osteochondritic calcification or ossification involving a phyllodes tumor. (D) Gross of histopathology confirms the presence of fluid-filled spaces (arrows), which surrounded leaf-like outgrowths of the phyllodes tumor. (Courtesy of Wendie A. Berg, MD, PhD, Lutherville, MD.)

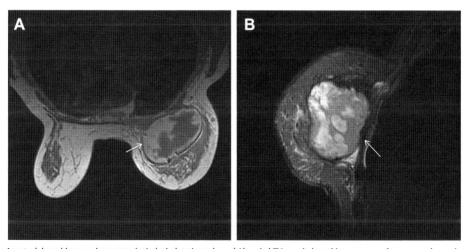

Fig. 60. Acute blood has a characteristic bright signal on (A) axial T1-weighted images and appears hypointense on (B) sagittal STIR images as in the case of a 77-year-old woman with a large hematoma (arrows) imaged 1 week after stereotactic core biopsy for DCIS. The seroma portion follows typical fluid signal characteristics (ie, hypointense on T1 and hyperintense on STIR images). (Courtesy of Wendie A. Berg, MD, PhD, Lutherville, MD.)

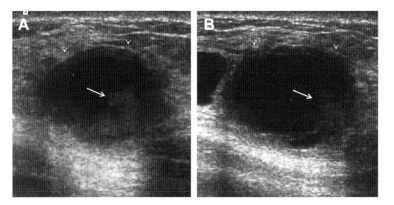

Fig. 61. A 50-year-old woman had a palpable mass in the right breast. (*A*) Transverse and (*B*) sagittal ultrasonographic images demonstrate a complex cystic and solid mass with thick wall (*arrowheads*) and possible intracystic mass (*arrows*). Ultrasound-guided 14-gauge core biopsy showed ruptured cyst with inflammation. (*Courtesy of* Wendie A. Berg, MD, PhD, Lutherville, MD.)

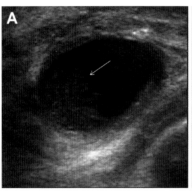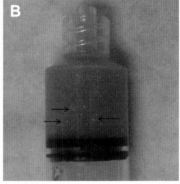

Fig. 62. A 42-year-old woman had screening MR imaging demonstrating a rim-enhancing mass. (*A*) Targeted ultrasonography showed a thick-walled cystic mass with possible intracystic mass (*arrow*). Ultrasound-guided aspiration was performed to resolution, showing (*B*) cloudy yellow fluid typical of benign cyst content and with visible cholesterol crystals (*arrows*). Because the fluid was typical of benign cyst content, it was discarded. Taking together imaging findings and results of aspiration, the mass is consistent with a ruptured or inflamed cyst. (*Courtesy of* Wendie A. Berg, MD, PhD, Lutherville, MD.)

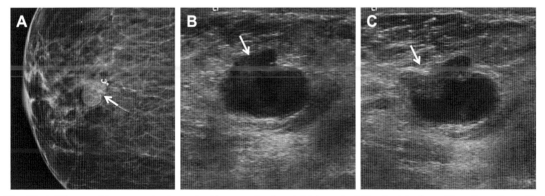

Fig. 63. A 76-year-old woman had a palpable mass in the right breast at the 9-o'clock position 1 cm from the nipple. (*A*) Spot compression CC mammogram demonstrates a circumscribed, gently lobulated mass with coarse calcification (*arrow*). Targeted (*B*) radial and (*C*) antiradial ultrasonography demonstrates an intracystic or thick-walled mass with angular margins (*arrows*). Biopsy showed DCIS in a papillary lesion. (*Courtesy of* Wendie A. Berg, MD, PhD, Lutherville, MD.)

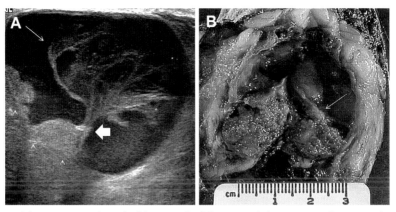

Fig. 64. A 75-year-old woman noted a palpable mass. On (A) targeted ultrasonography, a complex cystic and solid mass was noted with a frondlike appearance to the intracystic mass (*long arrow*). A vascular stalk (*short fat arrow*) was noted to the intracystic mass, and the wall was focally thickened (*arrowheads*). (B) Gross specimen demonstrates the intracystic mass (*arrow*). Histopathology showed in situ papillary carcinoma, which was focally invasive where the wall was thickened. (*Courtesy of* Dr Eva Gombos, Brigham and Women's Hospital, Boston, MA.)

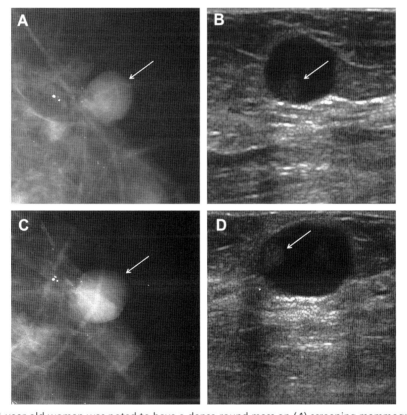

Fig. 65. An 81-year-old woman was noted to have a dense round mass on (A) screening mammography (*arrow*). (B) Targeted ultrasonography demonstrated a small intracystic mass (*arrow*). The mass was aspirated and was thought to resolve, but the mass was found to recur on 12-month follow-up (C) mammography and (D) ultrasonography (*arrows*). Biopsy was then performed, showing mucinous carcinoma (a special type of well-differentiated invasive ductal carcinoma). (*Courtesy of* Wendie A. Berg, MD, PhD, Lutherville, MD.)

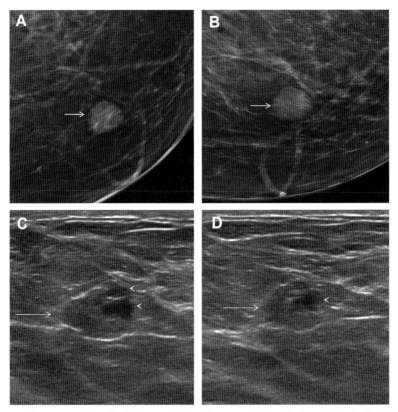

Fig. 66. A 45-year-old woman with prior history of fibroadenoma at 12-o'clock position in the left breast had an enlarging circumscribed mass in the lower inner left breast on screening (A) CC and (B) MLO (arrows). Targeted (C) radial and (D) antiradial ultrasonography demonstrated an isoechoic oval mass (arrows) with small eccentric cystic areas (arrowheads), that is, a complex cystic and solid mass. Ultrasound-guided 14-gauge core biopsy confirmed a complex fibroadenoma with usual duct hyperplasia and cystic areas. (Courtesy of Wendie A. Berg, MD, PhD, Lutherville, MD.)

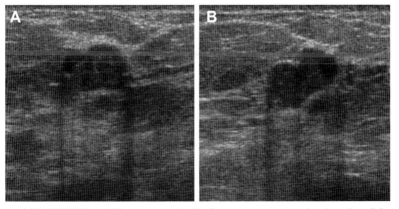

Fig. 67. A 75-year-old ACRIN 6666 participant was noted to have a complex predominantly solid mass on the third annual screening (A) radial and (B) antiradial ultrasonography. Ultrasound-guided core biopsy and excision showed benign papilloma. (Courtesy of Wendie A. Berg, MD, PhD, Lutherville, MD.)

diagnostic process (requiring rebiopsy). Core biopsy under ultrasound guidance is effective, with attention to sampling the solid components.[38] With thick-walled cystic lesions, the fluid often leaks out with the first core biopsy pass, and rarely loss of the fluid can make it difficult to see the residual lesion for additional samples. Use of coaxial technique (with a trochar) can facilitate taking additional samples. With small intracystic masses, which may become difficult to visualize once the fluid escapes, vacuum-assisted percutaneous biopsy can be helpful in assuring complete sampling. A clip should be placed whenever a lesion may be difficult to see after core biopsy or when correlation with mammographic or MR imaging findings is needed.

Careful correlation with histopathologic results is always appropriate. A result of benign papilloma on core biopsy generally merits excision because of an 8% to 14% risk of unsampled malignancy[39,40,41,42] and 17% to 22% risk of unsampled high-risk lesion,[39,40,41] with such upgrades more common with peripheral than central papillomas (near the nipple). In a 2008 abstract of 94 lesions excised after a diagnosis of benign papilloma on core biopsy, 12 (13%) were upgraded to malignancy with no significant differences in rates of upgrade to malignancy based on various factors: (a) 2 (14%) of 14 lesions biopsied with 11-gauge vacuum versus 10 (13%) of 80 biopsied with 14-gauge core, (b) 11 (14%) of 80 peripheral papillomas versus 1 (7%) of 14 central papillomas, (c) 0 of 6 incidental micropapillomas on core biopsy versus 12 (13%) of 89 targeted lesions, and (d) 11 (14%) of 81 with no residual imaging findings versus 1 (7%) of 13 with a residual lesion.[43] Any atypical core biopsy result should prompt excision because of an approximately 30% to 38% upgrade rate to malignancy at excision after a core biopsy result of atypical papilloma.[44,45]

SUMMARY

Experience from ACRIN 6666 shows that simple and complicated cysts are far more common than previously recognized, even in postmenopausal women not on hormone replacement therapy. Based on review of the literature and the results of ACRIN 6666, the vast majority of asymptomatic complicated cysts (also known as cysts with debris) and clustered microcysts can be dismissed as benign findings provided strict criteria are used; any suspicious change should prompt biopsy. Complex cystic and solid masses, with thick wall or thick septations, intracystic mass, or solid components, should prompt biopsy, with

36% of such lesions that are biopsied proving malignant. Most malignant intracystic masses are papillary DCIS. High-grade invasive ductal carcinoma can usually be distinguished from simple or complicated cysts by an indistinct margin, a thick wall, and/or solid components. The terminology for classification of cystic lesions other than simple cysts can be confusing, even among experienced radiologists. Precise use of existing and soon-to-be updated BI-RADS: ultrasonography[1] terminology for cystic lesions is encouraged both for proper management and to facilitate outcomes analysis.

ACKNOWLEDGMENTS

We thank Dr Ellen Mendelson, Feinberg School of Medicine, Northwestern University, Chicago, IL, USA for thoughtful review, and we also thank the many contributors of images detailed in the figure legends. The authors also thank the many site investigators, research associates, and participants in the ACRIN 6666 protocol.

REFERENCES

1. Mendelson EB, Baum JK, Berg WA, et al. Breast imaging reporting and data system, BI-RADS: ultrasound. 1st edition. Reston (VA): American College of Radiology; 2003.
2. Berg WA, Blume JD, Cormack JB, et al. Combined screening with ultrasound and mammography vs mammography alone in women at elevated risk of breast cancer. JAMA 2008;299(18):2151–63.
3. Available at: http://acrin.org/Portals/0/Protocols/6666/Protocol-ACRIN%206666%20Admin%20Update%2011.30.07.pdf. Accessed January 2, 2010.
4. Hilton SV, Leopold GR, Olson LK, et al. Real-time breast sonography: application in 300 consecutive patients. AJR Am J Roentgenol 1986;147(3):479–86.
5. Cyrlak D, Wong CH. Mammographic changes in postmenopausal women undergoing hormonal replacement therapy. AJR Am J Roentgenol 1993;161(6):1177–83.
6. Stomper PC, Van Voorhis BJ, Ravnikar VA, et al. Mammographic changes associated with postmenopausal hormone replacement therapy: a longitudinal study. Radiology 1990;174(2):487–90.
7. Brenner RJ, Bein ME, Sarti DA, et al. Spontaneous regression of interval benign cysts of the breast. Radiology 1994;193(2):365–8.
8. D'Orsi CJ, Bassett LW, Berg WA, et al. Breast Imaging reporting and data system, BI-RADS: mammography. 4th edition. Reston (VA): American College of Radiology; 2003.
9. Leung JW, Sickles EA. Multiple bilateral masses detected on screening mammography: assessment of

need for recall imaging. AJR Am J Roentgenol 2000; 175(1):23–9.

10. Berg WA, Blume J, Cormack JB, et al. Operator dependence of physician-performed whole breast US: lesion detection and characterization. Radiology 2006;241:355–66.

11. Itoh A, Ueno E, Tohno E, et al. Breast disease: clinical application of US elastography for diagnosis. Radiology 2006;239(2):341–50.

12. Barr RG. Real-time ultrasound elasticity of the breast: initial clinical results. Ultrasound Q 2010; 26(2):61–6.

13. Ginat DT, Destounis SV, Barr RG, et al. US elastography of breast and prostate lesions. Radiographics 2009;29(7):2007–16.

14. Hong AS, Rosen EL, Soo MS, et al. BI-RADS for sonography: positive and negative predictive values of sonographic features. AJR Am J Roentgenol 2005;184(4):1260–5.

15. Lamb PM, Perry NM, Vinnicombe SJ, et al. Correlation between ultrasound characteristics, mammographic findings and histological grade in patients with invasive ductal carcinoma of the breast. Clin Radiol 2000;55(1):40–4.

16. Bassett LW. Imaging of breast masses. Radiol Clin North Am 2000;38(4):669–91.

17. Morrogh M, Park A, Elkin EB, et al. Lessons learned from 416 cases of nipple discharge of the breast. Am J Surg 2010;200(1):73–80.

18. Leis HP Jr, Greene FL, Cammarata A, et al. Nipple discharge: surgical significance. South Med J 1988;81(1):20–6.

19. Berg W, Campassi C, Ioffe O. Cystic lesions of the breast: sonographic-pathologic correlation. Radiology 2003;227:183–91.

20. Buchberger W, DeKoekkoek-Doll P, Springer P, et al. Incidental findings on sonography of the breast: clinical significance and diagnostic workup. AJR Am J Roentgenol 1999;173:921–7.

21. Chang YW, Kwon KH, Goo DE, et al. Sonographic differentiation of benign and malignant cystic lesions of the breast. J Ultrasound Med 2007; 26(1):47–53.

22. Daly CP, Bailey JE, Klein KA, et al. Complicated breast cysts on sonography: is aspiration necessary to exclude malignancy? Acad Radiol 2008;15(5): 610–7.

23. Kolb TM, Lichy J, Newhouse JH. Occult cancer in women with dense breasts: detection with screening US– diagnostic yield and tumor characteristics. Radiology 1998;207(1):191–9.

24. Venta LA, Kim JP, Pelloski CE, et al. Management of complex breast cysts. AJR Am J Roentgenol 1999; 173(5):1331–6.

25. Gordon PB, Gagnon FA, Lanzkowsky L. Solid breast masses diagnosed as fibroadenoma at fine-needle aspiration biopsy: acceptable rates of growth at long-term follow-up. Radiology 2003; 229(1):233–8.

26. Harvey JA, Nicholson BT, Lorusso AP, et al. Short-term follow-up of palpable breast lesions with benign imaging features: evaluation of 375 lesions in 320 women. AJR Am J Roentgenol 2009;193(6): 1723–30.

27. Graf O, Helbich TH, Fuchsjaeger MH, et al. Follow-up of palpable circumscribed noncalcified solid breast masses at mammography and US: can biopsy be averted? Radiology 2004;233(3): 850–6.

28. Gizienski TA, Harvey JA, Sobel AH. Breast cyst recurrence after postaspiration injection of air. Breast J 2002;8(1):34–7.

29. Ikeda DM, Helvie MA, Adler DD, et al. The role of fine-needle aspiration and pneumocystography in the treatment of impalpable breast cysts. AJR Am J Roentgenol 1992;158(6):1239–41.

30. Ciatto S, Cariaggi P, Bulgaresi P. The value of routine cytologic examination of breast cyst fluids. Acta Cytol 1987;31(3):301–4.

31. Smith DN, Kaelin CM, Korbin CD, et al. Impalpable breast cysts: utility of cytologic examination of fluid obtained with radiologically guided aspiration. Radiology 1997;204(1):149–51.

32. Hindle WH, Arias RD, Florentine B, et al. Lack of utility in clinical practice of cytologic examination of nonbloody cyst fluid from palpable breast cysts. Am J Obstet Gynecol 2000;182(6):1300–5.

33. Mendelson EB. Evaluation of the postoperative breast. Radiol Clin North Am 1992;30(1):107–38.

34. Warner JK, Kumar D, Berg WA. Apocrine metaplasia: mammographic and sonographic appearances. AJR Am J Roentgenol 1998;170(5):1375–9.

35. Berg WA. Sonographically depicted breast clustered microcysts: is follow-up appropriate? AJR Am J Roentgenol 2005;185(4):952–9.

36. Framarino dei Malatesta ML, Piccioni MG, Felici A, et al. Intracystic carcinoma of the breast. Our experience. Eur J Gynaecol Oncol 1992;13(1 Suppl):40–4.

37. Liberman L, Bonaccio E, Hamele-Bena D, et al. Benign and malignant phyllodes tumors: mammographic and sonographic findings. Radiology 1996;198(1):121–4.

38. Doshi DJ, March DE, Crisi GM, et al. Complex cystic breast masses: diagnostic approach and imaging-pathologic correlation. Radiographics 2007; 27(Suppl 1):S53–64.

39. Jacobs TW, Connolly JL, Schnitt SJ. Nonmalignant lesions in breast core needle biopsies: to excise or not to excise? Am J Surg Pathol 2002;26(9): 1095–110.

40. Liberman L, Tornos C, Huzjan R, et al. Is surgical excision warranted after benign, concordant diagnosis of papilloma at percutaneous breast biopsy? AJR Am J Roentgenol 2006;186(5):1328–34.

41. Mercado CL, Hamele-Bena D, Oken SM, et al. Papillary lesions of the breast at percutaneous core-needle biopsy. Radiology 2006;238(3): 801–8.

42. Sakr R, Rouzier R, Salem C, et al. Risk of breast cancer associated with papilloma. Eur J Surg Oncol 2008;34(12):1304–8.

43. Sheridan TB, Berg WA, Warner JK, et al. Papillary lesions diagnosed by core needle biopsy of the breast: diagnostic pitfalls and management update. Paper presented at: USCAP 2008. Denver (CO), March 4, 2008.

44. Berg WA. Image-guided breast biopsy and management of high-risk lesions. Radiol Clin North Am 2004;42(5):935–46, vii.

45. Liberman L, Bracero N, Vuolo MA, et al. Percutaneous large-core biopsy of papillary breast lesions. AJR Am J Roentgenol 1999;172(2):331–7.

46. Omori LM, Hisa N, Ohkuma K, et al. Breast masses with mixed cystic-solid sonographic appearance. J Clin Ultrasound 1993;21(8):489–95.

47. Tea MK, Grimm C, Fink-Retter A, et al. The validity of complex breast cysts after surgery. Am J Surg 2009; 197(2):199–202.

Regional Lymph Node Staging in Breast Cancer: The Increasing Role of Imaging and Ultrasound-Guided Axillary Lymph Node Fine Needle Aspiration

Martha B. Mainiero, MD

KEYWORDS

- Breast cancer • Staging • Axilla • Ultrasound
- Fine needle aspiration • Biopsy

Axillary lymph node staging is a crucial component of breast cancer management, with the radiologist playing an increasing role. Historically, axillary lymph node staging was performed entirely through axillary lymph node dissection without using imaging or percutaneous diagnosis. However, more recently, less morbid techniques have been developed that require imaging guidance and necessitate that radiologists have an understanding of the anatomy, imaging appearance, and significance of abnormalities in the regional lymph node system of the breast. This article reviews the clinical significance and surgical staging of axillary metastatic involvement in breast cancer and then focuses on the use of axillary ultrasound and ultrasound-guided fine needle aspiration (USFNA) as a preoperative staging method. A brief discussion of internal mammary lymph node evaluation is also included.

SIGNIFICANCE AND ANATOMY OF AXILLARY LYMPH NODE METASTASIS IN BREAST CANCER

Once breast cancer is diagnosed, lymph node status is the most powerful indicator of long-term survival.[1] Although other features, such as tumor size, histologic grade, and hormone and Her2/neu receptor status, have predictive value, the status of the lymph nodes reflects the actual interaction of tumor aggressiveness and host resistance.[2] The number of lymph nodes involved, the extent of lymph node involvement within the individual nodes, and the location of involved lymph nodes also have prognostic significance. For instance, gross involvement of the lymph node by metastatic disease and extranodal extension of disease have a worse prognosis than microscopic metastatic disease. In addition, information on lymph node involvement not only is important for prognosis but also is used in treatment decision making.

The primary lymphatic drainage of the breast is to the axillary lymph nodes. Various names have been given to the groups of lymph nodes that constitute the axillary lymph node chain, although surgeons typically classify axillary nodes by their location relative to the pectoralis minor muscle. Level I nodes are lateral or inferior to the pectoralis minor, level II nodes are posterior to the pectoralis minor, and level III nodes are medial to the pectoralis minor (**Fig. 1**). Although involved level III nodes

Department of Diagnostic Imaging, Rhode Island Hospital, The Warren Alpert Medical School of Brown University, 593 Eddy Street, Providence, RI 02903, USA
E-mail address: mmainiero@lifespan.org

Radiol Clin N Am 48 (2010) 989–997
doi:10.1016/j.rcl.2010.06.010

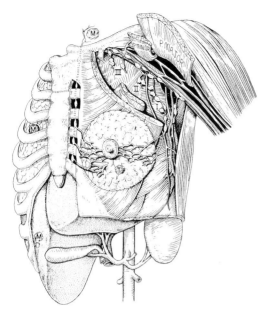

Fig. 1. Lymphatic drainage of the breast with roman numerals identifying axillary lymph node groups. Level I nodes are located lateral or inferior to the pectoralis minor, level II nodes are located deep to the muscle, and level III nodes are located medial to the muscle. M, metastatic supraclavicular node; T, primary tumor. *Reprinted from* Bland KI, Copeland EM, editors. The breast: comprehensive management of benign and malignant diseases. 4th edition. Philadelphia: Saunders Elsevier; 2009. p. 33; with permission.

are rarely present without involved level I or II nodes,[3,4] metastatic disease can "skip" to level II nodes without involving level I nodes in up to 25% of cases.[5] Most axillary metastases affect level I and II axillary lymph nodes, and contemporary axillary dissection involves removing level I and II nodes only.[6]

AXILLARY LYMPH NODE DISSECTION

Physical examination and mammography are unreliable in determining whether axillary lymph nodes are metastatic.[7,8] Axillary lymph node dissection (ALND) has been a standard part of breast cancer treatment since the advent of the radical mastectomy. Although it renders the most complete staging information and provides excellent local control of the axilla involved with metastatic disease, ALND is associated with significant morbidity, including lymphedema, decreased range of motion in the shoulder, and paresthesias. With earlier detection of breast cancer leading to fewer positive axillae, ALND has become a less-than-ideal modality for initial staging of the axilla. Sentinel lymph node biopsy

(SLNB), in which the first (sentinel) lymph node to drain the breast is identified and resected, was developed as an alternative to ALND for breast cancer in the 1990s after the technique was used successfully in melanoma.[9] SLNB is a less-invasive surgical technique, associated with less morbidity than ALND.

LYMPHOSCINTIGRAPHY

Injection of blue dye or a radioisotope into the breast maps the lymphatic drainage, and the sentinel lymph node is identified either through visual inspection, in the case of dye, or with a gamma camera or handheld gamma probe, in the case of Technetium-99m sulfur colloid injection. Although some surgeons will use blue dye alone to minimize expense, the lymphoscintigraphy procedure offers several advantages. The gamma camera's wide field of view of the entire chest allows visualization of both axillary and internal mammary nodal regions, and shows the three-dimensional distribution of lymph nodes. In addition, lymphoscintigraphy can alert the surgeon to surface contamination or dilated lymphatic channels, which may be mistaken for lymph nodes by the intraoperative handheld gamma probe.[10] Surgeons may use both dye and radiotracer to increase the success rate of finding the sentinel node.[11] Numerous technical considerations and protocols exist for injection and imaging during lymphoscintigraphy, which are reviewed elsewhere.[10]

SENTINEL LYMPH NODE BIOPSY

SLNB has become standard of care for clinicians experienced with the technique. SLNB is a technically challenging procedure, and the accuracy is related to the experience of the surgeon, both in total number and monthly number of cases performed.[12,13] In experienced hands, SLNB accurately predicts the status of the remainder of the axilla in greater than 95% of cases.[14–16] When SLNB is positive for metastatic disease, complete ALND is then performed for more detailed staging and to provide local control.

Although fewer lymph nodes are removed in SLNB than in ALND, the nodes removed are those most likely to be involved with tumor and are examined more rigorously by pathology with serial sectioning and immunohistochemistry. Removal of "hot" nodes downstream from the first sentinel node has been shown to decrease the false-negative rate of SLNB.[17–19]

The sentinel node may be examined intraoperatively with touch preparation, cytology smear, or frozen section, and an axillary dissection performed if evidence of metastatic disease is present. However, the sensitivity of these techniques is poor for micrometastases and, because of the concern about destroying tissue through intraoperative evaluation, many surgeons prefer to wait for definitive pathologic evaluation of the sentinel node and return the patient to the operating room for ALND if needed.[9]

The time-consuming, challenging nature of SLNB is a disadvantage, as is the need for a second surgery if the lymph nodes contain metastatic disease on permanent section. In addition, the procedure may be unsuccessful because of failure to visualize a sentinel node. Lack of radiotracer uptake and nonvisualization of the sentinel node may be from replacement of the node by tumor.[20] In addition, SLNB has a higher false-negative rate in patients who have undergone neoadjuvant chemotherapy.[21] Therefore, patients undergoing neoadjuvant chemotherapy often undergo SLNB before chemotherapy and will have to return to the operating room for breast surgery after chemotherapy. Given the disadvantages, an easier method that replaces SLNB is valuable.

AXILLARY ULTRASOUND

Although CT, MRI, and nuclear medicine techniques visualize the axillary lymph nodes, ultrasound is the most advantageous technique and has been the most used to characterize lymph nodes and detect axillary lymph node metastases.[7,22–25] Before SLNB, no real indication existed for routine ultrasound evaluation of the axilla for patients with breast cancer because these patients would undergo ALND for both diagnosis and treatment of metastatic disease in one operation. The advent of SLNB has resulted in the increased use of axillary ultrasound and the development of USFNA for preoperative diagnosis

of metastatic disease to minimize the number of operative procedures.[26–28] In addition, patients identified as having nodal disease preoperatively may be considered for enrollment in neoadjuvant chemotherapy protocols.[29]

A high-frequency (7.5 MHz and above) transducer provides the spatial resolution needed to identify and characterize lymph nodes adequately. The most important lymph node to at identify is the one most likely to be the sentinel node. Therefore, attention should be focused on the lower axilla near or just behind the lateral edge of the pectoralis major.[30]

Normal lymph nodes are oval in shape, typically having a long to short axis ratio of greater than 2, and have a wide echogenic fatty hilum and a thin cortex (**Fig. 2**A).[24] When normal lymph nodes are largely fatty replaced, the central echogenic hilum will actually become paradoxically hypoechoic because of the presence of relatively few vessels and mostly homogenous fat cells (see **Fig. 2**B).[31] One pitfall of axillary ultrasound is mistaking a large hypoechoic fatty hilum for a thickened hypoechoic cortex.

Size is not a useful criterion for distinguishing normal from abnormal axillary lymph nodes.[32,33] Reactive or fatty lymph nodes may be large enough to even be palpable and mistaken for metastatic disease. However, specific cortical and hilar morphologic changes seen on ultrasound have been shown to be predictive of malignancy, although different criteria have been used at different institutions to determine level of suspicion. As ultrasound of the axilla becomes more widely adopted, the criteria that are most useful in detecting metastatic disease are becoming more clearly defined.

The principal feature used in assessing axillary lymph nodes is the presence of cortical thickening, including cortical thickening that narrows or obliterates the fatty hilum.

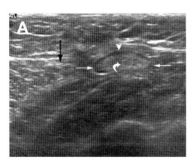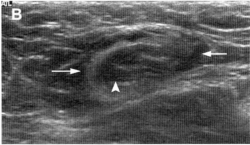

Fig. 2. Normal appearance of axillary lymph nodes on ultrasound. (*A*) This lymph node (*white arrows*), located adjacent to the pectoralis major muscle (*black arrow*) has a wide echogenic hilum (*curved arrow*) and a thin cortex (*arrowhead*). (*B*) A largely fatty-replaced lymph node (*arrows*) with a paradoxically hypoechoic hilum (*arrowhead*).

Although the normal vascular supply of a lymph node enters the hilum, the lymphatic channels enter through the cortex. When enough metastatic cells are deposited, the cortex becomes thicker. As the cortex is replaced and expanded by metastatic disease, the hilum becomes compressed and eventually absent. Therefore, the earliest changes seen on ultrasound will be focal thickening of the cortex, with the lymph node retaining a normal hilum (**Fig. 3**). Further involvement of the cortex will thicken the cortex more diffusely (**Fig. 4**). As the cortex enlarges, changes may occur in shape from outward bulging of the cortex, with the lymph node taking on a more lobulated appearance. Distortion, compression, or absence of the hilum is seen with large metastatic deposits from inward bulging of the involved cortex (**Fig. 5**). Decreased echogenicity of the cortex is also a feature of malignancy,[33] and completely replaced lymph nodes will be round and markedly hypoechoic, or even anechoic (**Fig. 6**). A round, anechoic lymph node may be mistaken for a cyst. This pitfall can be avoided by recognizing the typical lymph node location and using color Doppler to detect vascularity.

The presence of blood flow in a lymph node seen with color Doppler is not useful as a criterion to distinguish benign from malignant nodes, because both normal and abnormal nodes have hilar flow.[34,35] However, malignant lymph nodes are more likely to have nonhilar blood flow, in which the blood flow enters the cortex directly. This altered blood flow is presumably caused by engorgement of preexisting vessels as a consequence of hilar flow obstruction from metastatic disease.[36]

USFNA FOR PREOPERATIVE DIAGNOSIS OF NODAL DISEASE

Although ultrasound is sensitive for detecting metastatic disease to the axilla, overlap occurs in

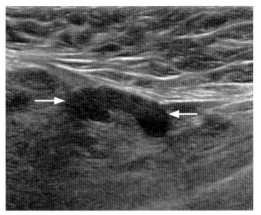

Fig. 4. Ultrasound image of a metastatic axillary lymph node (*arrows*) with diffuse cortical thickening.

the appearance of metastatic disease and normal or hyperplastic lymph nodes, limiting specificity. Adding fine needle aspiration to ultrasound allows a specific diagnosis of metastatic disease to be made that changes patient management. When metastatic disease to the axilla is diagnosed using USFNA as the initial staging procedure, the patient is spared SLNB and proceeds directly to ALND or neoadjuvant chemotherapy.[30,32,33,37–39]

The sensitivity of USFNA reported in the literature varies widely depending on patient selection criteria and the criteria for determining if a lymph node is abnormal. Reports of sensitivity range from 21% to 86%.[32,39] The wide range of sensitivities reflects the fact that USFNA is most sensitive in patients with more extensive lymph node involvement and less sensitive for the detection of small metastatic deposits (<5 mm) and micrometastases (<2 mm).[32,33] Patients with large primary tumors are more likely to have more extensive nodal disease that will alter the morphology of the lymph node and be more easily detected with

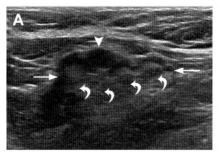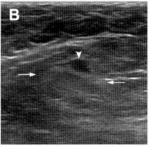

Fig. 3. Focal cortical thickening on ultrasound. (*A*) A metastatic lymph node (*arrows*) with suspicious cortical thickening (*arrowhead*). The large fatty hilum (*curved arrows*) is retained. (*B*) A metastatic lymph node (*arrows*) with one small focal area of cortical thickening (*arrowhead*).

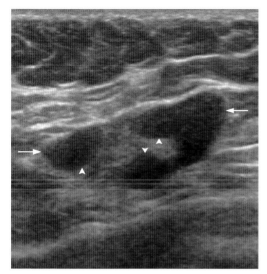

Fig. 5. Ultrasound image of a metastatic axillary lymph node (*arrows*) with distortion of the fatty hilum from focal cortical thickening in multiple areas (*arrowheads*).

ultrasound, and therefore USFNA will be more sensitive in this population. Koelliker and colleagues[33] reported a sensitivity of USFNA ranging from 56% in T1 tumors to 100% in T4 tumors. Similarly, the reported sensitivity of USFNA will vary depending on selection criteria based on the appearance of the axillary lymph nodes. When selecting only patients with abnormal-appearing lymph nodes, the sensitivity of the procedure to detect nodal disease has been in a more narrow range of 82% to 89%.[32,38,40,41] Most of the false-negative USFNA procedures in

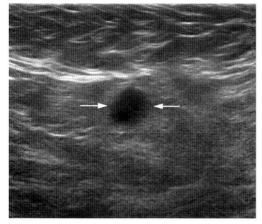

Fig. 6. Ultrasound image of a hypoechoic metastatic axillary lymph node (*arrows*) with a round shape and completely absent hilum.

this population will be in patients with metastatic deposits smaller than 5 mm and only one lymph node involved.[32] Expanding on their previous work as reported by Koelliker and colleagues,[33] in which USFNA was performed on all patients presenting for axillary ultrasound regardless of tumor size or lymph node appearance, the author's practice has been investigating the utility of USFNA in patients as a function of lymph node appearance and has found it to have a sensitivity of 11% for normal-appearing nodes, 44% for indeterminate nodes, and 93% for suspicious nodes (Martha B. Mainiero, MD, unpublished data).

Core needle biopsy (CNB) of axillary lymph nodes can be used as an alternative to fine needle aspiration.[42–46] Care must be taken to avoid the major vessels and nerves, and a biopsy device with a controllable needle action is safest, because the cutting cannula traverses tissue that has already been passed through by the needle.[45] The range of sensitivity of CNB for metastatic disease in the axilla ranges from 53% to 94%.[45,46] Unlike in the breast, in which a wide range of benign and malignant conditions require histology for diagnosis, the diagnosis of metastatic disease in the axilla can be made through identifying carcinoma cells on cytology without the need for histologic evaluation. Fine needle aspiration is less costly and less invasive than core biopsy, and core biopsy has the same problem as fine needle aspiration, with false-negatives in cases of small metastatic deposits.[42,45] In a comparison of fine needle aspiration and CNB of axillary nodes by Rao and colleagues,[40] in which the decision to perform fine needle aspiration or CNB was based on equipment availability and operator preference, the sensitivity of fine needle aspiration was 75% and the sensitivity of CNB was 82%. The author's practice concluded that given the consideration of cost, fine needle aspiration may allow equivalent sensitivity at lower cost. However, institutions without adequate cytology support or expertise may prefer to use ultrasound-guided core biopsy instead of fine needle aspiration.[45]

INDICATIONS FOR USFNA

Whether axillary ultrasound and USFNA should be performed on all patients with newly diagnosed breast cancer or only those at high risk for nodal disease is not firmly established. Because ultrasound and USFNA are not as sensitive as SLNB, patients will still need surgery when imaging or cytology results are negative. Patients who are most likely to be spared SLNB are, therefore, most likely to have a positive result on USFNA, either based on the high likelihood of having nodal disease because of characteristics of the primary tumor or because of the suspicious appearance of lymph nodes on ultrasound. Therefore, some authors suggest that the procedure can replace SLNB as the initial staging procedure in larger tumors only.[28]

In patients with smaller tumors or normal-appearing nodes, the technique will be less sensitive, but has been used to spare some patients SLNB, because USFNA is so much less time-consuming and invasive than SLNB.[33] Some authors recommend that USFNA should be part of the preoperative staging of all primary breast cancers.[37,41] The exact cutoff of what is an acceptable sensitivity to make the procedure worthwhile is still controversial and may require a cost-effective analysis.

Axillary ultrasound and USFNA are clearly indicated in patients with locally advanced disease. In a series of 27 axillae in 26 patients with a median primary tumor size of 4 cm, Oruwari and colleagues[47] reported a sensitivity of 100% and concluded that the technique is particularly useful in this population and should be used more frequently. Positive USFNA procedures in that series included two patients with normal-appearing lymph nodes. Patients with large primary tumors should have axillary ultrasound, and may benefit from USFNA even when lymph nodes appear normal because of the high prevalence of nodal disease. In addition, patients with large primary tumors are likely to be treated with neoadjuvant chemotherapy, and USFNA is particularly useful to establish a diagnosis of metastatic disease before chemotherapy is initiated.

USFNA is also indicated in patients with suspicious lymph nodes found on ultrasound. However, studies have used different criteria to determine whether a lymph node is suspicious enough to warrant fine needle aspiration.[30,32,33,38,42] Each ultrasound criterion has a different sensitivity and specificity for predicting nodal disease. Absence of a fatty hilum has been shown to be the most specific predictor of malignancy, but is not sensitive because it is a late finding.[33,45,48] Therefore, some measure of cortical thickening, either objective or subjective, must be used to determine whether USFNA is indicated if one hopes to detect most positive axillae preoperatively.

Based on an in vitro sonographic study, Bedi and colleagues[31] concluded that asymmetric focal hypoechoic cortical lobulation or a completely hypoechoic node (without a fatty hilum) should serve as guidelines for universal performance of USFNA. However, the appearance of the cortex is a subjective feature, and in practice, measuring the thickness of the cortex has been shown to provide the best compromise of sensitivity and specificity. Deurloo and colleagues[30] evaluated multiple nodal features, including cortex appearance and thickness, and found that the area under the receiver operating characteristic curve was highest (0.87) for maximum cortex thickness, and that a cutoff of 2.95 mm was the best indicator of when to perform USFNA. In a larger study also evaluating multiple nodal features, Choi and colleagues[48] found that a cortical thickness of greater than 3 mm was the best indicator to predict metastasis, with a higher sensitivity and specificity than eccentric or irregular nodular cortex. Abe and colleagues[45] reported a better sensitivity and specificity using 4 mm rather than 3 mm as the threshold.

The author's practice has found that using either a cortical thickness threshold of 3 mm or the presence of focal cortical thickening to be useful criteria for determining indication of USFNA. They previously reported the use of USFNA in patients with a wide range of primary tumor sizes and recommended further evaluation of the technique in a larger number of patients with smaller

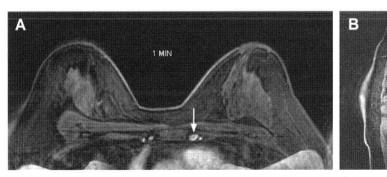

Fig. 7. Axial (*A*) and sagittal (*B*) MR images showing the parasternal location of a metastatic 7-mm internal mammary lymph node (*arrow*), immediately adjacent to the internal mammary vessels.

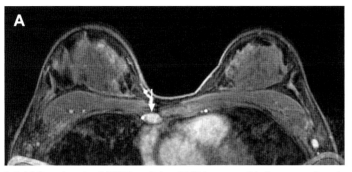
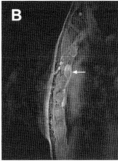

Fig. 8. Axial (A) and sagittal (B) T1-weighted MR images with fat saturation showing a metastatic 1.4-cm internal mammary lymph node (arrows).

tumors.[33] As they gained further experience, they have found that the low prevalence of metastatic disease in patients with invasive cancers smaller than 1 cm limits the utility of the procedure in this population, because the lymph nodes are rarely abnormal in this population. In patients with tumors 1 cm or larger, axillary ultrasound is worthwhile to assess the appearance of the axillary nodes, with USFNA indicated when lymph nodes meet selected criteria. In addition, the author's practice will perform USFNA of normal-appearing lymph nodes in patients with large tumors at very high risk for nodal disease.

INTERNAL MAMMARY LYMPH NODES

The internal mammary lymph node chain is another route of systemic dissemination in breast carcinoma, and the status of internal mammary nodes is also predictive of survival. The internal mammary nodes reside immediately adjacent, either medial or lateral, to the internal mammary artery and vein, parallel to the sternum and deep to costal cartilage (Fig. 7). The nodes most frequently involved in breast cancer are in the second to third intercostals spaces.[49] Abnormal internal mammary nodes can be seen on parasternal ultrasound, CT, and MRI.[49–51] Normal internal mammary nodes are very small and not visible on CT,[49] although they can often be seen on MR.[50] Kinoshita and colleagues[50] found that using a size criterion of 5 mm on MRI or greater had a 93.3% sensitivity and 89.3% specificity for predicting internal mammary node metastasis (Fig. 8).

Although most breast cancers that drain to the internal mammary nodes are located in the medial breast, tumor size and axillary nodal status are the most significant predictors of internal mammary nodal disease. Isolated involvement of internal mammary lymph nodes is low, with the rate of

internal mammary metastases in patients with a negative axilla reported to be 1% to 10%, with most series reporting less than 5%.[52]

SLNB of internal mammary drainage identified on lymphoscintigraphy is not routine but has been used to change management in patients with internal mammary node metastases.[53,54] When abnormal internal mammary nodes are identified through imaging, treatment regimens, particularly the radiation field, may be altered. In addition, if abnormal internal mammary nodes are detected through imaging, evaluation for more distant metastatic disease may be indicated, because internal mammary lymph node involvement is a poor prognostic sign.

SUMMARY

The status of axillary lymph nodes is a key prognostic indicator in patients with breast cancer and helps guide patient management. SLNB is increasingly being used as a less-morbid alternative to axillary lymph node dissection; however, when results are positive, axillary dissection is typically performed for complete staging and local control. Axillary ultrasound and USFNA are useful for detecting axillary nodal metastasis preoperatively and sparing patients SLNB, because patients with positive cytology on USFNA can proceed directly to axillary dissection or neoadjuvant chemotherapy. Internal mammary nodes are not routinely evaluated, but when the appearance of these nodes is abnormal on imaging, further treatment or metastatic evaluation may be necessary.

REFERENCES

1. Santillan AA, Kiluk JV, Cox CE. Assessment and designation of breast cancer stage. In: Bland KI, Copeland EM, editors. The breast: comprehensive

management of benign and malignant diseases. 4th edition. Philadelphia: Saunders Elsevier; 2009. p. 429–51.

2. Styblo TM, Wood WC. Clinically established prognostic factors in breast cancer. In: Bland KI, Copeland EM, editors. The breast: comprehensive management of benign and malignant diseases. 4th edition. Philadelphia: Saunders Elsevier; 2009. p. 455–62.

3. Veronesi U, Rilke F, Luini A, et al. Distribution of axillary node metastases by level of invasion. An analysis of 539 cases. Cancer 1981;59:682–7.

4. Rosen PP, Lesser ML, Kinne DW, et al. Discontinuous or "skip" metastases in breast carcinoma. Analysis of 12228 axillary dissections. Ann Surg 1983;197:276–83.

5. Pigott J, Nichols R, Maddox WA, et al. Metastases to the upper levels of the axillary nodes in carcinoma of the breast and its implications for nodal sampling procedures. Surg Gynecol Obstet 1984;158:255–9.

6. Chung MA. Therapeutic value of axillary node dissection and selective management of the axilla in small breast cancers. In: Bland KI, Copeland EM, editors. The breast: comprehensive management of benign and malignant diseases. 4th edition. Philadelphia: Saunders Elsevier; 2009. p. 953–69.

7. Pamilo M, Soiva M, Lavast EM. Real-time ultrasound, axillary mammography and clinical examination in the detection of axillary lymph node metastases in breast cancer patients. J Ultrasound Med 1989;8:115–20.

8. Sacre RA. Clinical evaluation of axillary lymph nodes compared to surgical and pathological findings. Eur J Surg Oncol 1986;12:169–73.

9. Chen SL, Iddings DM, Scheri RP, et al. Lymphatic mapping and sentinel node analysis: current concepts and applications. CA Cancer J Clin 2006;56:292–309.

10. Krynyckyi BR, Kim CK, Goyenechea MR, et al. Clinical breast lymphoscintigraphy: optimal techniques for performing studies, image atlas and analysis of images. Radiographics 2004;24:121–45.

11. Lucci A Jr, Kelemen PR, Miller C, et al. National practice patterns of sentinel lymph node dissection for breast carcinoma. J Am Coll Surg 2001;192:453–8.

12. Cox CE, Salud CJ, Cantor A, et al. Learning curves for breast cancer sentinel lymph node mapping based on surgical volume analysis. J Am Coll Surg 2001;193:593–600.

13. Cox CE, Furman B, Dupont EL, et al. Novel techniques in sentinel lymph node mapping and localization of nonpalpable breast lesions: the Moffitt experience. Ann Surg Oncol 2004;11:222S–6S.

14. Giuliano AE, Jones RC, Brennan M, et al. Sentinel lymphadenectomy in breast cancer. J Clin Oncol 1997;15:2345–50.

15. Krag D, Weaver D, Ashikaga T, et al. The sentinel node in breast cancer-a multicenter validation study. N Engl J Med 1998;339:941–6.

16. McMasters KM, Tuttle TM, Carlson DJ, et al. Sentinel lymph node biopsy for breast cancer: a suitable alternative to routine axillary dissection in multi-institutional practice when optimal technique is used. J Clin Oncol 2000;18:2560–6.

17. Wong SL, Edwards MJ, Chao C, et al. Sentinel lymph node biopsy for breast cancer: impact of number of sentinel nodes removed on false negative rate. J Am Coll Surg 2001;192:684–9.

18. Schrenk P, Rehberger W, Shamiyeh A, et al. Sentinel node biopsy for breast cancer: does the number of sentinel nodes removed have an impact on the accuracy of finding a positive node? J Surg Oncol 2002;80:130–6.

19. McCarter MD, Yeung H, Fey J, et al. The breast cancer patient with multiple sentinel nodes: when to stop? J Am Coll Surg 2001;192:692–7.

20. Brenot-Rossi I, Houvenaeghel G, Jacquemier J, et al. Nonvisualiztion of axillary sentinel node during lymphoscintigraphy: is there a pathologic significance in breast cancer? J Nucl Med 2003;44:1232–7.

21. Mamounas EP, Brown A, Anderson S, et al. Sentinel node biopsy after neoadjuvant chemotherapy in breast cancer: results from national surgical adjuvant breast and bowel project protocol B-27. J Clin Oncol 2005;23:2694–702.

22. Bruneton JN, Caramella E, Hery M, et al. Axillary node metastases in breast cancer: preoperative detection with ultrasound. Radiology 1986;158:325–6.

23. DeFreitas R Jr, Costa MV, Schneider SV, et al. Accuracy of ultrasound and clinical examination in the diagnosis of axillary lymph node metastasis in breast cancer. Eur J Surg Oncol 1991;17:240–4.

24. Vassallo P, Wernecke K, Roos N, et al. Differentiation of benign from malignant superficial lymphadenopathy: the role of high resolution US. Radiology 1992;183:215–20.

25. Tate JJ, Lewis V, Archer T, et al. Ultrasound detection of axillary lymph node metastases in breast cancer. Eur J Surg Oncol 1989;15:139–41.

26. Verbanck J, Vandewiele I, De Winter H, et al. Value of axillary ultrasonography and sonographically guided puncture of axillary nodes: a prospective study of 144 consecutive patients. J Clin Ultrasound 1997;25:53–6.

27. Bonnema J, van Geel AN, van Ooijen BV, et al. Ultrasound-guided aspiration biopsy for detection of nonpalpable axillary node metastases in breast cancer patients: new diagnostic method. World J Surg 1997;21:270–4.

28. De Kanter AY, van Eijck CH, van Geel AN, et al. Multicentre study of ultrasonographically guided axillary node biopsy in patients with breast cancer. Br J Surg 1999;86:1459–62.

29. Bedrosian I, Bedi D, Kuerer HM, et al. Impact of clinicopathological factors on sensitivity of axillary ultrasonography in the detection of axillary nodal metastases in patients with breast cancer. Ann Surg Oncol 2003;10:1025–30.

30. Deurloo EE, Tanis PJ, Gilhuijs KG, et al. Reduction in the number of sentinel lymph node procedures by preoperative ultrasonography of the axilla in breast cancer. Eur J Cancer 2003;39:1068–73.

31. Bedi DG, Krishnamurthy R, Krishnamurthy S, et al. Cortical morphologic features of axillary lymph nodes as a predictor of metastasis in breast cancer: in vitro sonographic study. AJR Am J Roentgenol 2008;191:646–52.

32. Krishnamurthy S, Sneige N, Bedi DG, et al. Role of ultrasound-guided fine-needle aspiration of indeterminate and suspicious axillary lymph nodes in the initial staging of breast carcinoma. Cancer 2002; 95:982–8.

33. Koelliker SL, Chung MA, Mainiero MB, et al. Axillary lymph nodes: US-guided fine-needle aspiration for initial staging of breast cancer-correlation with primary tumor size. Radiology 2008;246:81–9.

34. Walsh J, Dixon J, Chetty U, et al. Colour Doppler studies of axillary node metastases in breast carcinoma. Clin Radiol 1994;49:189.

35. Yang WT, Metreweli C. Colour Doppler flow in normal axillary lymph nodes. Br J Radiol 1998;71:381–3.

36. Yang WT, Chang J, Metreweli C. Patients with breast cancer: differences in color Doppler flow and grayscale US features of benign and malignant axillary lymph nodes. Radiology 2000;215:568–73.

37. Kuenen-Boumeester V, Menke-Pluymers M, de Kanter AY, et al. Ultrasound-guided fine needle aspiration cytology of axillary lymph nodes in breast cancer patients. A preoperative staging procedure. Eur J Cancer 2003;39:170–4.

38. Sapino A, Cassoni P, Zanon E, et al. Ultrasonographically-guided fine-needle aspiration of axillary lymph nodes: role in breast cancer management. Br J Cancer 2003;88:702–6.

39. Van Rijk MC, Deurloo EE, Nieweg OE, et al. Ultrasonography and fine-needle aspiration cytology can spare breast cancer patients unnecessary sentinel lymph node biopsy. Ann Surg Oncol 2005;13:31–5.

40. Rao R, Lilley L, Andrews V, et al. Axillary staging by percutaneous biopsy: sensitivity of fine-needle aspiration versus core needle biopsy. Ann Surg Oncol 2009;16:1170–5.

41. Jain A, Haisfield-Wolfe ME, Lange J, et al. The role of ultrasound-guided fine-needle aspiration of axillary nodes in the staging of breast cancer. Ann Surg Oncol 2007;15:462–71.

42. Damera A, Evans AJ, Cornford EJ, et al. Diagnosis of axillary nodal metastases by ultrasound-guided core biopsy in primary operable breast cancer. Br J Cancer 2003;89:1310–3.

43. Abdsaleh S, Azavedo E, Lindgen PG. Ultrasound-guided large needle core biopsy of the axilla. Acta Radiol 2004;45:193–6.

44. Topal U, Punar S, Tasdelen I, et al. Role of US-guided core needle biopsy of axillary lymph nodes in the initial staging of breast carcinoma. Eur J Radiol 2005;56:382–5.

45. Abe H, Schmidt RA, Kulkarni K, et al. Lymph nodes suspicious for breast cancer metastasis: sampling with US-guided 14-gauge core-needle biopsy-clinical experience in 100 patients. Radiology 2009; 250:41–9.

46. Britton PD, Coud A, Godward S, et al. Use of ultrasound-guided axillary node core biopsy in staging of early breast cancer. Eur Radiol 2009;19:561–9.

47. Oruwari JU, Chung MA, Koelliker S, et al. Axillary staging using ultrasound-guided fine needle aspiration biopsy in locally advanced beast cancer. Am J Surg 2002;184:307–9.

48. Choi YJ, Ko EY, Han B, et al. High-resolution ultrasonograpic features of axillary lymph node metastasis in patients with breast cancer. Breast 2009;18:119–22.

49. Scatarige JC, Boxen I, Smathers RL. Internal mammary lymphadenopathy: imaging of a vital lymphatic pathway in breast cancer. Radiographics 1990;10:857–70.

50. Kinoshita T, Odagiri K, Andoh K, et al. Evaluation of small internal mammary lymph node metastases in breast cancer by MRI. Radiat Med 1999;17: 189–93.

51. Ozdemir H, Atilla S, Ilgit ET, et al. Parasternal sonography of the internal mammary lymphatics in breast cancer: CT correlation. Eur J Radiol 1995;19:114–7.

52. Recht A. Radiotherapy and regional nodes. In: Bland KI, Copeland EM, editors. The breast: comprehensive management of benign and malignant diseases. 4th edition. Philadelphia: Saunders Elsevier; 2009. p. 1077–82.

53. Sacchini B, Bogen P, Galimberti V, et al. Surgical approach to internal mammary node lymph node biopsy. J Am Coll Surg 2001;193:703–13.

54. Madsen E, Gobardhan PD, Bongers V, et al. The impact on post-surgical treatment of sentinel lymph node biopsy of internal mammary lymph nodes in patients with breast cancer. Ann Surg Oncol 2007; 14:1486–92.

Controversies on the Management of High-Risk Lesions at Core Biopsy from a Radiology/ Pathology Perspective

Dianne Georgian-Smith, MD[a],*, Thomas J. Lawton, MD[b,c]

KEYWORDS

- Breast high-risk lesion • Lobular neoplasia • Papilloma
- Radial scar • Flat epithelial atypia (FEA)
- Breast core biopsy

PROLOGUE

Readers may feel less than satisfied when they discover that there is no consensus as to the appropriate recommendations for follow-up of risk lesions following percutaneous core biopsy. The significance of this article is in the details of the methodologies and results, and much less in the numbers. The overall goal is to emphasize the flaws in current studies.

Many of the studies do not control for inclusion, as well as exclusion, of surgical follow-up, which is being used as the gold standard. Even if surgical follow-up is performed, many studies lack imaging/ core biopsy/surgical biopsy/pathology concordance/discordance analyses. Meta-analyses of giant tables cannot make up for flawed methodologies with small numbers. The authors suggest that readers read between the numbers to capture the essence of where the current literature lies. The numbers are tabulated in Tables 1 to 4 in the Appendix. In 2010 there is not adequate data from which to make definitive decisions regarding treatment planning. We still can not agree on how to treat patients after a core biopsy diagnosis of any one of these high-risk lesions. Little progress has been made since the last time this topic was discussed in the 2004 *Radiologic Clinics of North America* by Berg.[1] Adding more retrospective reviews will take us no closer to discovering the truth, and yet such studies are ongoing.

The solution is a prospective, multi-institutional trial that is all-inclusive for patients to go to surgery without selection biases, that tracks all patients, has meticulous radiology/pathology/clinical correlation, and significant numbers. In many ways, it is rather shocking, almost depressing, to realize how little is known concerning this important topic in spite of decades of investigation, and how this trickles down to almost random health care for thousands of women. Clearly, there is no standard of care.[2]

INTRODUCTION

In the 2004 edition of the *Radiologic Clinics of North America*, Berg[1] reviewed the literature on the proposed management of several high-risk lesions diagnosed at core biopsy. The overall opinion at that time was to surgically excise all high-risk lesions diagnosed at core biopsy based

[a] Division of Breast Imaging, Department of Radiology, Brigham and Women's Hospital, Harvard Medical School, 75 Francis Street, RA 020, Boston, MA 02115, USA
[b] Seattle Breast Pathology Consultants, 117 East Louisa Street #185, Seattle, WA 98102, USA
[c] Clarient Inc, Aliso Viejo, CA, USA
* Corresponding author.
E-mail address: dgeorgiansmith@partners.org

Radiol Clin N Am 48 (2010) 999–1012
doi:10.1016/j.rcl.2010.06.004
0033-8389/10/$ – see front matter © 2010 Elsevier Inc. All rights reserved.

on retrospective data that documented varying frequencies of malignancy on follow-up. In the past 6 years, however, numerous studies have shown that for many of these high-risk lesions, subsequent surgical excision has revealed no cancers or at most a minimal percentage of cancer upgrades.

Two primary reasons for surgical follow-up after any nonmalignant core biopsy are possible: (1) underestimation of malignancy, and (2) radiology/pathology discordance in which the lesion was missed or the expected malignancy results were not obtained. With regard to the high-risk lesions, the debatable question is the former. The concept of underestimation of concurrent malignancy for atypical ductal hyperplasia (ADH) at core biopsy is well established,[3–5] even when the index radiographic lesion has been completely removed percutaneously.[6] How this concept translates into the management of other high-risk lesions, such as lobular carcinoma in situ (LCIS), atypical lobular hyperplasia (ALH), papillomas, radial scar, and flat epithelial atypia (FEA) remains debatable.

How to determine the accuracy of core sampling of a lesion is a question affecting radiology/pathology concordance beyond the scope of this article. In particular with benign or high-risk lesion core results, the radiologist should review the imaging of the procedure to: (1) determine whether the pathology results correlate accurately with the appearance of the lesion, and (2) document in the report the concordance/discordance and recommendation for appropriate follow-up.

The resulting conflicting data in the literature have placed health care professionals in the dilemma of not knowing how to best advise women regarding the need for surgical or clinical/imaging follow-up. Based on an informal survey by the authors that involved 10 academic breast radiologists and pathologists from around the country, it is clear that the issue of management of several high-risk lesions is still controversial.[2] The survey focused on 4 main high-risk lesions: lobular neoplasia (ALH and LCIS), benign papillomas, radial scar, and FEA (Table 1). Anecdotally, radiologists said that management depends on a given surgeon's preference, consequently varying within a given institution. These differences in personal opinions and lack of consensus in the medical community result in many women either being over treated with surgical excision or under treated and thereby missing a breast cancer. The authors review the literature since 2004 for the aforementioned 4 high-risk lesions highlighting both the radiology and pathology literature to illustrate the current trends in management. Now more than ever there

is a calling to prospectively study these specific histologic groups to determine more accurately the true risk of underestimation of malignancy and role of immediate surgical excision.

LOBULAR NEOPLASIA: LCIS AND ALH
Prevalence

Based on data from the Surveillance, Epidemiology and End Results (SEER) Cancer registry, the incidence of LCIS has increased 2.6-fold (95% confidence interval [CI] 2.3–2.9) from 1980 to 2001 likely related to the use of mammography.[7] Obtaining lobular neoplasia on core biopsy and facing the dilemma of what to do with these results is more frequent now than ever, as additional modes for core biopsy, such as magnetic resonance guidance, have developed in the last decade.

Pathology Definitions and Related Concerns

Lobular neoplasia is a term that encompasses ALH and LCIS. The cells of both ALH and LCIS are similar in appearance; the cells are small, uniform, discohesive, and generally lack nucleoli. It is the degree of the involvement of the lobular units that distinguishes these 2 entities. While there is disagreement in the literature as to specific criteria to distinguish LCIS from ALH, a widely accepted definition by Page and colleagues[8] requires for LCIS that at least 50% of the acinar units in a lobule be filled and distended by lobular neoplastic cells. The definition of distention was further quantified to require the presence of at least 8 lobular neoplastic cells spanning an individual acinar unit.[9] If a lobular unit does not fulfill these criteria, a diagnosis of ALH is made. Most pathologists recommend maintaining the 2 entities as separate given that follow-up studies show a lower rate in the incidence of the subsequent development of invasive carcinoma for ALH compared with LCIS.[8–12] Unfortunately, much of the core biopsy literature sums these results into lobular neoplasia. The reader should stay vigilant when comparing studies as to whether results are presented as lobular neoplasia or LCIS and ALH.

Recently, variants of LCIS have been described that do not fit this classic LCIS histopathology, including LCIS with central necrosis and pleomorphic LCIS.[13–17] Because of the small numbers of cases and lack of significant follow-up data, the natural history of these variants is not well established, but early data suggest that LCIS variants such as these may have a more aggressive behavior. Thus, many clinicians are recommending surgical biopsy when one of the variants of LCIS is present on core biopsy.

Table 1
Physician responses to a survey regarding need for surgical excision of high-risk lesions on core needle biopsy

Physician	ALH	LCIS	FEA	Radial Scar	Papilloma without Atypia
A (path)	No	No	Yes	No	No
B (path)	No	Yes	Yes	Yes	No
C (path)	Yes	Yes	Yes	Yes	No
D (path)	Yes	Yes	No	Yes	Yes
E (rad)	Yes	Yes	Yes	Yes	No
F (rad)	Yes	Yes	Yes	No	Yes
G (rad)	Yes	Yes	Yes	Yes	Yes
H (path)	No	No	Yes	No	No
I (rad)	Yes	Yes	Yes	No,	Yes
J (rad)	Yes	Yes	Yes	Yes	Yes

Incidental or Direct Sign of Radiographic Finding

A common belief is that lobular neoplasia is an incidental pathologic finding without radiographic correlate.[18–20] If always incidental, then all core results of lobular neoplasia would be discordant and warrant surgical excision. However, studies have shown that lobular neoplasia can be represented radiographically. Calcifications were directly indicative of LCIS in both the classic and pleomorphic forms,[13,18,21] and other studies have shown masses to correlate on both mammography[18,22] and sonography.[22]

One of the most complete evaluations in poster format was displayed at the 23rd Annual San Antonio Breast Cancer Symposium in 2000 by Tarjan and colleagues.[23] Their goal was to evaluate the incidence of lobular neoplasia as the direct sign of a mammographic or sonographic lesion. Out of 2280 consecutive core biopsies, there were 108 cases (4.7% incidence) of lobular neoplasia classified per mammographic lesion as mass, calcifications, asymmetric densities, or by sonographic finding of shadowing. In particular, the imaging and pathology were reviewed to determine whether the lobular neoplasia was the primary cause for the lesion or an incidental finding. There were 38 cases of primary lobular neoplasia (1.7% incidence) and 70 incidental cases. The primary cases were 32 calcifications and 6 masses.

The blanket statement that all lobular neoplasia is incidental is not accurate, and core pathology result of lobular neoplasia should not by itself direct recommendation for surgical follow-up.

Controversial Results Regarding Surgical Versus Imaging Follow-up

Many retrospective studies have looked at the presence of malignancy after surgical excision and/or imaging follow-up after core biopsy of lobular neoplasia. Most of the earlier studies were single institution with small numbers since prevalence is exceedingly low for lobular neoplasia, as well as for all high-risk lesions. Studies that recommended surgical follow-up reported malignancy rates of 14% (3/21),[24] 16% (1/6),[25] 20% (7/35),[26] 25% (5/20),[27] 37% (13/35),[28] and 50% (9/18).[29] These are reported individually, as opposed to a range, so that the reader can appreciate how small and inconsistent these ratios are from which much of the literature is derived. In addition, these malignancy rates are based on selected groups who underwent follow-up. Because not all of the patients with lobular neoplasia at core underwent immediate surgical excision or imaging follow-up, the results are skewed. As these studies are retrospective reviews, this selection is not controlled for, leading to significant flaws in the methodology and making generalizations to standard populations difficult at best.

A multi-institutional study from France found a malignancy rate of 19% (10/52) out of 52 undergoing surgery.[30] The largest study to date is by Brem and colleagues[31] who reviewed the core results from 14 institutions. Out of approximately 32,000 core biopsies, 278 (0.9%) were ALH and/or LCIS as the highest-grade lesion. Invasive carcinoma or ductal carcinoma in situ (DCIS) was found in 23% (38/164).

All of these studies[24–32] suggested surgical follow-up based on their rates of underestimation of malignancy. However, there are concerns with all of the studies, large and small, beyond lack of statistical significance, as has been commented on by Kopans.[33,34] Some studies used data only from immediate post–core biopsy surgical pathology, and others used both surgical pathology and imaging follow-up of variable lengths of time. Most importantly, most studies selected patients by some unknown method for immediate surgical excision. Were patients recommended for surgery because the radiologist believed that all lobular neoplasia is incidental and hence discordant with imaging? Were they selected because imaging was suspicious and hence discordant with pathology results? Or were they selected because of clinical reasons that were discordant with benign results? The corollary issue is that studies do not have data on the patients who were NOT excised or followed, and hence it is not known how those patients may have differed from the tracked cohort.

The study by Brem and colleagues[31] analyzed their facilities' data for radiology/pathology concordance/discordance, but noted that the definitions of discordance at each institution were not standardized. Some considered that a diagnosis of lobular neoplasia was incidental and therefore this result without any other pathologic diagnosis to explain the radiographic finding was cause for discordance. Other institutions did not specify their definitions of discordance. Nevertheless, out of the 82 concordant cases undergoing immediate surgery, 17% (N = 15) of cases underestimated malignancy, and out of the 74 discordant cases undergoing immediate surgery, 28% (N = 21) underestimated malignancy. So the investigators concluded that regardless of radiology/pathology concordance, surgical excision is warranted.

In contrast, more recent studies meticulously analyzed the issue of radiology/pathology concordance, and consequently concluded that immediate surgery was not indicated because of exceedingly low underestimation of malignancy. Menon and colleagues[35] reviewed in detail 47 cases of classic LCIS in which core biopsies were performed freehand in 8 cases, with ultrasound guidance in 14, and stereotactic in 25. Of the 8 malignant false-negative cases after immediate surgery (N = 25), 5 cases were missed masses and 2 were missed calcifications. The investigators do not break down the method of coring. Nagi and colleagues[36] analyzed 98 cases of lobular neoplasia and found an incidental minute focus of invasive lobular carcinoma at surgery in one case and DCIS mixed with LCIS in a second case. No other malignancies were found with imaging follow-up ranging from 1 to 8 years. These investigators concluded that immediate surgery was not warranted routinely and recommended careful imaging/pathology correlation.

The largest study with detailed review of the pathology results was a study by Hwang and colleagues.[37] The goal of this study was to accurately define specific morphology of lobular neoplasia at core biopsy that might be able to predict the presence of invasive carcinoma or DCIS. Over a decade, 333 core results of lobular neoplasia were collected, of which 41% (N = 136) went on to immediate surgery; 36% (49/136) of those cases were ADH with lobular neoplasia. Excluding these cases of ADH, malignancy was found at surgical excision in 23% (9/39) of cases of LCIS and 2% (1/48) of cases of ALH. These investigators continued their analyses of the malignant cases where others have stopped. Six of the 9 cases of LCIS were radiology/pathology discordant and the remaining 3 cases were nonclassic LCIS (LCIS with necrosis and pleomorphic LCIS). After excluding discordance and nonclassic LCIS cases, the upgrade was only 1%. Therefore, these investigators recommend imaging follow-up (not immediate surgery) for the classic form of LCIS after careful radiology/pathology review.

Development of Malignancy After Lobular Neoplasia Core Biopsy: Site Locations and Risk

An argument supporting follow-up in lieu of surgery is the observation that the risk for development of carcinoma in patients with prior biopsy of lobular neoplasia is bilateral and not necessarily at the core biopsy site. Chuba and colleagues[38] analyzed the SEER data to determine the laterality of invasive carcinoma occurring after LCIS in a study involving 4853 women. They excluded those with the diagnosis of invasive cancer within 1 year after lobular neoplasia to rule out synchronous disease. The minimum cumulative risk was 7.1% at 10 years for all patients regardless of form of prior biopsy. Form of biopsies were specified into 3 surgical categories: aspirate or core needle biopsies which defined "lesser surgery", partial mastectomy, and complete mastectomies. There were 178 patients in the subset who underwent lesser surgery and there was a 5.5% incidence of invasive cancer at 10 years. Acknowledged is the inherent decrease in sampling accuracy of fine-needle aspirates versus core biopsies. The significance, nevertheless, is that laterality for the entire cohort after surgical excision of lobular neoplasia was almost equal: 46% ipsilateral and 54% contralateral.[38] Page and Simpson[39] note that other studies have found the incidence of contralateral malignancy to be one-half that of the ipsilateral involved breast.

A study by Mulheron and colleagues[40] also arguing against immediate surgery found no carcinoma at final surgical excision in 12 out of 25 women with lobular neoplasia at core biopsy. Moreover, the *entire cohort* was followed for a mean 5.5 years. Five cancers developed (20%, 5/25): 3 who had undergone surgery and 2 who had been followed with imaging (P = .57). However, malignancy did not arise in the same quadrant as the location of the core in the imaging follow-up group. Immediate surgery neither identified concurrent carcinoma nor did it decrease the frequency of development of subsequent carcinoma. Similar results were reported[41] in a larger series of 50 patients with lobular neoplasia in which 0 malignancies were diagnosed in 21 immediate surgical excisions and 4 malignancies developed at a mean of 6 years, 1 of which was in the contralateral breast. The conclusion was that immediate surgical excision was not warranted, and that lobular neoplasia was only a risk marker for the development of bilateral invasive breast cancer.

BENIGN PAPILLOMAS

Papillomas are benign intraductal proliferations that often present in the subareolar region as a palpable mass, but can be multiple, peripherally located in the breast, and incidentally found on imaging. These growths are composed of fibrovascular cores lined by myoepithelial cells and an overlying layer of epithelium. Epithelial hyperplasia can arise within an otherwise benign papilloma, as can ADH (atypical papilloma) and DCIS. The criteria used for making a diagnosis of ADH within a papillary lesion are similar to those used in ducts outside a papillary lesion. However, the criteria distinguishing ADH versus DCIS arising in a papilloma are less well defined in the pathology literature.[42,43]

Consensus in the literature exists for surgical excision following core biopsy results for papilloma with *atypia* or *multiple* papillomas.[44,45] However, the literature is mixed with regard to the management after a core biopsy of a benign papilloma. As is noted in **Table 1**, 4 of the 5 radiologists and 1 out of 5 pathologists recommended surgical excision for benign papillomas. This shows an interesting disparity between radiologists and pathologists as well as the lack of agreement amongst specialized health care professionals.

Controversial Results Regarding Surgical Versus Imaging Follow-up

The faults previously noted in the retrospective reviews of lobular neoplasia also hold true

for benign papillomas. Some of the studies recommend surgical follow-up based on underestimation of concurrent malignancy whereas others do not recommend surgery. Studies with significant malignancy upgrades reported the following frequencies: 7% (4/56),[46] 10.5%, 9/86,[47] 17% (20/117),[48] and 29% (7/24).[49] Other studies of similar design reported low rates: 0% (0/25),[50] 0% (0/67),[51] and 0% (0/17).[52] Sydnor and colleagues[53] reported 1 case of malignancy out of 38 surgically removed and 25 tracked cases. However, the 1 malignant case was LCIS, and by current standards, most clinicians do not consider LCIS to be malignant. Investigators studying high-risk lesions, particularly papillomas and radial scars, have highlighted the differences in underestimation of results as they relate to core needle gauge and tru-cut, spring-loaded versus vacuum-assisted needles. Two studies suggested that removing a large amount of tissue at core biopsy improved the accuracy of the core results. Zografos and colleagues[54] used an 11-g needle and obtained a minimum of 24 core samples (range 24–96 cores). No cancers were present on follow-up. Carder and colleagues[55] tested the 11-g and 8-g vacuum-assisted probes (specifics as to number of cores not provided) against surgical excision for final assessment. No atypia or malignancies were noted at final pathology in the pure benign cases.

A shortcoming to all these studies is the lack of analyses of radiology/pathology concordance between the core and surgical pathology results. Liberman and colleagues,[56] however, addressed this parameter directly. There were 5 malignancies (4 DCIS, 1 invasive carcinoma) out of 35 concordant benign papillomas for a prevalence of 14% (5/35). Twenty-five cases went on to immediate surgical biopsy and 10 cases underwent a minimum of 2-year imaging surveillance. Out of the 5 cancers, there was growth or a new mass on mammography in 3 in the follow-up cohort (mean 18 months, range 7–22 months). A fourth patient developed bloody nipple discharge at 21 months. On further inspection of the fifth case of a patient who self-selected to undergo surgery 1 month after core biopsy, the DCIS was 1 cm distal to the site of the papilloma in which no residual papilloma was present at surgical excision. In summary, what seems at first glance to be a study of 14% underestimation of disease is actually a study of 0% upgrades in asymptomatic women with stable mammographic findings.

The importance of radiology/pathology concordance, or rather the lack thereof, is underscored in other studies as well. Ko and colleagues[57] reported 1 case of DCIS out of 42 sent to surgery because of radiology/pathology discordance. Mercado and colleagues[58] recommend surgical biopsy for all papillomas based on their reported upgrade of 21% (9/42) to DCIS *and* atypia. However, there were only 2 malignant cases, both DCIS, in which 1 was a case of pleomorphic calcifications and the second case was a new mass in a postmenopausal woman. If both of these patients had been excluded from final analysis because surgical excision would have been warranted based on factors other than the papilloma, zero cases upgraded to malignancy.

Other studies remarked that the malignancies were adjacent to the indexed papilloma and consequently incidental.[59–61] Sahasrabudhe and colleagues[62] reported 1 case of DCIS out of 19 benign papillomas involving 3 ductulolobular units in the same specimen as a 1-cm large papilloma. Their opinion was that 1 incidental lesion outside the papilloma should not mandate excision for all. The study by Bernik and colleagues[60] reported 7 out of 71 (10%) cases associated with malignancy and an additional 7 cases associated with atypia in the surrounding tissues, defined as "within 3 cm of the indexed papillary lesion," a distance that in some breasts may be in a different quadrant, and thus possibly unrelated.

These studies reflect neither inaccurate targeting nor an inability by the pathologist to diagnose a benign lesion. Should serendipitous occult malignancy dictate surgery for all patients with benign papillomas?

However, Bernik and colleagues[60] suggest, like Mercado and colleagues,[58] that surgical excision is indicated to rule out not only concurrent malignancy but also concurrent *atypia* given the argument that if the patient is found to have ADH, then the patient's risk for breast cancer increases, and she can be counseled for possible hormonal prevention treatment with tamoxifen or raloxifene. Hormonal treatment has been shown to reduce breast cancer risk by 70% and the duration benefit is 10 to 20 years after the completion of 5 years of tamoxifen. However, there is no evidence of survival benefit and hormonal treatment is not without its own risk. When diagnosed, it is not known how long patients have had ADH and who is going to go on to develop cancer (Judy Garber MD, Boston, MA, personal communication, January 2010). Therefore, the potential of finding atypia may not be justification for surgery after core biopsy of a benign papilloma.

Can Imaging Help Triage Patients into Surgery Versus Follow-up?

Several studies evaluated imaging features with core results as means to determine the need for surgery versus imaging follow-up. Ko and colleagues[57] reviewed in consensus with 2 radiologists the sonographic features of 69 papillomas (43 benign papillomas, 18 atypical papillomas, 7 intraductal papillary carcinomas, 1 invasive papillary carcinoma). They concluded that when there is imaging concordance using the American College of Radiology BI-RADS Ultrasound lexicon (4th edition)[63] applied to a benign core result, that further surgical excision is not needed.[57] In contrast, Lam and colleagues[64] did not find reliable radiographic features to distinguish benign from malignant when evaluating papillary lesions (papilloma, papillomatosis, sclerosing papilloma, atypical papilloma, and papillary carcinoma). Acknowledged are differences in papillary definitions possibly leading to contrasting results.

Two studies showed statistical significance between sizes of benign and malignant papillomas. Chang and colleagues[65] noted the mean size of 1.4 cm (malignant) versus 0.9 cm (benign) ($P = .039$), and Kil and colleagues[66] showed differences in size (>1.5 cm) as well as location within the breast, with atypical or malignant papillomas located more peripherally (defined as the posterior third of the breast on mammography or distal third of breast tissue circumferentially at sonography) than benign lesions ($P = .017$).

Larger studies corroborating these observations, as well as additional imaging features, would be helpful in predicting which patients to follow and which to refer to surgery.

RADIAL SCAR/COMPLEX SCLEROSING LESION

Radial scar and complex sclerosing lesion are terms used to describe a characteristic pathologic stellate lesion at low power containing a central elastotic stromal area often with entrapped benign ducts. At the periphery, ducts and glands radiate away from the central area. These ducts can contain usual type hyperplasia, atypical hyperplasia, even in situ carcinoma. By convention, radial scar refers to a lesion measuring 1 cm or less and complex sclerosing lesion refers to the same histology but for lesions greater than 1 cm.[67]

In the 2004 *Radiologic Clinics of North America* article by Berg,[1] the overall consensus was for surgical excision of radial scars on core biopsy when there was a mammographic finding of architectural distortion so as not to miss a possible tubular carcinoma, which is the main pathologic differential diagnosis. The study by Lopez-Medina and colleagues[68] highlights this point in that out of the 8 false-negative cases, 4 were tubular carcinomas, with the remaining 4 cases diagnosed as DCIS (N = 2) and infiltrating ductal carcinoma (N = 2). Nevertheless, the inability of pathologists to distinguish radial scar from tubular carcinoma has been exaggerated in the literature. The classic histologic findings of radial scar can be confused with invasive carcinoma both pathologically and by breast imaging. However, the entrapped glands within the central elastotic area of radial scars are benign and maintain their basal myoepithelial cell layer. Tubular carcinomas lose that cell layer and are thus invasive. Moreover, immunohistochemical stains, even on core biopsy, can be used to corroborate hemotoxylin and eosin interpretations. Therefore, if the center of the lesions and radiating fibers of the lesion have been included in core biopsies, the argument that pathologists cannot distinguish tubular cancer from radial scar is incorrect and should not dictate surgery.

Controversial Results Regarding Surgical Versus Imaging Follow-up

There is literature showing both high and low concurrent malignancy rates based on surgical and imaging follow-up after core biopsy of a radial scar. Becker and colleagues[69] reporting on a large, single institutional study of approximately 15,000 core biopsies, found 227 (1.4%) that included a radial scar at pathology. Of the 125 radial scars without atypia at core biopsy, there were 5 malignancies for a false-negative rate of 4% (5/125), the same percentage as reported by Brenner and colleagues's[70] multi-institutional study (4%, 5/128). In the literature, frequencies starting with studies advocating imaging follow-up are 0% (0/80)[71] and 0% (0/27)[72]; those advocating surgical follow-up are 8% (5/62),[73] 9%, (1/11),[25] and 22% (6/27).[68]

Some suggest that the gauge and number of cores markedly influence the accuracy of core biopsy results. The study by Becker and colleagues[69] was performed using a 14-g tru-cut needle in 176 lesions (average number of cores per lesion 6.1) and 11-g vacuum-assisted needle in 51 cases (average number of cores per lesion 32.1). In the cohort, 14-g core biopsy, there were 100 radial scars with benign pathology at core biopsy with 5 cancers (5%, 5/100) at subsequent immediate biopsy. In the cohort, 11-g vacuum-assisted probe, there were 25 cases of radial scar with benign pathology after core biopsy, and no malignancies were detected (0%, 0/25). This difference in needle gauge results was not statistically significant. The study by Resetkova and colleagues[71] specifically studied the 9- and 11-g vacuum-assisted probes. There were no malignancies in the entire cohort of 80

patients. The number of retrieved cores with the 11-g needle was 12 (±4) and with the 9-g needle was 9 (±3). Using a 14-g tru-cut needle, Cawson and colleagues[72] also had 0% malignancies on follow-up of 75 prospectively tracked radial scars. The investigators made the observation, as did Brenner and colleagues,[70] that the number of cores taken (≥5 cores) were more likely to have a correct diagnosis than if fewer were obtained, although this was not statistically significant (P = .09).[72]

The Importance of Radiology/Pathology Correlation

One study specifically observed the association of the core needle tracks at final surgical excision in relation to the indexed radial scar and associated malignancy. Douglas-Jones and colleagues[74] reviewed the 11 false-negative cases out of 281 core biopsies (3.9%) yielding radial sclerosing lesions at core biopsy that were malignant at final surgical pathology. In all cases, the needle tracks made by the core sampling were seen at final pathology. The tracks were observed to have missed the malignancy in all eleven cases by an average of 5 mm (range 1–20 mm) and less than 6 mm in 9/11 cases. This is an interesting observation, and may explain why those studies with a large number of cores were more accurate at final pathology.

Discordance between radiology and pathology may be not only because of inaccurate targeting but also because of incongruence between lesion morphology at imaging and that at pathology. The study by Linda and colleagues[73] may be an example of this. It is the first reported case of a false-negative radial scar using an 11-g vacuum-assisted needle. The radiographic finding was a group of benign- appearing punctate calcifications (Anna Linda MD, Udine, Italy, personal communication, January 2010) not associated with architectural distortion at mammography. The question that radiologists should ponder is whether a radial scar at pathology can manifest as only a cluster of calcifications at mammography. Because radiographs reflect what pathologists see at low-power microscopy, and because radial scars by definition must have a radial configuration of stroma, then can a pathology result of radial scar be concordant with only calcifications when no architectural distortion is present at mammography? In this scenario, is the radial scar therefore incidental? These questions are imperative when analyzing the pathology results with the imaging, and when determining the need for possible surgical follow-up. If a radial scar is deemed to be incidental after this review, is surgery warranted? The management of *incidental* radial scars is not certain, although the paper by Brenner and colleagues[70] reported no malignancies in 28 cases.

Pathology Controversy: ADH Versus DCIS

A tangential concern to issues of radiology/pathology concordance is the acknowledged subjectivity in pathology when diagnosing intraductal proliferative lesions. This controversy highlights that subjective criteria are often used to differentiate usual type ductal hyperplasia from ADH from DCIS. Interobserver variability studies in the pathology literature have shown this lack of consensus but have also indicated that rates of agreement can be improved with consistency in diagnostic criteria and with training of pathologists in those strict criteria.[75,76]

On this note it is interesting that Brodie and colleagues,[77] because of a personal upgrade malignancy rate of 34% for radial scar at core biopsy, questioned whether the results by Cawson and colleagues,[72] with an overall 7% (5/75) malignancy rate (including cases of pure radial scar as well as those associated with ADH/DCIS at core biopsy), reflected an interobserver variation in the diagnosis of ADH versus DCIS at pathology. In response, Cawson and colleagues[78] had half of the radial scars, not specifically selected, reviewed by another breast pathologist. Although there were no ADH cases (N = 27) that changed to DCIS, 30% of the ADH cases were down graded to "ductal epithelial hyperplasia of the usual type." Although no malignancies were missed, it is important that diagnoses of ADH, particularly if associated with high-risk lesions, be consistent and reproducible.

FLAT EPITHELIA ATYPIA

The term flat epithelial atypia was adopted by the World Health Organization Working Group on the Pathology and Genetics of Tumors of the Breast in 2003[79] to define a lesion of the terminal ductal lobular unit that was recognized more than 100 years ago and variably described as clinging carcinoma, atypical cystic lobules, columnar alteration with prominent apical snouts and secretions (CAPSS) with atypia, among others. In FEA, the often cystically dilated ducts are lined by one to several layers of monomorphic, but enlarged, round to oval cells with low-grade cytologic atypia. Although the cells are atypical, there are no architectural changes as seen in ADH or DCIS, such as micropapillary or cribriform growth patterns. As part of the spectrum of columnar cell changes, there may be "flocculant secretions in the lumini

of the acini" and these may calcify.[80] Numerous studies have shown an association between FEA and low-grade DCIS, lobular neoplasia, and tubular carcinoma.[81–88] Several good recent reviews cover the natural history of this lesion and its clinical significance.[89–91]

Mammographically, FEA usually presents as clustered, punctate, amorphous, or fine pleomorphic calcifications. Because the calcifications are secondary to secretions of calcium oxalate or calcium phosphate by the epithelium, the calcifications are small and amorphous if within the cystically dilated lobules. If the terminal ducts are involved, the calcifications may be fine, pleomorphic, conforming to the tubular structure of the ducts.[80]

Controversial Results Regarding Surgical Versus Imaging Follow-up

It is difficult to determine if there is an association between FEA and specific carcinomas because the literature presents conflicting results. The study by David and colleagues[92] in 2006 was one of the first to question the appropriate management of FEA after core biopsy. These investigators subdivided the atypical columnar cell changes, unlike current standards, into those with and without hyperplasia, as had been recommended by Schnitt.[89] Most pathologists now lump both categories into FEA. David and colleagues[92] found 7 cases of carcinoma for a rate of 17.5% (7/40), but only in the cases of FEA with hyperplasia, and only in cases in which the lesion measured 10 mm or greater. Surgical management was advocated for both groups of FEA cases. Other studies advocating surgery report malignancy rates of 14% (9/63),[93] 17% (2/12),[94] 20% (3/15),[95] and 21% (3/14).[96] Not surprisingly, there are also studies with no malignancy upgrades that recommend only imaging follow-up: 0% (0/41),[97] 0% (0/20),[98] and 0% (0/20).[99] In all 3 studies that noted no malignancy upgrades, the investigators used 11-g vacuum-assisted needles. The number of cores ranged from 6 to 8 for Senetta and colleagues[97] and 12 to 24 (mean 15) for Noel and colleagues.[99] In the third study, 74% (14/20) of the cases of calcifications were either entirely or almost completely removed by the vacuum-assisted needle.[98] The study by Martel and colleagues[93] has data with some of the longest follow-up. There were 63 cases of FEA out of a total of 1751 core biopsies (3.6%) followed for an average of 6.2 years (range 1–11 years). Nine malignancies developed (9/63, 14.3%) of which 7 were ipsilateral (time to detection, mean 3.7 years [range 2–9 years]) and 2 were contralateral (time to detection, 7 years). Significant, however, is that 2 of the 7 ipsilateral cases had undergone interval biopsies before the invasive carcinoma diagnosis, but after the FEA diagnosis, and these interval results showed FEA with ADH. It is possible that FEA reflects a slow neoplastic process that may or may not grow into a carcinoma, and hence is a high-risk marker.

In addition to the usual shortcomings of retrospective studies of low-prevalent lesions, the literature on FEA is confounded by lack of agreement in pathology on the definitions of atypia within columnar cell change. Davishian and colleagues[94] studied pathologist interobserver variability in the categories of atypia. Fifty-one cases of atypia, specifically ADH, ALH, and FEA, were distributed, without being identified, to 4 specialized breast pathologists for independent review. Following this review, they gathered for a tutorial session to review the general criteria of atypia on a second set of known cases. The study cases were then re-reviewed as a group to come to a consensus diagnosis for each of the 51 cases. The independent reviews were used to determine the interobserver agreement using kappa statistics. The consensus diagnosis was used to determine the diagnosis for upgrade after surgical excision. Overall, this group achieved a substantially high agreement with an overall kappa value of 0.79 (95% CI 0.69–0.89) and 0.85 for FEA. Two other studies corroborated their findings that interobserver agreement in cases of columnar cell change improved with training.[100,101]

In summary, since the 2003 World Health Organization consensus meeting,[79] studies have shown conflicting results in the frequency of concurrent malignancy at the time of core biopsy of FEA. The trend seems to show that if the core sampling involves large vacuum-assisted needles and a large number of cores such that the mammographic lesion is almost completely removed, then the risk of leaving undetected existing malignancy is extremely low to nonexistent. FEA does seem to be a significant risk factor that warrants close imaging surveillance at the least.

MAGNETIC RESONANCE IMAGING FOR HIGH-RISK LESION EVALUATION

Magnetic resonance (MR) imaging has been studied as a potential tool to determine preoperatively the presence or absence of concurrent malignancy with high-risk lesions. Linda and colleagues[102] gathered 79 cases of high-risk lesions (18 lobular neoplasia, 26 benign papillomas, 29 radial scar, 6 ADH) that had been evaluated preoperatively by MR imaging. It is their common practice to perform MR imaging within 2 weeks of core biopsy for high-risk lesions. For this study, the lesions were independently reviewed by 2 radiologists, blinded to the final pathology results, who categorized the lesions into suspicious or nonsuspicious for malignancy. The frequency of nonsuspicious per lesion was: 25/29 radial scars, 11/18 lobular neoplasia, and 15/26 papillary lesions for a total of 51/73 nonatypia high-risk lesions. There were no malignancies at surgical follow-up of the cases categorized as nonsuspicious.

Pediconi and colleagues[103] evaluated MR prospectively using a different methodology. Thirty spiculated masses suspected of being radial scars at mammography underwent preoperative MR imaging. The definition distinguishing radial scar from malignancy at mammography was not specifically noted other than the presence of "radiolucent lines between dense spicules" in 23/30 cases. There were 18/30 cases without enhancement at MR imaging, with no malignancy present at surgical excision. The remaining 12 enhancing lesions were malignant (DCIS or invasive carcinoma).

Two studies of high-risk lesions and MR imaging discuss MR-guided core biopsy. A small study by Sadaf and colleagues[104] in abstract form retrospectively looked at 135 MR-guided biopsies: 8 lobular neoplasias, 2 benign papillomas, 3 radial scars, and 2 FEA. In all cases the biopsies were considered to be successful with a 9-g vacuum-assisted core needle and there were no differences in the number of core samples obtained. There were no differences in the morphologies and kinetics, or lesion type (mass versus non-masslike) in the malignant and benign groups. The underestimation rate for lobular neoplasia was 3/6 (50%) and FEA 1/2 (50%). No cancers were found in benign papilloma (N = 2) or radial scars (N = 3). Orel and colleagues'[105] initial experience of MR core biopsy using a 9-g vacuum-assisted probe reported 85 lesions including 7 cases of lobular neoplasia and 3 radial scars; none had malignancy at surgical follow-up. Of the 4 papillomas diagnosed at MR-guided core biopsy, 3 underwent surgery without malignancy.

These small preliminary studies suggest that MR imaging may be helpful in determining the need for surgical or imaging follow-up after core biopsy. Larger studies are needed to determine if these findings can be generalized.

CONCLUDING REMARKS

This article raises more questions than answers, and sadly illustrates that there has been little progress since the last time this topic was discussed in the 2004 *Radiologic Clinics of North America*.[1] More retrospective studies will never give us the answer as to how to manage these high-risk lesions after core biopsy, regardless of the imaging modality used to guide sampling. Prospective trials that meticulously track the imaging and pathology for accurate radiology/pathology concordance are sorely needed. Patients who are not surgically followed for gold standard determination must also be tracked to determine if outcomes are similar to or different form those undergoing surgery. Pathologists need to come to consensus as to definitions of ALH versus LCIS, ADH versus DCIS arising within papillomas, and columnar cell change versus columnar cell change with atypia (FEA). These definitions need to be reproducible so that pathologists around the world can accurately apply these features.

We appeal to the radiology and pathology communities to collaborate and test prospective, radiology/pathology, hypothesis driven studies that could provide evidence-based data to guide us in the appropriate follow-up when core biopsy yields a high-risk lesion.

APPENDIX: UNDERESTIMATION RATES (2004–2009)

Table 1
Lobular neoplasia

Frequency	Reference
A: Low prevalence	
0% (0/12)	40
0% (0/21)	41
1% (1/87)	37,a
2% (2/98)	36
B: High prevalence	
4% (1/25)	35,b
14% (3/21)	24
16% (1/6)	25
19% (10/52)	30
20% (7/35)	26
23% (38/164)	31
25% (5/20)	27
37% (13/35)	28
50% (9/18)	29

[a] Adjusted for radiology-pathology discordance and non-classic LCIS.
[b] Adjusted for radiology-pathology discordance and a missed lesion at core biopsy.

Table 2
Benign papilloma

Frequency	Reference
A: Low prevalence	
0% (0/25)	50
0% (0/67)	51
0% (0/17)	52
0% (0/63)	53,a
0% (0/40)	54
0% (0/35)	56,b
0% (0/42)	58,c
0% (0/19)	62,d
2% (1/43)	57
B: High prevalence	
7% (4/56)	46
9% (9/104)	61
10% (7/71)	60
10.5% (9/86)	47
17% (20/117)	48
19% (15/80)	59
29% (7/24)	49

[a] Adjusted for LCIS classified benign at surgical pathology.
[b] Adjusted for asymptomatic patients with stable mammograms.
[c] Adjusted for radiology-pathology discordance and stable mammogram.
[d] Excluded incidental, minute focus DCIS.

Table 3
Radial scar

Frequency	Reference
A: Low prevalence	
0% (0/80)	71
0% (0/27)	72
0.7% (2/281)	74,a
B: High prevalence	
4% (5/125)	69
8% (5/62)	73
9% (1/11)	25
22% (6/27)	68

[a] Excluded 9 cases of missed lesion at core.

Table 4 FEA	
Frequency	**Reference**
A: Low prevalence	
0% (0/41)	97
0% (0/20)	98
0% (0/20)	99
B: High prevalence	
14% (9/63)	93
17% (2/12)	94
17.5% (7/40)	92
20% (3/15)	95
21% (3/14)	96

REFERENCES

1. Berg W. Image-guided breast biopsy and management of high-risk lesions. Radiol Clin North Am 2004;42:935–46.

2. Lawton TL, Georgian-Smith D. Excision of high-risk breast lesions on needle biopsy: is there a standard of core? AJR Am J Roentgenol 2009;192:W268.

3. Jackman RJ, Burbank F, Parker SH, et al. Atypical ductal hyperplasia diagnosed at stereotactic breast biopsy: improved reliability with 14-gauge, directional, vacuum-assisted biopsy. Radiology 1997;204:485–8.

4. Brem RF, Behrndt VS, Sanow L, et al. Atypical ductal hyperplasia: histologic underestimation of carcinoma in tissue harvested from impalpable breast lesions using 11-gauge stereotactically guided directional vacuum-assisted biopsy. AJR Am J Roentgenol 1999;172:1405–7.

5. Philpotts LE, Lee CH, Horvath LJ, et al. Underestimation of breast cancer with 11-gauge vacuum suction biopsy. AJR Am J Roentgenol 2000;175:1047–50.

6. Jackman RJ, Birdwell RL, Ikeda DM. Atypical ductal hyperplasia: can some lesions be defined as probably benign after stereotactic 11g vacuum-assisted biopsy, eliminating the recommendation for surgical excision? Radiology 2002;224:548–54.

7. Li C, Daling JR, Malone KE. Age-specific incidence rates of in situ breast carcinomas by histologic type 1980–2001. Cancer Epidemiol Biomarkers Prev 2005;14:1008–11.

8. Page DL, Dupont WD, Rogers LW, et al. Atypical hyperplastic lesions of the female breast. A long-term follow-up study. Cancer 1985;55(11):2698–708.

9. Simpson PT, Gale T, Fulford LG, et al. The diagnosis and management of pre-invasive breast disease: pathology of atypical lobular hyperplasia and lobular carcinoma in situ. Breast Cancer Res 2003;5(5):258–62.

10. Wheeler JE, Enterline HT, Roseman JM, et al. Lobular carcinoma in situ of the breast. Long-term follow-up. Cancer 1974;34(3):554–63.

11. Rosen PP, Kosloff C, Lieberman PH, et al. Lobular carcinoma in situ of the breast. Detailed analysis of 99 patients with average follow-up of 24 years. Am J Surg Pathol 1978;2(3):225–51.

12. Dupont WD, Page DL. Risk factors for breast cancer in women with proliferative breast disease. N Engl J Med 1985;312(3):146–51.

13. Georgian-Smith D, Lawton TJ. Calcifications of lobular carcinoma in situ of the breast: radiologic and pathologic correlation. AJR Am J Roentgenol 2001;176(5):1255–9.

14. Jacobs TW, Pliss N, Kouria G, et al. Carcinomas in situ of the breast with indeterminate features: role of E-cadherin staining in categorization. Am J Surg 2001;25(2):229–36.

15. Maluf HM, Swanson PE, Koerner FC. Solid low-grade in situ carcinoma of the breast: role of associated lesions and E-cadherin in differential diagnosis. Am J Surg Pathol 2001;25(2):237–44.

16. Sneige N, Wang J, Baker BA, et al. Clinical, histopathologic, and biologic features of pleomorphic lobular (ductal-lobular) carcinoma in situ of the breast: a report of 24 cases. Mod Pathol 2002;15(10):1044–50.

17. Fadare O, Dadmanesh F, Alvarado-Cabrero I, et al. Lobular intraepithelial neoplasia [lobular carcinoma in situ] with comedo-type necrosis: a clinicopathologic study of 18 cases. Am J Surg Pathol 2006;30(11):1445–53.

18. Philpotts LE, Shaheen NA, Jain KS, et al. Uncommon high-risk lesions of the breast diagnosed at stereotactic core-needle biopsy: clinical importance. Radiology 2000;216(3):831–7.

19. Rosen PP. Lobular carcinoma in situ and atypical lobular hyperplasia. In: Rosen PP, editor. Rosen's breast pathology. Philadelphia: Lippincott-Raven; 1997. p. 507–44.

20. Rebner M, Raju U. Noninvasive breast cancer. Radiology 1994;190:623–31.

21. Sapino A, Frigerio A, Peterse JL, et al. Mammographically detected in situ lobular carcinomas of the breast. Virchows Arch 2000;436(5):421–30.

22. Stein LF, Zisman G, Rapelyea JA, et al. Lobular carcinoma in situ of the breast presenting as a mass. AJR Am J Roentgenol 2005;184:1799–801.

23. Tarjan G, Wiley EL, Spilde J, et al. Image detected lobular neoplasia of breast: morphologic correlation with imaging lesions. Scientific poster presentations. 23rd Annual San Antonio Breast Cancer Symposium. San Antonio (TX), December 6–9, 2000.

24. Arpino G, Allred DC, Mohsin SK, et al. Lobular neoplasia on core-needle biopsy – clinical significance. Cancer 2004;101(2):242–50.

25. Zuiani C, Londero V, Bestagno A, et al. Proliferative high-risk lesions of the breast: contribution and limits of US guided core biopsy. Radiol Med 2005;110(5–6):589–602.

26. Margenthaler JA, Duke D, Monsees BS, et al. Correlation between core biopsy and excisional biopsy in breast high-risk lesions. Am J Surg 2006;192(4):534–7.

27. Mahoney MC, Robinson-Smith TM, Shaughnessy EA. Lobular neoplasia at 11-gauge vacuum-assisted stereotactic biopsy: correlation with surgical excisional biopsy and mammographic follow-up. AJR Am J Roentgenol 2006;187:949–54.

28. Londero V, Zuiani C, Linda A, et al. Lobular neoplasia: core needle breast biopsy underestimation of malignancy in relation to radiologic and pathologic features. Breast 2008;17(6):623–30.

29. Elsheikh TM, Silverman JF. Follow-up surgical excision is indicated when breast core needle biopsies show atypical lobular hyperplasia or lobular carcinoma in situ: a correlative study of 33 patients with review of the literature. Am J Surg Pathol 2005;29(4):534–43.

30. Lavoue V, Graesslin O, Classe JM, et al. Management of lobular neoplasia diagnosed by core needle biopsy: study of 52 biopsies with follow-up surgical excision. Breast 2007;16(5):533–9.

31. Brem RF, Lechner MC, Jackman RJ, et al. Lobular neoplasia at percutaneous breast biopsy: variables associated with carcinoma at surgical excision. AJR Am J Roentgenol 2008;190(3):637–41.

32. Anderson BO, Calhoun KE, Rosen EL. Evolving concepts in the management of lobular neoplasia. J Natl Compr Canc Netw 2006;4(5):511–22.

33. Kopans DB. Lobular neoplasia on core-needle biopsy – clinical significance. Cancer 2004;101(12):2902–3.

34. Kopans DB. LCIS found at core needle biopsy may not need surgical excision. AJR Am J Roentgenol 2008;191:W152.

35. Menon S, Porter GJ, Evans AJ, et al. The significance of lobular neoplasia on needle core biopsy of the breast. Virchows Arch 2008;452(5):473–9.

36. Nagi CS, O'Donnell JE, Tismenetsky M, et al. Lobular neoplasia on core needle biopsy does not require excision. Cancer 2008;112(10):2152–8.

37. Hwang H, Barke LD, Mendelson EB, et al. Atypical lobular hyperplasia and classic lobular carcinoma in situ in core biopsy specimens: routine excision is not necessary. Mod Pathol 2008;21:1208–16.

38. Chuba PJ, Hamre MR, Yap J, et al. Bilateral risk for subsequent breast cancer after lobular carcinoma-in-situ: analysis of surveillance, epidemiology, and end results data. J Clin Oncol 2005;23(24):5534–41.

39. Page DL, Simpson JF. What is atypical lobular hyperplasia and what does it mean for the patient? J Clin Oncol 2005;23(24):5432–3.

40. Mulheron B, Gray RJ, Pockaj BA, et al. Is excisional biopsy indicated for patients with lobular neoplasia diagnosed on percutaneous core needle biopsy of the breast? Am J Surg 2009;198(6):792–7.

41. Sohn VY, Arthurs ZM, Kim FS, et al. Lobular neoplasia: is surgical excision warranted? Am Surg 2008;74(2):172–7.

42. Page DL, Salhany KE, Jensen RA, et al. Subsequent breast carcinoma risk after biopsy with atypia in a breast papilloma. Cancer 1996;78(2):258–66.

43. Collins LC, Schnitt SJ. Papillary lesions of the breast: selected diagnostic and management issues. Histopathology 2008;52(1):20–9.

44. Lewis JT, Hartmann LC, Vierkant RA, et al. An analysis of breast cancer risk in women with single, multiple, and atypical papilloma. Am J Surg Pathol 2006;30(6):665–72.

45. Harjit K, Willsher PC, Bennett M, et al. Multiple papillomas of the breast: is current management adequate? Breast 2006;15:777–81.

46. Sakr R, Rouzier R, Salem C, et al. Risk of breast cancer associated with papilloma. Eur J Surg Oncol 2008;34:1304–8.

47. Rizzo M, Lund MJ, Oprea G, et al. Surgical follow-up and clinical presentation of 142 breast papillary lesions diagnosed by ultrasound-guided core-needle biopsy. Ann Surg Oncol 2008;15(4):1040–7.

48. Shin HJ, Kim HH, Kim SM, et al. Papillary lesions of the breast diagnosed at percutaneous sonographically guided biopsy: comparison of sonographic features and biopsy methods. AJR Am J Roentgenol 2008;190:630–6.

49. Tseng HS, Chen YL, Chen ST, et al. The management of papillary lesion of the breast by core needle biopsy. Eur J Surg Oncol 2009;35:21–4.

50. Agoff SN, Lawton TJ. Papillary lesions of the breast with and without atypical ductal hyperplasia: can we accurately predict benign behavior from core needle biopsy? Am J Clin Pathol 2004;122(3):440–3.

51. Arora N, Hill C, Hoda SA, et al. Clinicopathologic features of papillary lesions on core needle biopsy of the breast predictive of malignancy. Am J Surg 2007;194(4):444–9.

52. Carder PJ, Garvican J, Haigh I, et al. Needle core biopsy can reliably distinguish between benign and malignant papillary lesions of the breast. Histopathology 2005;46:320–7.

53. Sydnor MK, Wilson JD, Hijaz TA, et al. Underestimation of presence of breast carcinoma in papillary lesions initially diagnosed at core-needle biopsy. Radiology 2007;242(1):58–62.

54. Zografos GC, Zagouri F, Sergentanis TN, et al. Diagnosing papillary lesions using vacuum-assisted breast biopsy: should conservative or surgical management follow? Onkologie 2008;31: 653–6.

55. Carder PJ, Khan T, Burrows P, et al. Large volume "mammotome" biopsy may reduce the need for diagnostic surgery in papillary lesions of the breast. J Clin Pathol 2008;61:923–33.

56. Liberman L, Tornos C, Huzjan R, et al. Is surgical excision warranted after benign, concordant diagnosis of papilloma at percutaneous breast biopsy? AJR Am J Roentgenol 2006;186:1328–34.

57. Ko ES, Cho N, Cha JH, et al. Sonographically-guided 14 gauge core needle biopsy for papillary lesions of the breast. Korean J Radiol 2007;8(3): 206–11.

58. Mercado CL, Hamele-Bena D, Oken SM, et al. Papillary lesions of the breast at percutaneous core-needle biopsy. Radiology 2006;238(3):801–8.

59. Skandarajah AR, Field L, Yuen Larn Mou A, et al. Benign papilloma on core biopsy requires surgical excision. Ann Surg Oncol 2008;15(8):2272–7.

60. Bernik SF, Troob S, Ying BL, et al. Papillary lesions of the breast diagnosed by core needle biopsy: 71 cases with surgical follow-up. Am J Surg 2009; 197(4):473–8.

61. Jaffer S, Nagi C, Bleiweiss IJ. Excision is indicated for intraductal papilloma of the breast diagnosed on core needle biopsy. Cancer 2009;115(13): 2837–43.

62. Sahasrabudhe N, Beetles U, Coyne J. Accuracy of needle core biopsies in the diagnosis of papillary breast lesions. Histopathology 2006;49:91.

63. BI-RADS® - Ultrasound American College of Radiology (ACR) breast imaging reporting and data system atlas (BI-RADS® atlas). 1st edition. Reston (VA): American College of Radiology; 2003.

64. Lam WW, Chu WC, Tang AP, et al. Role of radiologic features in the management of papillary lesions of the breast. AJR Am J Roentgenol 2006; 188:1322–7.

65. Chang JM, Moon WK, Cho N, et al. Ultrasound detected benign papilloma diagnosed at percutaneous breast biopsy: upgrade rate at surgical excision. Scientific session SSK01-05 [abstract]. Radiological Society of North America 95th Scientific Assembly and Annual Meeting. Chicago (IL), November 29 to December 4, 2009. p. 521.

66. Kil WH, Cho EY, Kim JH, et al. Is surgical excision necessary in benign papillary lesions initially diagnosed at core biopsy? Breast 2008; 17:258–62.

67. Page D, Anderson T. Radial scars and complex sclerosing lesions. Page D. In: Anderson T, editor. Diagnostic histopathology of the breast. Edinburgh (UK): Churchill Livingston; 1987. p. 89–103.

68. Lopez-Medina A, Cintora E, Mugica B, et al. Radial scars diagnosed at stereotactic core-needle biopsy: surgical biopsy findings. Eur Radiol 2006; 16:1803–10.

69. Becker L, Trop I, David J, et al. Management of radial scars found at percutaneous breast biopsy. Can Assoc Radiol J 2006;57(2):72–8.

70. Brenner RJ, Jackman RJ, Parker SH, et al. Percutaneous core needle biopsy of radial scars: when is excision necessary? AJR Am J Roentgenol 2002; 179:1179–84.

71. Resetkova E, Edelweiss M, Albarracin CT, et al. Management of radial sclerosing lesions of the breast diagnosed using percutaneous vacuum-assisted core needle biopsy: recommendations for excision based on seven years' of experience at a single institution. Breast Cancer Res Treat 2008. [Epub ahead of print].

72. Cawson JN, Malara F, Kavanagh A, et al. Fourteen-gauge needle core biopsy of mammographically evident radial scars: is excision necessary? Cancer 2003;97(2):345–51.

73. Linda A, Zuiani C, Furlan A, et al. Radial scars without atypia diagnosed at image-guided needle biopsy: how often is associated malignancy found at subsequent surgical excision, and do mammography and sonography predict which lesions are malignant? AJR Am J Roentgenol 2010;194(4):1146–51.

74. Douglas-Jones AG, Denson JL, Cox AC, et al. Radial scar lesions of the breast diagnosed by needle core biopsy: analysis of cases containing occult malignancy. J Clin Pathol 2007;60(3):295–8.

75. Rosai J. Borderline epithelial lesions of the breast. Am J Surg Pathol 1991;15(3):209–21.

76. Schnitt SJ, Connolly JL, Tavassoli FA, et al. Interobserver reproducibility in the diagnosis of ductal proliferative breast lesions using standardized criteria. Am J Surg Pathol 1992;16(12):1133–43.

77. Brodie C, O'Doherty A, Quinn C. Fourteen-gauge needle core biopsy of mammographically evident radial scars: is excision necessary? [letter to the editor]. Cancer 2004;100(3):652–3.

78. Cawson JN, Hill P, Henderson M. Fourteen-gauge needle core biopsy of mammographically evident radial scars: is excision necessary? Cancer 2004; 100(3):653–4 Author reply letter to the editor.

79. Tavassoli FA, Hoefler H, Rosai J, et al. Intraductal proliferative lesions. In: Tavassoli FA, Devillee P, editors. World Health Organization classification of tumors of the breast and female genital organs. Lyon (France): IARC Press; 2003. p. 63–75.

80. Pandey S, Kornstein MJ, Shanke W, et al. Columnar cell lesions of the breast: mammographic findings

with histopathologic correlation [special issue]. Radiographics 2007;27(Suppl 1):79–89.

81. Goldstein NS, O'Malley BA. Cancerization of small ectatic ducts of the breast by ductal carcinoma in situ cells with apocrine snouts: a lesion associated with tubular carcinoma. Am J Clin Pathol 1997; 107(5):561–6.

82. Oyama T, Maluf H, Koerner F. Atypical cystic lobules: an early stage in the formation of low-grade ductal carcinoma in situ. Virchows Arch 1999;435(4):413–21.

83. Rosen PP. Columnar cell hyperplasia is associated with lobular carcinoma in situ and tubular carcinoma. Am J Surg Pathol 1999;23(12):1561.

84. Brogi E, Oyama T, Koerner FC. Atypical cystic lobules in patients with lobular neoplasia. Int J Surg Pathol 2001;9(3):201–6.

85. Bratthauer GL, Tavassoli FA. Assessment of lesions coexisting with various grades of ductal intraepithelial neoplasia of the breast. Virchows Arch 2004;444(4):340–4.

86. Abdel-Fatah TM, Powe DG, Hodi Z. High frequency of coexistence of columnar cell lesions, lobular neoplasia, and low grade ductal carcinoma in situ with invasive tubular carcinoma and invasive lobular carcinoma. Am J Surg Pathol 2007;31(3): 417–26.

87. Collins LC, Achacoso NA, Nekhlyudov L, et al. Clinical and pathologic features of ductal carcinoma in situ associated with the presence of flat epithelial atypia: an analysis of 543 patients. Mod Pathol 2007;20(11):1149–55.

88. Leibl S, Regitnig P, Moinfar F. Flat epithelial atypia (DIN 1a, atypical columnar change): an under diagnosed entity very frequently coexisting with lobular neoplasia. Histopathology 2007;50(7):859–65.

89. Schnitt SJ. The diagnosis and management of preinvasive breast disease: flat epithelial atypia – classification, pathologic features and clinical significance. Breast Cancer Res 2003;5(5):263–8.

90. Lerwill MF. Flat epithelial atypia of the breast. Arch Pathol Lab Med 2008;132(4):615–21.

91. Moinfar F. Flat ductal intraepithelial neoplasia of the breast: a review of diagnostic criteria, differential diagnoses, molecular-genetic findings, and clinical relevance – it is time to appreciate the Azzopardi concept!. Arch Pathol Lab Med 2009;133(6):879–92.

92. David N, Labbe-Devilliers C, Moreau D, et al. Lesions de metaplasie cylindriques atypiques (MCA) diagnostiquees par macrobiopsies assistees par aspiration: opportunite d'une exerese chirugicale? J Radiol 2006;87(11):1671–7 [in French].

93. Martel M, Barron-Rodriguez P, Ocal IT, et al. Flat DIN (flat epithelial atypia) on core needle biopsy: 63 cases identified retrospectively among 1,751

core biopsies performed over an 8-year period (1992–1999). Virchows Arch 2007;451:883–91.

94. Darvishian F, Singh B, Simsir A, et al. Atypia on breast core needle biopsies: reproducibility and significance. Ann Clin Lab Sci 2009;39(3):270–6.

95. Ingegnoli A, D'Aloia C, Frattaruolo A, et al. Flat epithelial atypical and atypical ductal hyperplasia: carcinoma underestimation rate. Breast J 2009; 13:1–5.

96. Kunju LP, Kleer CG. Significance of flat epithelial atypia on mammotome core needle biopsy: should it be excised? Hum Pathol 2007;38(1):35–41.

97. Senetta R, Campanino PP, Mariscotti G, et al. Columnar cell lesions associated with breast calcifications on vacuum-assisted core biopsies: clinical, radiographic, and histologic correlations. Mod Pathol 2009;22:762–9.

98. Piubello Q, Parisi A, Eccher A, et al. Flat epithelial atypia on core needle biopsy: which is the right management? Am J Surg Pathol 2009;33(7): 1078–84.

99. Noel JC, Buxant F, Engohan-Aloghe C. Immediate surgical resection of residual microcalcifications after a diagnosis of pure flat epithelial atypia on core biopsy: a word of caution. Surg Oncol 2009. [Epub ahead of print].

100. Tan PH, Ho BC, Selvarajan S, et al. Pathological diagnosis of columnar cell lesions of the breast: are there issues of reproducibility? J Clin Pathol 2005;58:705–9.

101. O'Malley FP, Mohsin SK, Badve S, et al. Interobserver reproducibility in the diagnosis of flat epithelial atypia of the breast. Mod Pathol 2006; 19:172–9.

102. Linda A, Zuiani C, Bazzocchi M, et al. Borderline breast lesions diagnosed at core needle biopsy: can magnetic resonance mammography rule out associated malignancy? Preliminary results based on 79 surgically excised lesions. Breast 2008;17: 125–31.

103. Pediconi F, Occhiato R, Venditti F, et al. Radial scars of the breast: contrast enhanced magnetic resonance mammography appearance. Breast J 2005;11(1):23–8.

104. Sadaf A, Bukhanov K, McCready DR, et al. High risk breast lesions diagnosed with MRI guided vacuum-assisted breast biopsy (MRgVABB): can underestimation be predicted? [abstract SSK01-09] Radiological Society of North America 95th Scientific Assembly and Annual Meeting. Chicago (IL), November 29 to December 4, 2009. p. 522–3.

105. Orel SG, Rosen M, Mies C, et al. MR imaging-guided 9-gauge vacuum-assisted core-needle breast biopsy: initial experience. Radiology 2006; 238(1):54–61.

Breast MR Imaging: Current Indications and Advanced Imaging Techniques

Susan Weinstein, MD[a], Mark Rosen, MD, PhD[b],*

KEYWORDS

- Breast cancer • Magnetic resonance imaging • Diffusion
- Spectroscopy

Breast cancer is the most common solid tumor diagnosed in women. The American Cancer Society estimates that in 2009 there will be 192,000 new cases of breast cancer diagnosed,[1] and that some 40,000 women will die from breast cancer in 2009. In the past decades, strides have been made in breast cancer screening. Improved awareness and screening have resulted in early diagnosis, which in turn has resulted in improved survival rates in women diagnosed with breast cancer. Before mammographic screening, intraductal carcinoma (DCIS) represented 2% of breast cancers. Nowadays, DCIS makes up approximately 20% of breast cancers diagnosed, primarily screen-detected disease. While multiple screening trials have shown the benefits of screening mammography, there are limitations to x-ray mammography. The overall sensitivity of mammography is approximately 85%.[2] However, the sensitivity of mammography varies by breast density. In the fatty breast, the sensitivity of mammography is excellent, and has been reported to be in the percentage range of the high 90's. In the dense breast, however, the sensitivity is much lower, closer to 50%.[3,4] In populations who are at extremely high risk for breast cancer, such as the BRCA1/2 mutation carriers, the sensitivity is reportedly even lower.[5] Given the inherent limitations in x-ray mammography, efforts have been made to develop adjunctive imaging techniques, including screening ultrasound, gamma-specific breast imaging, breast tomosynthesis, dedicated breast computed tomography (CT), and breast magnetic resonance (MR) imaging. Some of these techniques, such as tomosynthesis and dedicated breast CT, are currently research tools and are not approved by the Food and Drug Administration (FDA) at the time publication. In this article, the authors address the current indications and advanced imaging applications of breast MR imaging.

The use of gadolinium contrast in breast MR imaging to detect cancer was first reported in 1989.[6,7] Since then, the technology has significantly improved, with high image signal to noise ratios (SNR) and faster scanning speed. Since the initial studies, breast MR imaging is now widely used in a variety of clinical settings. One of the most common uses is local staging in patients with recent diagnosis of breast cancer, where MR imaging may be used to evaluate for multifocal or multicentric tumor as well as chest wall invasion. At the time of the ipsilateral breast evaluation, the contralateral breast may be imaged and screened for clinically and mammographically occult breast cancer. Other indications for breast MR imaging include screening in high-risk women who have a greater than 20% to 25% lifetime risk

[a] Division of Breast Imaging, Department of Radiology, University of Pennsylvania School of Medicine, 1 Silverstein Building, 3400 Spruce Street, Philadelphia, PA 19104, USA
[b] Division of Body MRI, Department of Radiology, University of Pennsylvania School of Medicine, 1 Silverstein Building, 3400 Spruce Street, Philadelphia, PA 19104, USA
* Corresponding author.
E-mail address: mark.rosen@uphs.upenn.edu

Radiol Clin N Am 48 (2010) 1013–1042
doi:10.1016/j.rcl.2010.06.011

for breast cancer. MR imaging may also be used to evaluate clinically concerning nipple discharge, to evaluate an indeterminate mammographic abnormality, to monitor response to neoadjuvant chemotherapy in patients with locally advanced breast cancer, and to evaluate patients who present with axillary lymph node metastasis with negative mammographic and clinical breast evaluation.

In this article the authors cover basic breast MR imaging techniques as well as more advanced MR imaging applications, including image acceleration, diffusion-weighted imaging (DWI), spectroscopy, and 3-Tesla (T) imaging. The common clinical uses of breast MR imaging are reviewed. Finally, the controversies related to breast MR imaging are discussed.

BACKGROUND

The formation of neovascularity by the malignant tumor serves as the basis for breast cancer detection by MR imaging. With the use of gadolinium-based intravenous contrast agents, the sensitivity of MR imaging for invasive breast cancer approaches 100%. The neovasculature of cancers does not resemble blood vessels found in normal tissue or benign lesions. These new blood vessels have increased permeability (ie, "leakiness") resulting in rapid tumor uptake of contrast and early enhancement on MR imaging. In many, but not all breast cancers, this leaky vasculature also results in early washout of contrast. The rapid early uptake and subsequent washout of contrast produces a dynamic enhancement pattern that helps to differentiate malignant from benign enhancing breast lesions.

Just as breast density limits the sensitivity of mammography, the degree of background or physiologic glandular enhancement limits the sensitivity of MR imaging. This background physiologic enhancement may "mask" enhancing cancers on MR imaging, just as dense breast tissue may obscure a cancer of the same density at mammography. The degree of background enhancement, quantified by the volume and the intensity of enhancing glandular tissue, is categorized as "minimal" (<25% volumetric enhancement), "mild" (25%–50% volumetric enhancement), "moderate" (50%–75% volumetric enhancement), or "marked" (>75% volumetric enhancement) (Fig. 1). To minimize physiologic enhancement, it is recommended that premenopausal women be imaged between days 7 and 14 of the menstrual cycle.[8] Although this may be possible for screening MR imaging studies, it may not be feasible to postpone imaging until days 7 to 14 of the subsequent menstrual cycle

in patients with recently diagnosed breast cancer referred for preoperative MR imaging for local staging.

Many benign lesions such as lymph nodes, fibroadenomas, papillomas, radial scars, abscesses, and fat necrosis may also enhance following gadolinium administration (Figs. 2 and 3), as can risk-marker lesions such as lobular carcinoma in situ or atypical ductal hyperplasia, and benign proliferative and fibrocystic changes. Thus, whereas the sensitivity of MR imaging has been reported to be high, in the range of 71% to 100%,[9] the specificity of MR imaging is reported to be lower, often in the range of 60% to 70%.[10–13] In prospective and retrospective screening studies, the reported positive predicted value (PPV) of MR biopsies ranges from 17% to 89%.[3,14–21] In addition, the sensitivity of MR imaging for intraductal carcinoma in situ (DCIS) was initially reported to be lower,[22–27] especially for lower-grade DCIS lesions presenting as mammographic calcifications. However, MR imaging is highly sensitive (98%) in detecting high-grade intraductal carcinoma, and may detect DCIS lesions that are not detected by conventional mammography.[28]

BASIC MR TECHNIQUES FOR BREAST CANCER IMAGING

Since the early development of breast MR imaging, numerous technical developments, variations, and innovations have been described and often debated. Given the dynamic nature of MR imaging technology and the rapid pace of advances in hardware and software, any description of standard breast MR imaging techniques or protocols is by nature a reflection of the current state of the technology and the science as applied by breast imagers. This section describes the basic features of a breast MR imaging protocol common to nearly all imaging facilities. Subsequent sections describe newer innovations that are under evaluation but have not, to date, become routinely applied to MR imaging for breast cancer evaluation.

Breast MR Imaging Coils and Patient Positioning

All breast MR imaging is performed with the patient in the prone position, lying on a dedicated breast "coil." The coil contains 2 separate depressions, or wells, in which the breasts lie dependently. Housed within these depressions are the electronic receiver coils, which detect the weak magnetic signals from the breast that arise during the MR imaging examination.

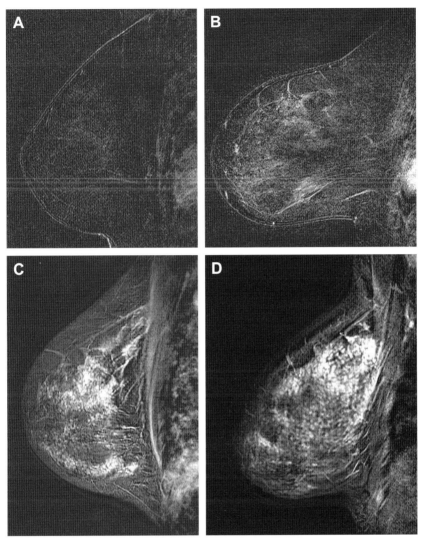

Fig. 1. Patterns of glandular enhancement. Subtraction sagittal MR imaging images in women without focal enhancing lesions demonstrate degree and patterns of background enhancement. (*A*) Minimal glandular enhancement. (*B*) Mild glandular enhancement. (*C*) Moderate glandular enhancement. (*D*) Marked glandular enhancement.

Prone patient positioning minimizes the effects of respiratory motion on images, and helps to move the breasts away from the chest wall and the resulting artifacts from cardiac and respiratory movement. However, optimal breast MR imaging requires careful patient positioning to assure that the breasts are optimally seated within the coil areas. Patient comfort is vital, as the breast MR imaging examination can last 30 minutes or longer, and any patient discomfort is likely to manifest as movement during or between scans. Intravenous access for contrast administration should be placed ahead of time and secured to a power injector, so as to minimize any interaction between technologist and patient (which may lead to

inadvertent patient motion) once the examination has begun.

All coil manufacturers use a similar basic design of 2 individual wells for the left and right breast. Coil designs vary in the number and placement of the receive coils that detect the MR imaging signals for reconstructing the images. Breast coils may function with as few as 2 receiver coils (one for each breast). More often, combinations of coils—ranging in number from 4 to up to 32—are available.[29] Choice of breast coil for MR imaging will depend on availability for each magnet manufacturer and field strength. In general, breast coils with a larger number of individual receive channels will provide

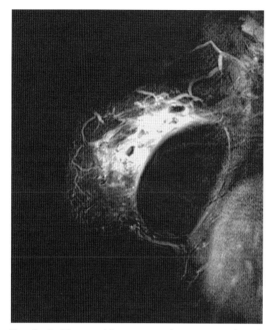

Fig. 2. A 36-year-old woman who presented with right breast pain. Saline implants are present that were placed several years previously. Bilateral MR imaging demonstrated an asymmetric area regional area of enhancement. Given the asymmetry and the intense enhancement, the finding was felt to be suspicious for malignancy. Core needle biopsy revealed an organizing abscess with periductal inflammation.

higher imaging SNR[30,31] and greater adaptability for advanced imaging techniques.[32–34] However, standard 4-channel coils can provide very robust performance. Other factors in evaluating a breast

coil are durability, patient comfort, and ease of access to the breast for MR imaging–guided interventions.

MR Imaging Field Strength

Breast MR imaging has been reported at low field strengths (ie, 1.0 T and less).[35–38] However, the current recommendations require that breast MR imaging be performed at 1.5 T or higher. The higher field strength enables the acquisition of high-resolution imaging with adequate SNR, and enables the use of fat suppression. Imaging at 3.0 T provides an opportunity for even greater improvement in SNR, increased image resolution, and faster imaging.[39–42] However, to date no studies have demonstrated conclusively that advantages of breast MR imaging at 3 T mandate its use over 1.5 T imaging, and 1.5 T remains the norm for breast MR imaging applications in many centers.

Imaging Protocols

Gadolinium-enhanced T1-weighted imaging
Innumerable variations in imaging protocols have been described in the literature. Common to all breast MR imaging protocols for cancer evaluation is the use of small molecular weight gadolinium-based contrast agents to depict enhancing lesions on T1-weighted (T1W) imaging. Imaging should be done with adequate resolution so that the morphologic features of the enhancing lesions are clearly demonstrated. Higher imaging matrices (at least 256 × 256 pixels, but often 512 × 256 or higher)

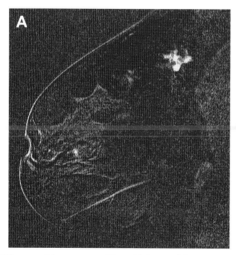
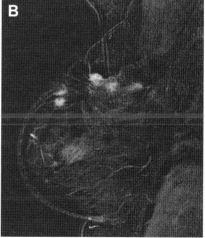

Fig. 3. A 66-year-old woman with a history of breast cancer. (A) The patient's original cancer is shown in the subtraction MR imaging image. The patient subsequently had lumpectomy followed by radiation therapy. (B) Two years later, the patient had an MR imaging that showed multiple areas of irregular enhancement. The appearance was felt to be highly suspicious for malignancy. Percutaneous biopsy revealed fat necrosis. The patient subsequently underwent excisional biopsy, which confirmed the diagnosis.

allow for improved in-plane resolution. Three-dimensional imaging is generally preferred to facilitate the use of thin slices without interslice gaps.

The T1W imaging should be done before and immediately following intravenous bolus contrast administration, with imaging performed as rapidly as possible post contrast to ensure that the early phase of enhancement (ie, the time window between maximal enhancement of malignant lesions and the subsequent more delayed enhancement of background breast parenchyma and benign lesions) is sampled. For this reason gradient echo sequences, which are faster than spin echo sequences, are used.

Most practitioners recommend that imaging be undertaken in the first 1 to 2 minutes after contrast administration, with additional acquisitions continued for a total of 4 to 8 minutes to define the dynamic enhancement pattern of enhancing lesions. However, to depict the morphology of enhancing breast lesions optimally, high-spatial-resolution imaging is required, a feature that limits the achievable temporal resolution with standard MR imaging techniques. Bilateral imaging is strongly recommended so that asymmetries in breast enhancement may be appreciated. However, simultaneous bilateral imaging, depending on the protocol used, can place additional restrictions on the spatial and/or temporal image resolution of the dynamic T1W sequence.

The breast MR radiologist must factor in these issues when designing the breast imaging protocol on their MR system. Recommended guidelines for breast MR imaging from the American College of Radiology (ACR) include[43]:

- Simultaneous bilateral imaging
- Temporal resolution
  5 minutes or less (single postcontrast image)
  3 minutes or less (for multiphase kinetic analysis)
- Minimal spatial resolution:
  ≤ 1 mm (in-plane)
  ≤ 3 mm (slice thickness).

Other aspects of gadolinium-enhanced imaging that must be chosen include the plane of imaging and the use of fat suppression. The ACR guidelines encourage the use of fat-suppression techniques to augment the contrast between enhancing and nonenhancing tissues and to improve the dynamic range of the T1W images. The use of subtraction techniques between pre- and postcontrast imaging may also be used to optimize the depiction of enhancing lesions. However, other practitioners

have championed nonfat-suppressed T1W imaging, which can reduce scan times and avoid fat-suppression artifacts, relying solely on subtraction of the precontrast images from the postcontrast images to highlight enhancing lesions.

Imaging plane is also an important feature of breast MR imaging protocols. In many cases, the use of ultrathin (≤ 1 mm) slices to achieve (near-)isotropic voxels may lead to unacceptably poor image SNR and/or inadequate temporal resolution. As result, with the use of anisotropic voxels, the plane of acquisition becomes the optimal viewing orientation of the dynamic gadolinium-enhanced imaging. Sagittal or axial planes of acquisition are therefore preferred, as these planes allow for better depiction of the ductal organization of the breast glandular tissue than does the coronal plane. Sagittal imaging provides the opportunity for much higher in-plane resolution because of the small imaging field of view (FOV) obtainable. However, simultaneous bilateral sagittal imaging is challenging on some software systems, may require longer imaging times, and can lead to inadvertent exclusion of breast tissue in the axillary region. Axial imaging is therefore often used for bilateral breast MR imaging, although the larger FOV places practical limits on in-plane resolution (generally on the order of 1 mm per pixel).

Implementation of the dynamic enhanced imaging requires careful monitoring by the MR imaging technologist. The intravenous line should be in place and secured to a power injector before the examination begins. Precontrast T1W imaging should be checked carefully to ensure adequate breast coverage and lack of severe artifacts. Postcontrast imaging should begin immediately after the intravenous gadolinium bolus (0.1 mmol Gd/kg) and saline flush are completed. The optimal timing of the initial postcontrast scan relative to the end of contrast injection depends on the rapidity of scanning. In general, scanning is begun once the contrast bolus is complete, during saline flush. However, for very rapid imaging, initiation of the scan sequence before the end of the saline flush may produce an initial postcontrast image that is acquired too early, before malignant lesions are optimally enhanced.

Non-gadolinium-enhanced sequences
In addition to the standard dynamic gadolinium-enhanced T1W imaging, the breast MR imaging examination is generally supplemented with a T2-weighted (T2W) sequence. T2W imaging

can depict nonenhancing structures that correlate to mammographic or palpable findings, including simple or complex cysts, and dilated retroareolar ducts. T2W imaging can also help characterize certain benign lesions such as fibroadenomas, which may have a characteristic appearance on T2W images (**Fig. 4**).[44,45]

If fat-suppressed T1W imaging is performed before and after gadolinium administration, inclusion of a nonfat-suppressed T1W image before gadolinium administration may provide improved morphologic depiction of certain enhancing lesions, such as fat necrosis or lymph nodes (**Fig. 5**).[46,47] Nonfat-suppressed T1W imaging may also depict to better advantage lesions such as angiolipomas and hamartomas.[48,49]

Nephrogenic fibrosing sclerosis

In 2007, the FDA issued a warning for the administration of gadolinium-containing contrast agents in patients with renal insufficiency.[50] These new guidelines were a response to reported association[51,52] between gadolinium administration and nephrogenic fibrosing sclerosis (NSF), a disorder of progressive skin and organ fibrosis, which in severe cases can lead to significant morbidity and mortality. Although frequency of the association varies with different contrast agents, all gadolinium-based agents pose a risk. However, the association between gadolinium and NSF was only seen in patients with severe renal insufficiency, suggesting a link between circulation times of gadolinium and the disorder. At the time of writing, the FDA guidelines[50] recommend that gadolinium administration be avoided in any patient with severe renal insufficiency, defined as an estimated glomerular filtration rate (GFR) of ≤ 30 mL/min/1.73 m^2, and that dosage not exceed the standard 0.1 mmol/kg gadolinium.

ADVANCED MR IMAGING TECHNIQUES IN BREAST CANCER
Breast MR Imaging at 3 T

With the advent of 3-T imaging, many investigators began to explore the options that breast imaging at this higher field would allow. At present, all major vendors provide breast coils for use at 3 T, many of which have features such as multicoil arrangements that are optimized for parallel imaging. In general, the signal of MR imaging increases by the square of the field strength, while the noise increases linearly with field strength. Thus, 3-T breast MR imaging in theory provides twice the SNR of 1.5-T breast MR imaging. Another factor that comes into play at 3 T is the lengthening of tissue T1 relaxation times, a phenomenon that can be parlayed into greater tissue contrast if appropriate parameter adjustments are made. Also, the higher field strength at 3 T increases the separation, or spectral dispersion, between lipid and water, providing improved opportunities for more efficient fat suppression while increasing the resolution of MR spectroscopy.

Despite these advances, to date no large prospective trial has demonstrated a conclusive clinical advantage of 3-T breast MR imaging over that performed at 1.5 T. A multisite clinical trial testing such a hypothesis would be challenging to perform, and current data from the literature rely mostly on small single-site studies detailing experiences of imaging at 3 T. However, a few studies have directly compared 1.5-T and 3-T imaging. Kuhl and colleagues[42] found higher

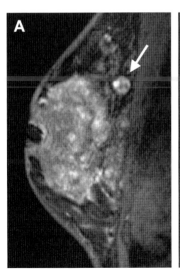 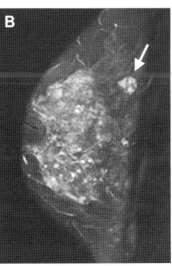

Fig. 4. Characteristic T2W image of a fibroadenoma. (*A*) Post-gadolinium image demonstrates a focal enhancing lesion in the upper posterior breast (*arrow*), with nonenhancing septations, a morphology highly characteristic of fibroadenoma. (*B*) The corresponding T2W image is shown (*arrow*), demonstrating a high signal intensity lesion with dark septations, correlating well with the gadolinium-enhanced image. High T2W signal in solid lesions may be a useful adjunctive finding of benignity, especially when the pattern of dark internal septations on both image sets is demonstrated, as is shown here.

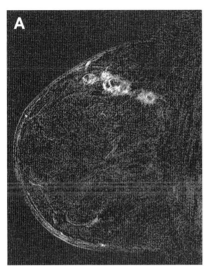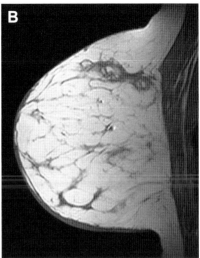

Fig. 5. Usefulness of nonfat-suppressed T1 imaging. MR imaging of a women with prior history of breast reduction, and new palpable findings in the superior breast. (*A*) Subtraction post-gadolinium image demonstrates multiple irregular avidly enhancing foci. Note that geometric pattern of enhancing foci does not correspond to normal ductal morphology. (*B*) T1 nonfat-suppressed spin echo image at the same location confirms the presence of central fat within these foci, a finding pathognomonic for fat necrosis.

diagnostic confidence for lesion depiction at 3 T than at 1.5 T, though performance depended on optimized imaging parameters. However, downsides of 3-T breast imaging, such as greater B1 field inhomogeneity,[53] have been noted. As such, translating the benefits of 3-T breast MR imaging to improvements in clinical performance will require more than higher-quality images. Rather, more robust acquisition techniques that result in improvements in the specificity and accuracy of breast lesion characterization are required to realize the potential clinical benefit of 3-T breast MR imaging.

Temporal Versus Spatial Resolution

As discussed earlier, the breast MR radiologist must make choices between spatial resolution, temporal resolution, and optimal volume coverage. The physics of MR imaging presents obstacles that prevent one from achieving an imaging protocol that optimally satisfies all of these diverging demands. Very thin slice imaging to achieve isotropic voxels requires longer imaging times, which risks missing the early phase of post-gadolinium enhancement when the contrast between malignant and benign lesions is greatest. The use of sagittal imaging plane allows for smaller imaging FOVs, thus dramatically increasing the in-plane resolution. However, sagittal imaging requires a larger number of slices for bilateral breast examinations, thus lengthening the time of imaging. Conversely, very rapid imaging (on the

order of 5–15 seconds per image) can be achieved, but only if one uses lower resolution imaging (such that lesion morphology is compromised), or focuses imaging on only a portion of one breast (a solution that is impractical for routine clinical implementation). As such, one cannot with conventional imaging sequences achieve optimal techniques in all aspects of spatial/temporal resolution and volume coverage.

Given these technical limits, much debate has arisen over the influence of both temporal and spatial resolution on the accuracy of breast MR imaging. Some early researchers advocated using temporal resolution as low as 12 seconds with single-slice techniques for optimal temporal kinetic evaluation of breast lesions.[54] Others have shown that reducing temporal resolution to 45 seconds does not impair kinetic curve analysis.[55] On the other hand, very rapid imaging allows for more quantitative pharmacologic modeling of breast lesion enhancement kinetics,[56,57] a process that may require extremely high (on the order of 2–3 seconds) temporal resolution.

Initial reports of the *morphologic* approach to breast MR imaging lesion characterization used a high-resolution imaging protocol with in-plane resolution of approximately 0.3 mm/pixel but temporal resolution of approximately 2 minutes per scan.[58,59] Conversely, researchers using a more *dynamic* method, but with less image resolution (approximately 1.5 mm/pixel) also achieved acceptable accuracy in breast lesion charactareization.[6,60] However, few researchers have tackled the "temporal-versus-spatial" dilemma head on. Kuhl and colleagues[61] examined a cohort of patients with repeat MR imaging on separate days, directly comparing high-spatial- and high-temporal-resolution protocols. These investigators noted that the accuracy of the dynamic enhancement pattern analysis suffered when imaging was run at lower temporal resolution. However, overall diagnostic accuracy was improved with the lower-temporal resolution protocol because of improved depiction of lesion morphology. In a multisite study in which patients underwent sequential spatially- and temporally-optimized imaging studies on separate days,[62] the combination of morphologic and dynamic enhancement patterns of enhancing lesions was found to be superior to either a purely kinetic or morphologic model for characterizing benign and malignant lesions.

Parallel Imaging

Parallel imaging makes use of the geometric arrangement of MR receiver coils to impart spatial information to the image reconstruction process. Spatial representation of MR signals normally derives from frequency and phase encoding, processes that occur through the use of magnetic gradients during signal acquisition. In the case of phase encoding, repetitive cycles of excitation and signal emission from the excited protons are required to encode spatial localization of signals in all 3 dimensions, adding to the acquisition time, especially for high-resolution imaging. However, if one uses the spatial information derived from the geometric arrangement of surface coils, one can reduce the number of phase encoding steps by a factor of 2 or more. This reduction allows for a proportional reduction in imaging time. As such, a $2\times$ factor in parallel imaging results in the acquisition of an image in half the time when compared with the same image acquired without parallel imaging, and $3\times$ parallel imaging in a 67% reduction in imaging time. In practice, the actual time saved is somewhat less, as additional phase encoding steps are often needed to optimize the parallel imaging acquisition.

In order for parallel imaging to work optimally, the overlap in the spatial information from the different receive coils must be minimized, an effect that cannot always be achieved in MR imaging based on constraints of anatomy and coil design. However, in breast MR, the anatomic and coil geometries are ideal for parallel imaging (**Fig. 6**A). Because there are 2 phase-encode directions in 3-dimensional gradient echo imaging, one can in theory employ parallel imaging in each of these directions, further multiplying the acceleration of the imaging. In the idealized schematic shown in **Fig. 6**B, an eightfold reduction in image time is achieved. In practice, acceleration factors greater than two- to threefold are difficult to achieve, as higher acceleration in parallel imaging comes at a cost of lower SNR and increased artifacts. Many researchers advocate the use of 3-T scanners for breast imaging, with the understanding that the higher imaging SNR of the 3-T system may provide greater latitude in the use of larger parallel imaging acceleration factors.

Keyhole and Non-Cartesian Imaging Methods

In routine MR imaging, raw data is derived from the excited protons as they precess about the main magnetic field and induce current in the MR receiver coils. This induced current is digitized into bits of data, which constitute the components of k-space. To derive enough raw data to produce a high-resolution 3-dimensional imaging set, a comparable amount of raw data must be acquired and placed into specified locations, or bins, within k-space. The central portion of k-space contains information on image contrast, whereas the more peripheral edges of k-space encode data that are transformed into information on fine-structure and edges (ie, resolution). The manner in which k-space is "filled" is a topic of ongoing research and inquiry. Traditionally, k-space was filled one line at a time, requiring a complete data set in 2 (or 3) dimensions before a single high-resolution image or image set could be created. This process creates practical limits on temporal resolution of multiphase imaging. Images derived from only a partial set (usually the central aspect) of the k-space data can be acquired more rapidly, but suffer from poorer spatial resolution.

Researchers have explored numerous ways to accelerate the process of k-space filling for rapid multiphase imaging without sacrificing volume coverage or spatial resolution. These "keyhole" techniques replenish only the central aspect of k-space during dynamic imaging, enabling more rapid imaging by "borrowing" the data that defines the edges of the anatomic images from earlier or later acquisitions. Keyhole imaging was initially proposed for MR angiography acquisitions,[63] and has been applied to dynamic T1W enhanced breast imaging.[64] However, this method often produces artifacts when applied to breast imaging, where the imaged objects are small and demonstrate only modest contrast with adjacent tissues.[65,66]

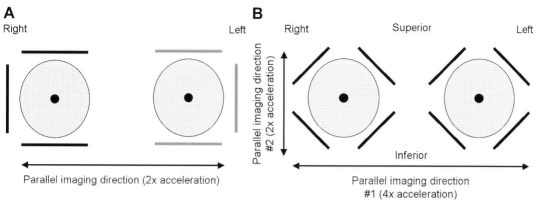

Fig. 6. Coil geometries and parallel imaging in breast MR imaging. (*A*) A hypothetical 2-channel breast MR imaging coil in the coronal projection. Phase encode direction is right to left in an axial acquisition. The geometric separation of the coils and anatomy is optimal for parallel imaging with a 2× acceleration factor. (*B*) A hypothetical 8-channel coil is demonstrated, allowing the operator to make use of parallel imaging in the primary phase encoding (left-right) direction, as well as the secondary phase (slice) encoding direction. In this example, acceleration factors of up to 8× can be entertained. However, the anatomic and geometric separation of coils and anatomy are not as distinct as in the 2× acceleration example (*A*), which may lead to degraded image quality.

Other methods for accelerating the pace at which multiple dynamically enhanced images can be obtained include non-Cartesian methods that do not traverse k-space in an orderly linear fashion. Techniques such as spiral[67] or radial[34,68] imaging have been successfully employed for temporally accelerated breast MR imaging. Because these techniques can control the number of times the central aspect of k-space is sampled, they can be leveraged for more rapid temporal image generation, similar to the keyhole techniques, while maintaining effective spatial resolution. Each of these techniques requires "resampling" of the raw data to create the Cartesian (xyz) structure of k-space required for the creation of an image with regular rectangular voxels. Errors in this resampling step introduce artifacts that differ from those encountered in traditional Cartesian imaging and are unique to the type of k-space sampling employed. Nevertheless, in some settings non-Cartesian imaging may limit or alter motion artifacts, resulting in improved image quality (**Fig. 7**).

MR Spectroscopy

In vivo MR spectroscopy (MRS) is a technique whereby water (and variably) lipid magnetic signals are suppressed to reveal the weaker signals from hydrogen atoms within small molecular weight metabolites. Only metabolites that are present in sufficient concentration (on the order of 1 mM or greater) are normally visible in routine MR spectroscopy. Each metabolite will resonate at a slightly different frequency, depending on the chemical nature of the molecule. The MR spectrum is thus presented along a linear axis of frequencies, with different metabolites located at characteristic locations along the frequency axis. Because frequency is a function of magnetic field, MR spectra are generally plotted by chemical shift, where the chemical shift is represented as a percentage shift in the frequency (in "parts per million," or ppm) from the resonance frequency of a reference molecule; this allows for standardization of metabolite position independent of actual magnetic field. The relative metabolite concentrations in a given tissue can be approximated by the heights of the various MRS signals (absolute metabolite concentrations are more difficult to calculate, and are currently only performed in research settings).

In clinical MRS, data are presented either as single-voxel or multivoxel formats. In multivoxel spectroscopy (which has been employed in other clinical MRS examinations, but not as frequently in breast MRS), an array of voxels of similar sizes are acquired to evaluate for metabolic differences within lesions or organs. In single-voxel (SV-)MRS, the operator selects a 3-dimensional box of variable size, outside of which the MRS signal is suppressed. A single MR spectrum, representing the metabolite profile of that volume of tissue, is obtained. In theory, a box of any dimension may be prescribed for SV-MRS. In practice, minimal voxel sizes of approximately 1 cm³ or more are required to produce spectra with adequate SNR in a reasonable time frame. An area or lesion of

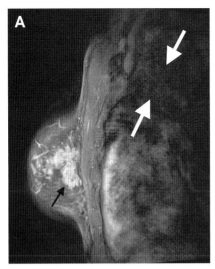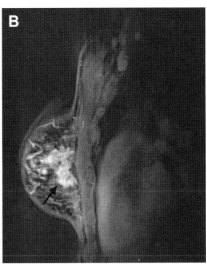

Fig. 7. Comparison between Cartesian and radial image acquisition. Medial left breast mass representing known cancer in a 45-year-old woman. Sagittal post-gadolinium fat-suppressed image acquired with standard Cartesian (A) or radial (B) k-space acquisition, demonstrating portion of the spiculated mass (*small black arrow*). Image quality is similar. However, motion effects (such as superior to the heart, *white arrows* in A) are less evident on radial image set. Fine streaking in the radial image can be observed in the spaces superior and inferior to the breast on the radial images. Fat suppression appears improved in the radial image, reflecting altered contrast due to method of k-space sampling. Radial imaging provided with support from Siemens Healthcare, Germany.

interest typically is outlined by the radiologist or technologist after the dynamic gadolinium acquisition. The SV-MRS examination is then performed. Depending on the voxel size, signal averaging for 4 to 6 minutes is required to produce an MRS spectrum of sufficient SNR.

In breast MR imaging, the hallmark of the spectroscopic examination is the detection of choline and its derivatives (collectively referred to as "total choline," or tCho), at 3.2 ppm. Choline, a molecule required for fatty acid synthesis during cell membrane production, is present in elevated concentrations in most malignant tissues. Detection of choline and choline-related compounds at 3.2 ppm on a SV-MRS examination has been used as a sign of increased likelihood of malignancy (**Fig. 8**). Methods for defining tCho detection vary. Some researchers advocate qualitative visual assessment, whereas others report the depiction of a tCho peak height that is greater that 2 times the adjacent spectral noise level. Still others report more quantitative measures that require standardization of the tCho peak area to that of unsuppressed water.[69]

Elevated tCho has been shown more frequently in malignant than in benign enhancing breast lesions.[70–74] The use of MRS as an adjunctive examination to enhanced MR imaging may provide added specificity in defining malignant breast lesions.[75] While MRS may be more easily applied to mass lesions than to nonmass lesions,

Bartella and colleagues[76] found 100% sensitivity of tCho depiction by MRS for malignant nonmass enhancements, and found that the PPV for suspicious enhancing nonmass lesions might have increased from 20% to 63% if MRS criteria were incorporated into the diagnostic algorithm. However, as the detectability of tCho in malignant lesions on MRS may be related to tumor biologic features,[77] most researchers suggest that MRS be used as an adjunctive rather than primary method for characterizing indeterminate enhancing lesions.

Diffusion-Weighted Imaging

Diffusion represents the random (Brownian) motion of water that occurs in tissue. The application of specialized pairs of magnetic gradients decreases the relative MR signal intensity of each tissue in proportion to the amount of free diffusion of its water molecules. Diffusion-weighted imaging (DWI) can be performed via the application of a single set of diffusion gradients in a single orientation. More typically, diffusion gradients in different directions are employed, and the resulting directionally averaged tissue signal is compared with the tissue signal intensity in the absence of any gradients. For a given diffusion gradient strength, the amount of signal loss of water molecules in tissue is exponentially proportional to degree of diffusion, resulting in the ability

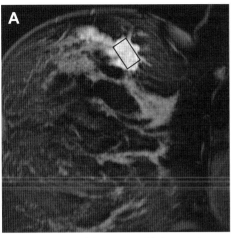
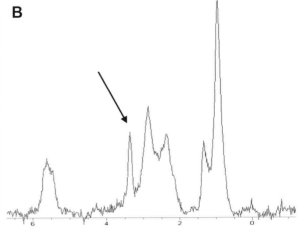

Fig. 8. A 42-year-old woman with known breast cancer. (*A*) MR imaging demonstrates lobular enhancing cancer in upper posterior left breast. Boxed region shows area prescribed for MR spectroscopy. (*B*) MR spectrum demonstrates tCho peak (*arrow*) characteristic of malignant breast lesions.

for one to calculate the "apparent diffusion coefficient" (or ADC) of a tissue on a pixel-by-pixel basis based on the equation:

$$SI^B = SI^0 * \exp(- B * ADC)$$

where SI^0 represents signal intensity without diffusion gradients applied, SI^B the signal intensity with diffusion gradients applied, B the strength of the diffusion gradient (in s/mm²), and ADC the apparent diffusion coefficient of the tissue (in mm²/s). If diffusion gradients of various strengths are applied, curve fitting can be performed to calculate ADC. In research settings, DWI with multiple B values has been used to define different ADCs at lower and higher B values, thought to represent contributions of rapid tissue signal loss from internal vascular flow and slower signal loss from true Brownian motion in tissue, respectively.

DWI is generally applied with T2-weighted echo-planar imaging (EPI), a technique that allows for extremely rapid imaging to limit the time of the DWI portion of the examination and reduce effects of patient motion. However, EPI is complicated by high sensitivity to local magnetic field variations, and potentially severe image distortion. Newer more robust diffusion imaging methods linked to fast spin echo or balanced gradient echo sequences remain experimental. When DWI is performed, one or more sets of diffusion-weighted images can be produced and viewed. In addition, an ADC pixel map can be calculated from the component diffusion-weighted images produced from 2 or more DWI sets.

Invasive breast cancers demonstrate more restricted diffusion (lower ADC) than does

normal breast tissue or benign breast lesions (**Fig. 9**).[78–80] As such, DWI may be helpful in identifying malignant lesions when dynamic enhanced gadolinium imaging is equivocal. Given the reduced diffusivity of water in invasive cancers, these lesions will be relatively bright on diffusion-weighted images. However, benign lesions with high intrinsic T2 signal intensity may remain bright on DWI, due to the phenomenon of "T2 shine-through" (**Fig. 10**). As such, most investigators recommend the use of ADC quantification rather than DWI inspection for breast lesion characterization. The use of optimized ADC cutoff was shown to improve breast lesion characterization without decreasing sensitivity,[81] with a potential reduction in the number of negative biopsies. However, ADC values and optimal cutoffs for benign/malignant differentiation may depend on the B value combination used.[82] Furthermore, experience with DWI at 3 T is more limited,[40,83] although useful discrimination between benign and malignant tumors at 3 T has been demonstrated.[84]

CLINICAL APPLICATIONS OF MAGNETIC RESONANCE IMAGING IN BREAST CANCER
Local Cancer Staging

One of the most common uses for MR imaging is in the patient with recent diagnosis of breast cancer. MR imaging has the ability to map primary tumor size, define unsuspected additional foci of tumor, and to screen for clinically occult cancer in the contralateral breast. MR imaging can better estimate primary tumor size,[85] allowing for appropriate surgical planning. MR imaging is also

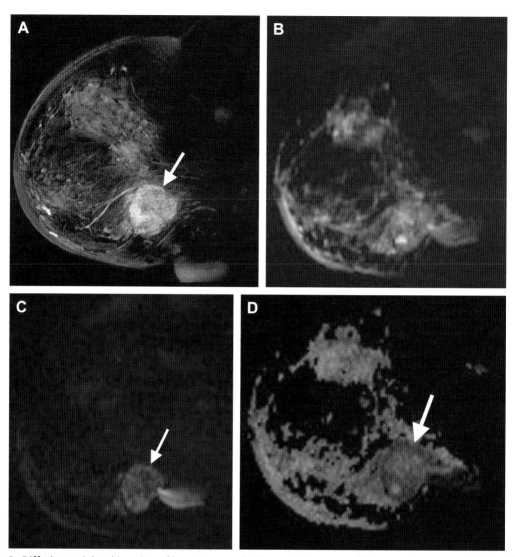

Fig. 9. Diffusion-weighted imaging of breast cancer. A 61-year-old woman with known large cancer in the right breast. (*A*) Post-gadolinium sagittal image of the right breast demonstrates a large slightly heterogeneously enhancing round mass in the inferior breast (*arrow*), representing known cancer. (*B*) Diffusion-weighted images with B = 0 and (*C*) B = 600 demonstrate that the lesion is isointense to breast parenchyma on the B = 0 imaging, but is hyperintense on the B = 600 image (*arrow* in *C*), reflecting restricted diffusion. Apparent diffusion coefficient (ADC) map in (*D*) demonstrates darker intensity of the lesion (*arrow*), confirming the restricted diffusion of this cancer.

better able than mammography to depict primary tumor margins in invasive lobular cancers,[86] and can lower reexcision rates in this subgroup of women.[87]

Prevalence of multicentric disease

In women with clinically localized breast cancer, there is often unsuspected multicentric disease. Rosen and colleagues[88] simulated lumpectomy in patients with suspected unifocal disease using 203 mastectomy specimens and evaluated for residual or multifocal disease. For primary tumors less then 2 cm, there was residual cancer in 26% of the patients increasing to 38% for tumors greater than 2 cm. For cancers located in the sub-areolar region, residual cancer was present 80% of the time after a simulated partial mastectomy. Holland and colleagues[89] produced similar results in evaluating the mastectomy specimen of 314 patients with T1 and T2 breast cancers. The

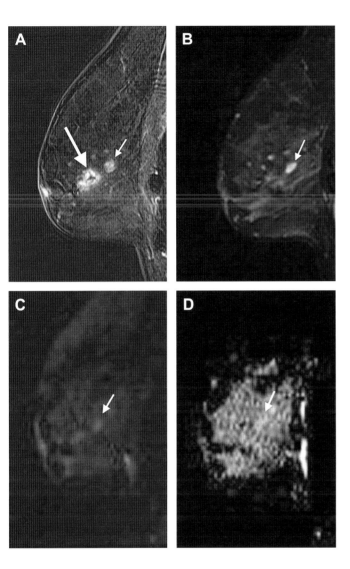

Fig. 10. Diffusion-weighted imaging (DWI) of benign lesion, with T2 shine-through effect. A 46-year-old woman with newly diagnosed invasive breast cancer, with additional enhancing lesion noted on staging MR imaging study. (A) Sagittal post-gadolinium image demonstrates postoperative changes from needle localization and surgical excision of known cancer in the anterior breast (*large arrow*). More posteriorly, an additional rounded enhancing mass (*small arrow*) is seen. The mass is bright on T2W imaging (*small arrow* in B), and was also bright on B = 0 DWI (not shown). Diffusion-weighted images with B = 600 (C) demonstrates the mass to be hyperintense to breast tissue (*small arrow*). However, apparent diffusion coefficient (ADC) map in (D) demonstrates the mass (*small arrow*) to be isointense to background breast parenchyma, suggesting nonrestricted diffusion. MR-guided biopsy revealed a fibroadenoma.

investigators found additional cancer foci within 2 cm of the known cancer in 20% of specimens. In 43% of cases, the tumor was greater than 2 cm away from the primary tumor.

The findings of additional distant disease foci within mastectomy specimens of patients with clinically localized disease were initially cited as an argument against the use of breast conservation therapy.[88–90] Without postoperative radiation therapy, local treatment failure rates can be as high as 40%.[91–93] However, it has since been demonstrated that adjuvant radiation therapy significantly lowers the local recurrence rate,[94] providing strong evidence that radiation can successfully treat residual disease not excised during surgery. Nevertheless, the reported local recurrence rates after breast conservation therapy with whole breast radiation vary, as high as 10% in some series, although lower in other studies.[95,96] Whereas later local "recurrences" may result from the emergence of a new primary cancer, early local breast cancer recurrence (within 2–3 years) is likely due to residual disease not eradicated by adjuvant radiation and chemotherapy.

Detection of disease extent by imaging

Multiple studies have shown that in the patient recently diagnosed with breast cancer, MR imaging can detect additional foci of cancer that are mammographically and clinically occult.[11,26,97–102] The prevalence of MR imaging-detected multifocal or multicentric disease in patients with clinically localized tumors varies widely, ranging from 12% to 88%.[13,103–106]

Multimodality imaging comparisons in local breast cancer staging generally demonstrate the superiority of MR imaging for detecting additional tumor foci. Berg and colleagues[100] investigated the diagnostic accuracy of clinical breast examination, mammography, whole breast sonography, and MR imaging in estimating tumor extent in 111 patients with known breast cancer. In total, 177 malignant foci were detected. The investigators found ultrasound and MR imaging to be more sensitive in the evaluation for invasive cancer, especially in patients with dense breasts. However, no one modality was detected all 177 malignancies. The addition of whole breast sonography to clinical breast examination and mammography detected additional cancers, changing surgical management in 17 of 96 patients. Subsequent addition of MR imaging added additional suspicious findings in 29 of 96 patients. Berg and colleagues also found that the addition of sonography after an MR imaging examination did not result in additional cancer yield. The combination of mammography, MR imaging, and clinical breast examination yielded the greatest sensitivity, with detection of all 177 cancers.

MR imaging for preoperative mapping
A preoperative MR image may assist the surgeon in mapping out disease extent prior to definitive surgery (**Fig. 11**). Bedrosian and colleagues[107] assessed 267 patients with known cancer who underwent MR imaging evaluation prior to definitive surgery. All patients had a complete conventional imaging evaluation. In 69 patients, suspicious findings were seen on MR, requiring biopsy. Pathology confirmed malignancy in 49 of 69 patients (71%). In addition, 44 patients who were felt to be candidates for breast conservation therapy based on conventional imaging were converted to mastectomy based on findings seen only on MR imaging after pathologic confirmation.

Although radiation has the potential to treat small residual foci, the mean size of secondary cancers detected on MR imaging is 1 cm, with many representing high-grade disease, findings similar to those of mammographically detected second foci in women with palpable primary cancers.[97,108] It is conceivable that these cancers—partially treated by radiation therapy—may be the cause of early local failure of breast conservation therapy. However, to date no prospective studies have validated the concept that preoperative MR imaging, with its potential to detect unsuspected multicentric and multifocal disease, may reduce the incidence of local treatment failure after breast conservation therapy.

Assessing for pectoral muscle and chest wall invasion
In patients with large cancers or cancers that are located in the posterior breast, the status of the pectoralis muscle and chest wall may be

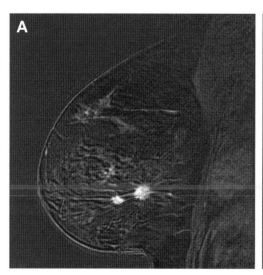 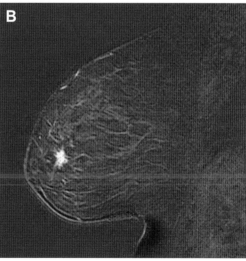

Fig. 11. A 54-year-old woman who palpated a left breast mass. Sonography and mammography revealed an irregular, approximately 1-cm mass. Biopsy confirmed a well-differentiated invasive ductal carcinoma. An MR image was obtained before definitive therapy. MR imaging showed additional enhancing masses spanning several centimeters, greater in extent than had been suspected on mammography and sonography. (*A*) Sagittal post-gadolinium subtraction image shows 2 adjacent masses. MR-guided biopsy confirmed malignancy. (*B*) MR imaging screening of the contralateral breast demonstrated an unsuspected suspicious enhancing lesion Biopsy revealed a poorly differentiated invasive ductal carcinoma. The contralateral tumor was morphologically distinct form the ipsilateral lesions, confirming its metachronous nature.

evaluated on MR imaging. Both mammography and sonography are limited in the evaluation of the extent of posterior disease in deep tumors, a determination that may also be difficult on clinical examination. The key imaging finding associated with pectoral muscle invasion appears to be abnormal enhancement of the muscle on post-gadolinium images (**Fig. 12**), a finding with sensitivity of 100% and specificity of 93% to 100%.[109,110] The obliteration of the fat plane anterior to the pectoralis muscle alone, without increased muscle enhancement, does not predict muscle invasion on pathologic evaluation (**Fig. 13**). Deeper degrees of chest wall invasion are rarer, but can be depicted readily by MR imaging.

Detection of synchronous contralateral cancers
The incidence of synchronous contralateral breast cancer, detected clinically or by imaging, is estimated to be approximately 1% to 7% (**Fig. 14**).[111,112] Even in the setting of negative mammography and sonography, there are multiple reports of MR imaging–detected contralateral breast cancers in women,[13,113–118] with incidence rates generally between 3% and 4% in most series.

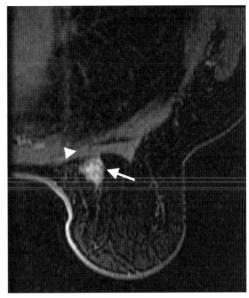

Fig. 13. A 71-year-old woman with prior left breast cancer, status post lumpectomy and radiation therapy, with new mammographic abnormality in the posterior left breast distant from the original lumpectomy site. Post-gadolinium axial MR image demonstrates irregular enhancing mass (*arrow*) abutting the pectoralis muscle (*arrowhead*) without intervening fat, but with no muscle enhancement. Biopsy revealed invasive carcinoma. Mastectomy demonstrated clear surgical margins posteriorly with no pectoralis muscle invasion.

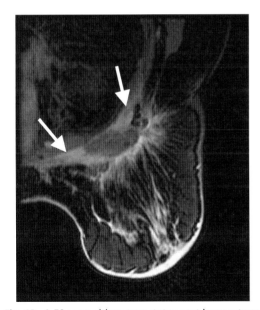

Fig. 12. A 59-year-old woman status post lumpectomy for invasive cancer 2 years previously, without subsequent radiation therapy, presented with increasing contraction at the surgery site. The patient had declined to have radiation therapy. Post-gadolinium axial image demonstrates large irregular enhancement extending from the prior lumpectomy site into the muscle (*arrows*). Biopsy confirmed recurrent tumor.

Liberman and colleagues[115] analyzed 223 women with recently diagnosed breast cancer who had contralateral MR imaging screening examinations. The patients enrolled in the study had negative mammograms and clinical breast examinations within 6 months of the MR imaging study. Twelve cancers (12/223) were detected, with a cancer detection rate of 5%. There were 6 invasive carcinomas and 6 cases of ductal carcinoma in situ.

The first multicenter prospective trial to address the contralateral MR imaging screening question was performed by the International Breast Magnetic Resonance Consortium (IBMC).[117] The 108 patients recruited for the study had a recent diagnosis of unilateral breast cancer, and negative mammograms and clinical breast examinations within 90 days of the contralateral MR imaging screening. Five women were excluded, leaving 103 women in the final analysis. Biopsy was recommended in 12 of 103 women (12%) yielding 4 cancers, all invasive. The PPV of positive MR was 4 out of 12 (33%). The average size of the 4 cancers was 13.2 mm (range 8–17 mm).

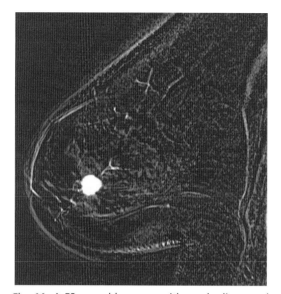

Fig. 14. A 53-year-old woman with newly diagnosed right breast cancer presenting as a 3-cm area of calcifications. Contralateral MR imaging screening evaluation of the left breast revealed an avidly enhancing irregular mass in the anterior breast. Core needle biopsy revealed a moderately differentiated invasive ductal carcinoma with associated DCIS. At excision, the mass measured 1.2 cm.

The largest prospective contralateral MR imaging screening trial to date was sponsored by the ACR Imaging Network.[118] The final analysis included 969 women, in whom 30 (3.1%) cancers that were mammographically and clinically occult were detected. Biopsy was performed in 12.5% (121) of women, with a PPV of 24.8% (30/121). There were 12 DCIS and 18 invasive carcinomas. The average size of the invasive carcinoma was 10.9 mm. The cancer detection rate in the study was not related to breast density or menopausal status.

The detection and treatment of a synchronous tumor allows for informed surgical decision making when considering reconstruction options, especially if tissue reconstruction is being considered. Abdominal tissue flaps, such as the transverse rectus abdominis muscle flap, may be performed only once. If a second flap is needed at a later date, tissue will need to be harvested from elsewhere, such as the latissimus dorsi, or implant reconstruction will become necessary. In addition, if chemotherapy is necessary the patient would only need treatment once for bilateral synchronous cancers, not twice as would be the situation for metachronous cancers.

Follow-Up After Positive Surgical Margins

In patients with positive margins after initial excision, breast MR imaging may aid in the assessment of how much residual disease is present before the patient returns to the operating room. Depending on the extent of disease seen on the MR imaging, the findings may assist the surgeon in planning the appropriate surgical procedure, potentially minimizing the number of reexcisions required to obtain clear pathologic margins. Postoperative MR imaging may be performed shortly after surgery, and is generally well tolerated during this time period. A thin rim of benign-appearing enhancement may be seen around the biopsy cavity, and is not in general suspicious for residual cancer (**Fig. 15**A). At times, nodular or thicker rim enhancement may be seen (**Fig. 15**B), in which case it may be difficult to differentiate between enhancing granulation tissue and residual tumor. However, more extensive enhancement extending from the biopsy cavity is generally a sign of residual tumor (**Fig. 15**C). Furthermore, residual microscopic disease may not be visible by MR imaging. Therefore, at all times postoperative MR imaging should be correlated with the pathologic status of the surgical margins at the time of lumpectomy. In situations where cancer detection was based on abnormal mammographic calcifications, a postsurgical mammogram may be necessary to evaluate for residual calcifications, as a negative postlumpectomy MR imaging examination does not exclude the presence of residual intraductal carcinoma.

Evaluation of Patients with an Occult Primary Cancer

Presentation of clinically and mammographically occult breast cancer with a positive axillary lymph node is an uncommon event, accounting for less than 1% of diagnosed breast cancers. Traditionally the surgical treatment of choice has been mastectomy and axillary node dissection. Even after mastectomy, the primary cancer was found only one-third of the time on pathologic evaluation. In addition, studies have found no survival difference between women who did and did not have mastectomy.

In many cases, MR imaging can depict the site of primary cancer not revealed by mammography or clinical breast examination (**Fig. 16**). Reports of MR imaging-detected primary cancers in patients presenting with positive axillary lymph nodes were initially published in the late 1990s.[119–123] The reported MR imaging sensitivity varies from 25% to 100%. The largest series was by Buchanan and colleagues[124] in 2005, who

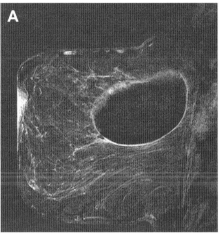 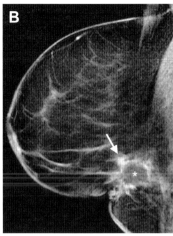 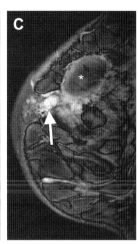

Fig. 15. Examples of postbiopsy MR imaging findings. (A) Sagittal post-gadolinium subtraction image demonstrates a large postbiopsy seroma with thin uniform rim of enhancement. Findings are typical for early postsurgical changes and do not suggest residual disease. (B) Sagittal post-gadolinium image in a different patient status post excisional biopsy for invasive cancer and close anterior margin on pathology. Excisional cavity is seen (asterisk) with nodular area of enhancement (arrow) interpreted as suspicious for residual carcinoma. Pathology at reexcision demonstrated no residual tumor. (C) Sagittal post-gadolinium image in another patient, with positive surgical margins after lumpectomy for invasive cancer. Postoperative MR imaging revealed an enhancing irregular nodule (arrow) slightly distant from the anterior margin of the seroma cavity (asterisk). Reexcision revealed residual invasive disease.

reported a 59% detection rate in 162 patients. Once the primary cancer is detected on MR imaging, the suspicious area may be biopsied under MR guidance. The patient may then be a candidate for breast conservation therapy. If MR imaging fails to demonstrate the primary cancer, the patient is offered the option of mastectomy with or without reconstruction or whole breast radiation, followed by systemic therapy.

When there is a suspicious lesion on MR imaging that is occult on mammography and physical examination, targeted ultrasound is often performed in an attempt to identify the lesion and localize it for biopsy. If the lesion is identified by ultrasonography, biopsy under this modality is performed, as the authors find that ultrasound-guided biopsies are better tolerated by patients, and are faster to perform than MR imaging–guided biopsy. It is imperative that the sonographic-MR imaging correlation be made to confirm that the lesion seen on MR imaging correlates with that seen on sonography.

When ultrasonography fails to demonstrate the lesion, biopsy can be performed under MR imaging, either by MR imaging–guided core biopsy or MR imaging–guided needle localization followed by surgical excision. One major drawback to MR imaging–guided biopsies is the lack of ability to confirm lesion removal. Unlike mammographically guided localization and excisional biopsies, the there is no way to confirm excision

of the MR imaging localized lesions, as specimens cannot be viewed under MR imaging to demonstrate lesion enhancement. Similarly, it is not possible to confirm appropriate sampling during MR imaging–guided core biopsies, other than to use parenchyma landmarks to document that the appropriate area has been sampled (**Fig. 17**). Nevertheless, MR-guided biopsies have gained acceptance and provide acceptable rates of diagnostic accuracy.[125,126]

Evaluation of Nipple Discharge

Unilateral spontaneous nipple discharge that is bloody, clear, or serosanguinous may be a clinical manifestation of breast cancer. Following evaluation of physical examination, imaging is performed in attempts to identify an anatomic cause of the discharge. Depending on the age of the patient, mammography may be used as the first-line imaging test to assess for any unsuspected masses or calcifications. Sonographic evaluation of the periareolar area may also be performed, noting that most intraductal origins accounting for the discharge are located within several centimeters of the nipple. Occasionally an intraductal mass may be seen by ultrasonography, although often the sonographic evaluation will be negative. Galactography is now less commonly used for evaluation of nipple discharge.

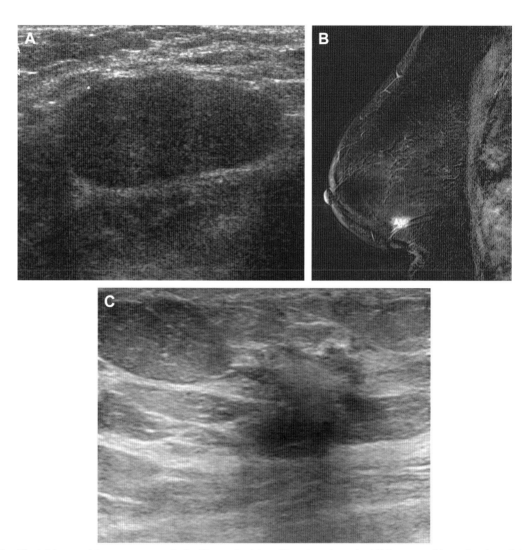

Fig. 16. A 74-year-old woman presented with a palpable axillary lymph node. (*A*) Sonographic evaluation of the left axilla shows an oval solid mass. A fine-needle aspiration demonstrated adenocarcinoma. A breast primary was not seen on mammography. (*B*) Bilateral MR imaging study shows a spiculated enhancing mass in the lower outer quadrant. (*C*) The mass was visible on targeted ultrasound and the patient subsequently had an ultrasound-guided core needle biopsy, which revealed invasive lobular carcinoma.

Mammography, ultrasonography, and galactography may all be limited in the evaluation of nipple discharge, while cytologic evaluation of the discharge fluid has been associated with both false-positive and false-negative results.[127] As such, MR imaging is now often used for assessing the patient with nipple discharge. Numerous reports have shown that MR imaging may detect both benign[128] and malignant[129–132] etiologies of nipple discharge that are occult on clinical breast examination and on conventional imaging (Fig. 18). In one study[131] the positive predictive value of MR imaging in patients presenting with clinically concerning nipple discharge was 56%,

compared with 19% for galactography. MR imaging also had a high negative predictive value of 87%. However, as MR imaging was not able to detect all cancers in these women, surgical ductal exploration may still be required in some cases.

Based on these findings, MR imaging has replaced galactography in many institutions. As opposed to galactography, which will only assess one ductal system, MR imaging is able to globally evaluate the clinically symptomatic breast as well as the contralateral side, to assess for symmetry of ductal structures and enhancement. In addition, MR imaging is able to differentiate nonenhancing

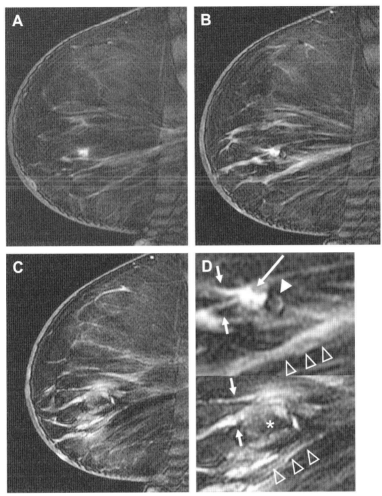

Fig. 17. Use of parenchymal landmarks during MR imaging–guided biopsy. A 53-year-old woman, 1 year status post lumpectomy and radiation for invasive carcinoma, with new mammographic density in the central breast seen on only one view. MR imaging revealed corresponding enhancing lesion. Targeted ultrasound was negative. (*A*) Post-gadolinium sagittal image during MR imaging–guided vacuum core biopsy re-demonstrated enhancing lesion. Sheath placement (*B*) and postbiopsy images (*C*) are shown. Blow-up of the lesion area is shown in (*D*) before (*top*) and after (*bottom*) biopsy. Enhancing lesion is shown by a long arrow. Biopsy sheath is shown by a white arrowhead. After biopsy, seroma is demonstrated (*asterisk*). Adequacy of lesion sampling is confirmed by identical position of seroma and lesion relative to strands of hyperintense parenchyma (*short white arrows* and *outlined arrowheads*). Pathology revealed invasive carcinoma.

intraductal debris from enhancing masses such as papillomas and DCIS, bearing in mind that not all DCIS will enhance on MR.

Evaluation of Inconclusive Mammographic or Sonographic Findings

MR imaging may be used as a problem-solving tool when equivocal results are obtained after clinical evaluation and complete conventional imaging workup of palpable or screen-detected abnormalities. However, MR imaging should not be used as a substitute for an incomplete conventional imaging workup. A thorough mammographic and sonographic evaluation should be performed before recommending MR imaging. One situation when MR imaging may be helpful is in the case of focal mammographic asymmetry, or a mammographic density seen only on one view with no sonographic correlate. In one study,[133] this was the most common indication for supplemental MR imaging, with a cancer incidence of 5.2% and a PPV of MR imaging of 40%. If the corresponding lesion enhances, MR imaging may help to

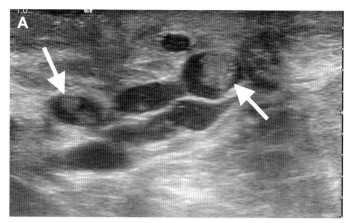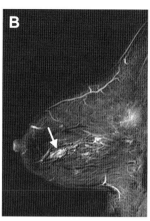

Fig. 18. A 32-year-old woman with a history of bloody nipple discharge and a negative mammogram. (*A*) Sonographic evaluation of the subareolar regions revealed small filling defects within the ducts (*arrows*). (*B*) MR imaging was obtained prior to excisional biopsy and shows a linear area of ductal enhancement (*arrow*) extending to the posterior breast. Excisional biopsy revealed intraductal carcinoma, intermediate nuclear grade.

characterize the lesion, and provide guidance for biopsy or targeted ultrasonography. Although the sensitivity of MR imaging for invasive cancer is high, a suspicious finding on conventional imaging should not preclude biopsy based on a negative MR imaging.

MR Imaging and Neoadjuvant Chemotherapy

In patients with inoperable locally advanced breast cancer, neoadjuvant chemotherapy is necessary prior to definitive surgery. Neoadjuvant therapy may also be administered for advanced but operable disease in patients who otherwise would require mastectomy but who desire breast conservation. In such cases, systemic therapy is given in an attempt to shrink the tumor[134,135] in order to allow for more limited surgery.

Given that MR imaging has been shown to be the most precise imaging technique for determining extent of disease, MR imaging is recommended prior to neoadjuvant therapy to document the exact extent of disease, to facilitate comparison with posttreatment imaging, and to enable accurate preoperative planning. MR imaging is also important to screen for clinically and mammographically occult contralateral disease, so as to ensure that an occult contralateral cancer does not undergo partial treatment with systemic therapy, only to recur later.

During neoadjuvant chemotherapy, it is necessary to monitor patients for nonresponse so that alterations in the treatment plan may be made. However, monitoring response to the chemotherapy by clinical examination may be difficult, as fibrotic change may mask tumor response. There are also limitations to following tumor

response by mammography or ultrasound. Breast MR imaging is ideal for following patients treated with neoadjuvant chemotherapy, as it is more robust than mammography and clinical examination for detection of residual viable tumor. As MR imaging is dependent on tumor vascularity, nonviable necrotic tissue will not enhance. Decreasing size of abnormal enhancement on MR imaging correlates well with response to chemotherapy.[136–139] However, the response to chemotherapy may not simply relate to changes in the amount of enhancing tissue on MR imaging, as the morphologic pattern of enhancement change may indicate the degree of treatment response.

MR imaging has been shown to be superior to clinical breast examination and mammography for depicting the presence and extent of residual viable tumor following completion of neoadjuvant therapy.[140–143] As such, MR imaging should be routinely used in preoperative planning after neoadjuvant chemotherapy. It should be noted that tumor response follows certain morphologic patterns. Disease that begins as a large focal mass tends—when responsive to chemotherapy—to shrink in a concentric pattern (**Fig. 19**), facilitating conversion from modified radical mastectomy to lumpectomy. Conversely, chemosensitive advanced breast cancers that present as irregular areas or multicentric enhancing regions tend to regress in a pattern that may leave multiple small tumor foci at completion of therapy (**Fig. 20**). In such cases, careful correlation with the preoperative MR imaging is required for adequate surgical planning to ensure excision of all residual disease.

A negative MR image following neoadjuvant therapy does not ensure complete pathologic

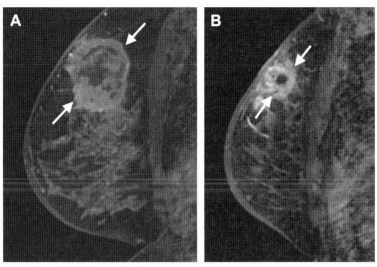

Fig. 19. Concentric shrinkage of locally advanced breast cancer. (*A*) A 45-year-old woman with invasive cancer presenting as a focal mass (*arrows*) in the superior left breast. (*B*) After completion of neoadjuvant chemotherapy, the mass (*arrows*) has shrunk to less than half its initial size, allowing for more localized surgery.

response, as microscopic foci of viable tumor may not enhance on MR imaging. As such, posttreatment surgery is still required, even when clinical examination and MR imaging do not reveal macroscopic residual disease. The authors advocate placement of a clip prior to neoadjuvant therapy, which will facilitate localizing the original tumor site for excisional biopsy if there is complete

imaging response. However, clip location should be correlated with sites of any macroscopic tumor revealed on MR imaging, because of unpredictable patterns of tumor shrinkage in response to systemic therapy (**Fig. 21**).

While MR imaging can be used to monitor the responsiveness of tumor to neoadjuvant chemotherapy, tumor shrinkage is not generally seen until

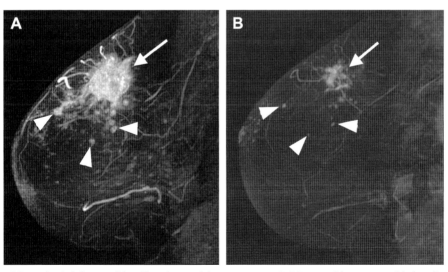

Fig. 20. Multicentric shrinkage of locally advanced breast cancer. A 36-year-old woman with locally advanced breast cancer. (*A*) Sagittal maximum intensity projection (MIP) of the post-gadolinium subtraction MR image before neoadjuvant therapy demonstrates a dominant superior mass (*arrow*) with multiple satellite nodules (*arrowheads*) in the central and anterior breast. (*B*) At the completion of neoadjuvant therapy, sagittal MIP image demonstrates significant shrinkage of the dominant mass (*arrow*). However, the distant satellite nodules, though also smaller, persist as enhancing foci (*arrowheads*). Concern for persistent multicentric disease led to mastectomy over lumpectomy. Pathology revealed 1.5-cm residual cancer, with sub-centimeter foci of additional cancer medial and anterior to the dominant mass.

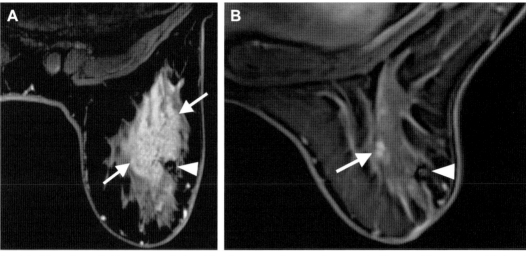

Fig. 21. Alteration of clip-tumor relationship after neoadjuvant therapy. A 48-year-old woman with locally advanced invasive cancer. (A) Axial post-gadolinium image before neoadjuvant therapy demonstrates large infiltrating mass (*arrows*) occupying a majority of the central and lateral posterior breast. Image artifact (*arrowhead*) from a marker clip placed during ultrasound-guided biopsy at an outside institution can be seen at the lateral aspect of the mass. (B) After completion of neoadjuvant therapy, a small residual focus of abnormal enhancement (*arrow*) is seen in the central breast. However, the clip artifact (*arrowhead*) remains in the lateral breast, far distant from the focus of residual enhancement. Post-chemotherapy mammogram (not shown) demonstrated extensive residual calcifications, which were bracketed by needle localization. Pathology revealed extensive intraductal carcinoma, with small 0.7-cm focus of residual invasive disease.

after at least several cycles of therapy. Studies have suggested that computer-assisted volumetric analysis may be superior to simple linear tumor lengths for documenting early treatment changes, especially for irregular or multifocal/multicentric lesions.[144] However, even volumetric responses may not be a sensitive marker of early treatment response. Conversely, the quantitative evaluation of tCho on MRS may serve as a marker for early therapy response.[145–147] These reports have shown that in patients destined to be complete pathologic responders, a decrease in the tCho peak may be seen as early as 24 hours after the initial does of chemotherapy.[146] Another report did not detect significant differences in tCho values after the first dose of chemotherapy between complete responders and noncomplete responders,[147] but did define tCho midway through therapy to be a better predictor of response. However, in a multivariate analysis, the investigators found the tumor size at mid therapy to be the overall best predictor of pathologic response.

HIGH-RISK BREAST SCREENING BY MR IMAGING

Whereas the lifetime risk of breast cancer for a woman is as high as 1 in 8, for a woman who is a genetic mutation carrier the lifetime risk can be as high as 80%.[148,149] In addition to a significantly higher lifetime risk, these women tend to develop more aggressive cancers at an earlier age. Multiple studies have reported mammographically occult breast cancer detected by MR imaging in high-risk populations.[3,14–21,150] Therefore, surveillance by MR imaging, as an adjunct to screening mammography, is necessary in this high-risk population.

Kriege and colleagues[3] screened 1909 women (358 were known BRCA carriers) with greater than 15% lifetime risk for breast cancer comparing clinical breast examination (CBE) every 6 months, annual mammography, and MR imaging. The sensitivity and specificity of each of the examinations for invasive cancer were as follows: CBE (17.9%, 98.1%), mammography (33.3%, 95.0%) and MR imaging (79.5%, 89.8%). Although MR imaging had higher sensitivity in detecting invasive cancer, it was at the cost of slightly decreased specificity.

In the United Kingdom, Leach and colleagues[14] screened 649 women with either a strong family history of breast cancer or who were known BRCA1/2 or TP53 mutation carriers. The women were screened with mammography and MR imaging. There were 35 cancers diagnosed in 649 women: 19 were only seen on MR imaging,

6 only on mammography, 8 on both mammography and MR imaging, with 2 interval cases not initially identified on any modality. The sensitivity and specificity, respectively, for MR imaging was 77% and 81%, and for mammography 40% and 93%. The combined sensitivity of both MR imaging and mammography was 94%. Thirteen of the 35 cancers were diagnosed in BRCA1 carriers, and it is in this group that MR imaging sensitivity was the greatest (92% for MR imaging versus 23% for mammography).

Kuhl and colleagues[150] prospectively screened 529 asymptomatic high-risk women, detecting 43 cancers: 34 invasive and 9 DCIS. There was 1 interval cancer. The sensitivity and specificity of MR imaging was 91% and 97.2%, respectively, and for mammography 33% and 96.8%, respectively. In the known BRCA1 and BRCA2 mutation carriers, the sensitivity of MR imaging and mammography were, respectively, 100% and 25%, with MR imaging detecting 14 invasive cancers as well as 5 intraductal cancers in these high-risk women.

Canadian results also confirm the higher sensitivity of MR imaging compared with mammography. Warner and colleagues[16] screened 236 women detecting 22 cancers (6 invasive and 6 DCIS). The sensitivity and specificity were respectively 77% and 95.4% for MR imaging, and 33% and 99.8% for mammography.

Comparison of multimodality imaging techniques in high-risk populations has also been performed. Film screen mammogram, digital mammogram, whole breast ultrasound, and MR imaging were evaluated in 609 high-risk women in a screening setting.[151] The patients underwent each imaging modality separately (including separate initial interpretations), and the cancer yield of each distinct modality was evaluated. The overall cancer yield was 3%. By modality, the cancer yield was as follows: film screen mammography 1%, digital mammography 1.2%, whole breast ultrasound 0.5%, and MR imaging 2.1%. Whole breast sonography had the lowest sensitivity and cancer yield, although the screening study was performed by dedicated breast imagers at a teaching institution. The investigators found the addition of MR imaging to mammography resulted in the greatest incremental cancer yield.

Based on multiple studies, the sensitivity of MR imaging ranges from 71% to 100% compared with 16% to 40% for mammography,[9] with more recent studies reporting that MR imaging can even detect mammographically occult DCIS. However, there are drawbacks to MR imaging. The higher sensitivity of MR imaging is at the cost of a higher biopsy rate and lower specificity. In addition, although it has been demonstrated that MR imaging detects clinically and mammographically occult cancer, there is a lack of data demonstrating that screening MR imaging will result in improved survival for these patients. A large randomized study with mortality as the end point would be needed to answer such a question, but such a study would be difficult to perform, entailing accrual of a very large numbers of women at an extremely high study cost. Furthermore, as it is well established that MR imaging can detect mammographically and clinically occult cancer in the high-risk population, it may be difficult to recruit women into the non–MR imaging arm of a randomized prospective study.

Based on available data, the American Cancer Society screening guidelines include annual MR imaging screening for women with known BRCA1 or BRCA2 mutations, untested first-degree relatives of a known mutation carrier, and women with a greater than 20% to 25% lifetime risk-based assessment models. Based on expert consensus opinion, annual MR imaging is also recommended for patients (and first-degree relatives of patients) with Cowden, Bannayan-Riley-Ruvalcaba, or Li-Fraumeni syndromes, and for women who received radiation therapy to the chest between the ages of 10 and 30 years. At this time, it is felt that there is inconclusive evidence regarding screening of women with a personal history of breast cancer, lobular carcinoma in situ, atypical lobular hyperplasia, atypical ductal carcinoma, dense breast tissue, and lifetime risk level of 15% to 20%. MR imaging is not recommended for women with a less than 15% lifetime risk of breast cancer.

BREAST MR IMAGING CONTROVERSIES

Criticisms about MR imaging include the potential high false-positive rate, leading to unnecessary biopsies, and the clinical relevance of the MR imaging–detected secondary cancers. There are many factors that contribute to the false-positive rate. One is the interobserver variability of readers interpreting MR imaging studies,[152,153] a finding also observed in mammogram interpretations.[154] It is hoped that as experience with breast MR imaging increases, the false-positive rate will decrease. In the screening setting, the recall rate decreases with subsequent rounds of screening.[15,155] Comparison studies will decrease the recall rate, as is seen with mammography. The ACR Breast Imaging Reporting and Data System,[156] last published in 2003, includes a lexicon for breast MR imaging. The next edition of this lexicon is expected by 2011. As the lexicon and the imaging guidelines become standardized, this will aid in decreasing the variations in technique and interpretation.

Another common criticism of MR imaging is the clinical relevance of the cancer that is detected. Prior studies reporting pathologic evaluation of the mastectomy specimen of patients eligible for breast conservation therapy have shown tumor separate from the known primary tumor in 20% to 80% of patients.[88,89,157] The presence of unsuspected residual tumor on pathology was, in the past, used as an argument against breast conservation therapy. The results of 6 randomized studies, however, have shown there is no difference in survival between breast conservation therapy and mastectomy. The local recurrence after breast conservation therapy at 10 years is low, at less than 10% in patients with negative surgical margins.[158] It has been argued that whole breast radiation "controlled" the microscopic residual disease that may have been present. However, there are limitations to what radiation will treat. Studies have shown the average size of a clinically and mammographically occult incidental breast cancer detected by MR imaging is 1 cm. A 1-cm cancer found on MR imaging may behave no differently to a 1-cm cancer found on mammography, and it is accepted that radiation will often fail to adequately treat residual cancers of that size. It is these patients with substantial additional foci of cancer who therefore may fail breast conservation therapy. In addition, as increasingly localized treatments, such as partial breast radiation, gain in popularity, MR imaging will likely play a greater role in treatment planning.

Mastectomy rates have been rising after a decline in the 1990s. The reasons for the increase in the mastectomy rates are not clear. The increase may be partly attributed to the recognition of genetic susceptibility for breast cancer, the discovery of the BRCA1 and BRCA2 genes, and the increasing availability of gene testing for high-risk patients. While the number of gene-positive patients alone would not account for the increased mastectomy rate, patients not documented to be mutation carriers may still opt for prophylactic mastectomy, because these patients are aware that a negative test for the most common BRCA mutations does not exclude the possible presence of another, less common germline mutation when there is no documented mutation in the family.

Some researchers attribute the increase in mastectomy rates to the increasing use of MR imaging. MR imaging is highly sensitive in detecting breast cancer, but it does have lower specificity, not dissimilar to mammography. A

retrospective study was done at the Mayo Clinic evaluating the trends in the mastectomy rates at this institution.[159] After a decline in mastectomy rates of 45% in 1997 to 31% in 2003, they increased from 2003 to 2006. The investigators found that the mastectomy rates were higher in women who had MR imaging (54%), although the mastectomy rate also increased in women who did not undergo MR imaging (36%). The investigators were not able explain why there was a sharper increase in the mastectomy rate in women who had MR imaging studies.

Another reason for the overall increase in the mastectomy rates is that there are now elegant reconstruction options that can be performed at the time of the mastectomy, ranging from tissue flaps to implant reconstruction or a combination of both. In a study by Alderman and colleagues,[160] the patients who were informed about the reconstruction options were 4 times more likely to consider mastectomy over breast conservation therapy.

Finally, there is now evidence from multiple studies that MR imaging detects clinically and mammographically occult breast cancer. This improved detection of occult secondary malignant foci by MR imaging would in theory allow for improved surgical management. However, in a recently published randomized multisite trial,[161] preoperative MR imaging did not reduce the reexcision rate in women with clinically localized breast cancer. Furthermore, while one retrospective study has demonstrated fewer local recurrences in breast conservation therapy patients who underwent preoperative MR imaging,[162] there are currently no published prospective randomized studies demonstrating improvement in long-term local recurrence rates with preoperative MR imaging. As such, the role of preoperative MR imaging in women with clinically localized breast cancer remains controversial.

SUMMARY

Breast MR imaging has brought about a revolution in breast imaging, and continues to evolve and improve technically. From its nascent period when the first contrast-enhanced MR imaging was performed, breast MR imaging use has grown substantially, with multiple clinical scenarios whereby MR imaging is now routine for screening, diagnosis, or staging of disease. There are still limitations to the technology; it is expensive and not as widely available as mammography. Deficiencies with specificity remain a challenge to the breast imaging community, and controversies regarding the best indication for clinical use remain. As breast MR imaging techniques and practice evolve and the role of breast MR imaging is refined and redefined, firmer clinical indications for breast MR imaging will likely emerge, and the uses of MR imaging will continue to expand.

REFERENCES

1. Jemal A, Siegel R, Ward E, et al. Cancer statistics, 2009. CA Cancer J Clin 2009;59:225–49.

2. Kerlikowske K, Carney PA, Geller B, et al. Performance of screening mammography among women with and without a first-degree relative with breast cancer. Ann Intern Med 2000;133(11):855–63.

3. Kriege M, Brekelmans CT, Boetes C, et al. Efficacy of MRI and mammography for breast-cancer screening in women with a familial or genetic predisposition. N Engl J Med 2004; 351(5):427–37.

4. Mandelson MT, Oestreicher N, Porter PL, et al. Breast density as a predictor of mammographic detection: comparison of interval- and screen-detected cancers. J Natl Cancer Inst 2000;92(13):1081–7.

5. Kuhl CK. The "coming of age" of nonmammographic screening for breast cancer. JAMA 2008; 299(18):2203–5.

6. Kaiser WA, Zeitler E. MR imaging of the breast: fast imaging sequences with and without Gd-DTPA. Preliminary observations. Radiology 1989;170(3 Pt 1):681–6.

7. Heywang SH, Wolf A, Pruss E, et al. MR imaging of the breast with Gd-DTPA: use and limitations. Radiology 1989;171(1):95–103.

8. Kuhl CK, Bieling HB, Gieseke J, et al. Healthy premenopausal breast parenchyma in dynamic contrast-enhanced MR imaging of the breast: normal contrast medium enhancement and cyclical-phase dependency. Radiology 1997; 203(1):137–44.

9. Saslow D, Boetes C, Burke W, et al. American Cancer Society guidelines for breast screening with MRI as an adjunct to mammography. CA Cancer J Clin 2007;57(2):75–89.

10. Bluemke DA, Gatsonis CA, Chen MH, et al. Magnetic resonance imaging of the breast prior to biopsy. JAMA 2004;292(22):2735–42.

11. Orel SG, Schnall MD. MR imaging of the breast for the detection, diagnosis, and staging of breast cancer. Radiology 2001;220(1):13–30.

12. Boetes C, Barentsz JO, Mus RD, et al. MR characterization of suspicious breast lesions with a gadolinium-enhanced TurboFLASH subtraction technique. Radiology 1994;193(3):777–81.

13. Fischer U, Kopka L, Grabbe E. Breast carcinoma: effect of preoperative contrast-enhanced MR imaging on the therapeutic approach. Radiology 1999;213(3):881–8.

14. Leach MO, Boggis CR, Dixon AK, et al. Screening with magnetic resonance imaging and mammography of a UK population at high familial risk of breast cancer: a prospective multicentre cohort study (MARIBS). Lancet 2005; 365(9473):1769–78.

15. Kuhl CK, Schmutzler RK, Leutner CC, et al. Breast MR imaging screening in 192 women proved or suspected to be carriers of a breast cancer susceptibility gene: preliminary results. Radiology 2000;215(1):267–79.

16. Warner E, Plewes DB, Hill KA, et al. Surveillance of BRCA1 and BRCA2 mutation carriers with magnetic resonance imaging, ultrasound, mammography, and clinical breast examination. JAMA 2004;292(11):1317–25.

17. Podo F, Sardanelli F, Canese R, et al. The Italian multi-centre project on evaluation of MRI and other imaging modalities in early detection of breast cancer in subjects at high genetic risk. J Exp Clin Cancer Res 2002;21(Suppl 3):115–24.

18. Tilanus-Linthorst MM, Obdeijn IM, Bartels KC, et al. First experiences in screening women at high risk for breast cancer with MR imaging. Breast Cancer Res Treat 2000;63(1):53–60.

19. Morris EA, Liberman L, Ballon DJ, et al. MRI of occult breast carcinoma in a high-risk population. AJR Am J Roentgenol 2003;181(3):619–26.

20. Lehman CD, Blume JD, Weatherall P, et al. Screening women at high risk for breast cancer with mammography and magnetic resonance imaging. Cancer 2005;103(9):1898–905.

21. Lehman CD, Isaacs C, Schnall MD, et al. Cancer yield of mammography, MR, and US in high-risk women: prospective multi-institution breast cancer screening study. Radiology 2007;244(2):381–8.

22. Orel SG, Mendonca MH, Reynolds C, et al. MR imaging of ductal carcinoma in situ. Radiology 1997;202(2):413–20.

23. Boetes C, Mann RM. Ductal carcinoma in situ and breast MRI. Lancet 2007;370(9586):459–60.

24. Bazzocchi M, Zuiani C, Panizza P, et al. Contrast-enhanced breast MRI in patients with suspicious microcalcifications on mammography: results of a multicenter trial. AJR Am J Roentgenol 2006; 186(6):1723–32.

25. Ikeda O, Nishimura R, Miyayama H, et al. Magnetic resonance evaluation of the presence of an extensive intraductal component in breast cancer. Acta Radiol 2004;45(7):721–5.

26. Menell JH, Morris EA, Dershaw DD, et al. Determination of the presence and extent of pure ductal carcinoma in situ by mammography and magnetic resonance imaging. Breast J 2005;11(6):382–90.

27. Neubauer H, Li M, Kuehne-Heid R, et al. High grade and non-high grade ductal carcinoma in situ on dynamic MR mammography: characteristic findings

for signal increase and morphological pattern of enhancement. Br J Radiol 2003;76(901):3–12.

28. Kuhl CK, Schrading S, Bieling HB, et al. MRI for diagnosis of pure ductal carcinoma in situ: a prospective observational study. Lancet 2007; 370(9586):485–92.

29. Partridge SC. Future applications and innovations of clinical breast magnetic resonance imaging. Top Magn Reson Imaging 2008;19(3):171–6.

30. Ikeda T, Monzawa S, Komoto K, et al. Performance assessment of phased-array coil in breast MR imaging. Magn Reson Med Sci 2004;3(1):39–43.

31. Konyer NB, Ramsay EA, Bronskill MJ, et al. Comparison of MR imaging breast coils. Radiology 2002;222(3):830–4.

32. Han M, Beatty PJ, Daniel BL, et al. Independent slab-phase modulation combined with parallel imaging in bilateral breast MRI. Magn Reson Med 2009;62(5):1221–31.

33. Orlacchio A, Bolacchi F, Rotili A, et al. MR breast imaging: a comparative analysis of conventional and parallel imaging acquisition. Radiol Med 2008;113(4):465–76.

34. Dougherty L, Isaac G, Rosen MA, et al. High frame-rate simultaneous bilateral breast DCE-MRI. Magn Reson Med 2007;57(1):220–5.

35. Calabrese M, Brizzi D, Carbonaro L, et al. Contrast-enhanced breast MR imaging of claustrophobic or oversized patients using an open low-field magnet. Radiol Med 2009;114(2):267–85.

36. Rubinstein WS, Latimer JJ, Sumkin JH, et al. Prospective screening study of 0.5 Tesla dedicated magnetic resonance imaging for the detection of breast cancer in young, high-risk women. BMC Womens Health 2006;6:10.

37. Paakko E, Reinikainen H, Lindholm EL, et al. Low-field versus high-field MRI in diagnosing breast disorders. Eur Radiol 2005;15(7):1361–8.

38. Daniel BL, Butts K, Glover GH, et al. Breast cancer: gadolinium-enhanced MR imaging with a 0.5-T open imager and three-point Dixon technique. Radiology 1998;207(1):183–90.

39. Pinker K, Grabner G, Bogner W, et al. A combined high temporal and high spatial resolution 3 Tesla MR imaging protocol for the assessment of breast lesions: initial results. Invest Radiol 2009;44(9): 553–8.

40. Matsuoka A, Minato M, Harada M, et al. Comparison of 3.0-and 1.5-tesla diffusion-weighted imaging in the visibility of breast cancer. Radiat Med 2008;26(1):15–20.

41. Kuhl CK. Breast MR imaging at 3T. Magn Reson Imaging Clin N Am 2007;15(3):315–20, vi.

42. Kuhl CK, Jost P, Morakkabati N, et al. Contrast-enhanced MR imaging of the breast at 3.0 and 1.5 T in the same patients: initial experience. Radiology 2006;239(3):666–76.

43. Available at: http://www.acr.org/SecondaryMain MenuCategories/quality_safety/guidelines/breast/ mri_breast.aspx; 2008. Accessed October 3, 2010.

44. Ballesio L, Savelli S, Angeletti M, et al. Breast MRI: are T2 IR sequences useful in the evaluation of breast lesions? Eur J Radiol 2009;71(1):96–101.

45. Kuhl CK, Klaschik S, Mielcarek P, et al. Do T2-weighted pulse sequences help with the differential diagnosis of enhancing lesions in dynamic breast MRI? J Magn Reson Imaging 1999;9(2):187–96.

46. Taboada JL, Stephens TW, Krishnamurthy S, et al. The many faces of fat necrosis in the breast. AJR Am J Roentgenol 2009;192(3):815–25.

47. Daly CP, Jaeger B, Sill DS. Variable appearances of fat necrosis on breast MRI. AJR Am J Roentgenol 2008;191(5):1374–80.

48. Testempassi E, Ishi C, Yamada T, et al. Case report: breast hamartoma: MR findings. Radiat Med 1995; 13(4):187–9.

49. Killian JK, Merino M, Bondy C, et al. MRI of angiolipoma of the breast in Turner's syndrome. AJR Am J Roentgenol 2004;183(6):1843–4.

50. Available at: http://www.fda.gov/NewsEvents/ Newsroom/PressAnnouncements/2007/ucm108919. htm. 2007. Accessed October 3, 2010.

51. Grobner T, Prischl FC. Gadolinium and nephrogenic systemic fibrosis. Kidney Int 2007;72(3):260–4.

52. Grobner T. Gadolinium—a specific trigger for the development of nephrogenic fibrosing dermopathy and nephrogenic systemic fibrosis? Nephrol Dial Transplant 2006;21(4):1104–8.

53. Kuhl CK, Kooijman H, Gieseke J, et al. Effect of B1 inhomogeneity on breast MR imaging at 3.0 T. Radiology 2007;244(3):929–30.

54. Stack JP, Redmond OM, Codd MB, et al. Breast disease: tissue characterization with Gd-DTPA enhancement profiles. Radiology 1990;174(2): 491–4.

55. El Khouli RH, Macura KJ, Barker PB, et al. Relationship of temporal resolution to diagnostic performance for dynamic contrast enhanced MRI of the breast. J Magn Reson Imaging 2009;30(5): 999–1004.

56. Li X, Huang W, Yankeelov TE, et al. Shutter-speed analysis of contrast reagent bolus-tracking data: preliminary observations in benign and malignant breast disease. Magn Reson Med 2005;53(3):724–9.

57. Huang W, Li X, Morris EA, et al. The magnetic resonance shutter speed discriminates vascular properties of malignant and benign breast tumors in vivo. Proc Natl Acad Sci U S A 2008;105(46): 17943–8.

58. Nunes LW, Schnall MD, Orel SG, et al. Breast MR imaging: interpretation model. Radiology 1997; 202(3):833–41.

59. Nunes LW, Schnall MD, Orel SG. Update of breast MR imaging architectural interpretation model. Radiology 2001;219(2):484–94.

60. Kuhl CK, Mielcareck P, Klaschik S, et al. Dynamic breast MR imaging: are signal intensity time course data useful for differential diagnosis of enhancing lesions? Radiology 1999;211(1):101–10.

61. Kuhl CK, Schild HH, Morakkabati N. Dynamic bilateral contrast-enhanced MR imaging of the breast: trade-off between spatial and temporal resolution. Radiology 2005;236(3):789–800.

62. Schnall MD, Blume J, Bluemke DA, et al. Diagnostic architectural and dynamic features at breast MR imaging: multicenter study. Radiology 2006; 238(1):42–53.

63. Korosec FR, Frayne R, Grist TM, et al. Time-resolved contrast-enhanced 3D MR angiography. Magn Reson Med 1996;36(3):345–51.

64. Perman WH, Heiberg EV, Herrmann VM. Half-Fourier, three-dimensional technique for dynamic contrast-enhanced MR imaging of both breasts and axillae: initial characterization of breast lesions. Radiology 1996;200(1):263–9.

65. Plewes DB, Bishop J, Soutar I, et al. Errors in quantitative dynamic three-dimensional keyhole MR imaging of the breast. J Magn Reson Imaging 1995;5(3):361–4.

66. Bishop JE, Santyr GE, Kelcz F, et al. Limitations of the keyhole technique for quantitative dynamic contrast-enhanced breast MRI. J Magn Reson Imaging 1997;7(4):716–23.

67. Han M, Daniel BL, Hargreaves BA. Accelerated bilateral dynamic contrast-enhanced 3D spiral breast MRI using TSENSE. J Magn Reson Imaging 2008;28(6):1425–34.

68. Chan RW, Ramsay EA, Cunningham CH, et al. Temporal stability of adaptive 3D radial MRI using multidimensional golden means. Magn Reson Med 2009;61(2):354–63.

69. Baek HM, Yu HJ, Chen JH, et al. Quantitative correlation between (1)H MRS and dynamic contrast-enhanced MRI of human breast cancer. Magn Reson Imaging 2008;26(4):523–31.

70. Jacobs MA, Barker PB, Argani P, et al. Combined dynamic contrast enhanced breast MR and proton spectroscopic imaging: a feasibility study. J Magn Reson Imaging 2005;21(1):23–8.

71. Kim JK, Park SH, Lee HM, et al. In vivo 1H-MRS evaluation of malignant and benign breast diseases. Breast 2003;12(3):179–82.

72. Kvistad KA, Bakken IJ, Gribbestad IS, et al. Characterization of neoplastic and normal human breast tissues with in vivo (1)H MR spectroscopy. J Magn Reson Imaging 1999; 10(2):159–64.

73. Gribbestad IS, Singstad TE, Nilsen G, et al. In vivo 1H MRS of normal breast and breast tumors using a dedicated double breast coil. J Magn Reson Imaging 1998;8(6):1191–7.

74. Roebuck JR, Cecil KM, Schnall MD, et al. Human breast lesions: characterization with proton MR spectroscopy. Radiology 1998;209(1):269–75.

75. Bartella L, Morris EA, Dershaw DD, et al. Proton MR spectroscopy with choline peak as malignancy marker improves positive predictive value for breast cancer diagnosis: preliminary study. Radiology 2006;239(3):686–92.

76. Bartella L, Thakur SB, Morris EA, et al. Enhancing nonmass lesions in the breast: evaluation with proton (1H) MR spectroscopy. Radiology 2007;245(1):80–7.

77. Chen JH, Baek HM, Nalcioglu O, et al. Estrogen receptor and breast MR imaging features: a correlation study. J Magn Reson Imaging 2008;27(4): 825–33.

78. Guo Y, Cai YQ, Cai ZL, et al. Differentiation of clinically benign and malignant breast lesions using diffusion-weighted imaging. J Magn Reson Imaging 2002;16(2):172–8.

79. Kinoshita T, Yashiro N, Ihara N, et al. Diffusion-weighted half-Fourier single-shot turbo spin echo imaging in breast tumors: differentiation of invasive ductal carcinoma from fibroadenoma. J Comput Assist Tomogr 2002;26(6):1042–6.

80. Kuroki Y, Nasu K, Kuroki S, et al. Diffusion-weighted imaging of breast cancer with the sensitivity encoding technique: analysis of the apparent diffusion coefficient value. Magn Reson Med Sci 2004;3(2):79–85.

81. Partridge SC, DeMartini WB, Kurland BF, et al. Quantitative diffusion-weighted imaging as an adjunct to conventional breast MRI for improved positive predictive value. AJR Am J Roentgenol 2009;193(6):1716–22.

82. Pereira FP, Martins G, Figueiredo E, et al. Assessment of breast lesions with diffusion-weighted MRI: comparing the use of different b values. AJR Am J Roentgenol 2009;193(4):1030–5.

83. Lo GG, Ai V, Chan JK, et al. Diffusion-weighted magnetic resonance imaging of breast lesions: first experiences at 3 T. J Comput Assist Tomogr 2009; 33(1):63–9.

84. Bogner W, Gruber S, Pinker K, et al. Diffusion-weighted MR for differentiation of breast lesions at 3.0 T: how does selection of diffusion protocols affect diagnosis? Radiology 2009;253(2):341–51.

85. Wasif N, Garreau J, Terando A, et al. MRI versus ultrasonography and mammography for preoperative assessment of breast cancer. Am Surg 2009; 75(10):970–5.

86. Mann RM, Veltman J, Barentsz JO, et al. The value of MRI compared to mammography in the assessment of tumour extent in invasive lobular carcinoma of the breast. Eur J Surg Oncol 2008;34(2):135–42.

87. Mann RM, Loo CE, Wobbes T, et al. The impact of preoperative breast MRI on the re-excision rate in invasive lobular carcinoma of the breast. Breast Cancer Res Treat 2010;119(2):415–22.

88. Rosen PP, Fracchia AA, Urban JA, et al. "Residual" mammary carcinoma following simulated partial mastectomy. Cancer 1975;35(3):739–47.

89. Holland R, Veling SH, Mravunac M, et al. Histologic multifocality of Tis, T1-2 breast carcinomas. Implications for clinical trials of breast-conserving surgery. Cancer 1985;56(5):979–90.

90. Faverly DR, Hendriks JH, Holland R. Breast carcinomas of limited extent: frequency, radiologic–pathologic characteristics, and surgical margin requirements. Cancer 2001;91(4):647–59.

91. Fisher B, Anderson S, Redmond CK, et al. Reanalysis and results after 12 years of follow-up in a randomized clinical trial comparing total mastectomy with lumpectomy with or without irradiation in the treatment of breast cancer. N Engl J Med 1995; 333(22):1456–61.

92. Veronesi U, Luini A, Galimberti V, et al. Conservation approaches for the management of stage I/II carcinoma of the breast: Milan Cancer Institute Trials. World J Surg 1994;18(1):70–5.

93. Veronesi U, Luini A, Del Vecchio M, et al. Radiotherapy after breast-preserving surgery in women with localized cancer of the breast. N Engl J Med 1993;328(22):1587–91.

94. Fisher B, Anderson S, Bryant J, et al. Twenty-year follow-up of a randomized trial comparing total mastectomy, lumpectomy, and lumpectomy plus irradiation for the treatment of invasive breast cancer. N Engl J Med 2002;347(16):1233–41.

95. Wapnir IL, Anderson SJ, Mamounas EP, et al. Prognosis after ipsilateral breast tumor recurrence and locoregional recurrences in five National Surgical Adjuvant Breast and Bowel Project node-positive adjuvant breast cancer trials. J Clin Oncol 2006; 24(13):2028–37.

96. Solin LJ, Orel SG, Hwang WT, et al. Relationship of breast magnetic resonance imaging to outcome after breast-conservation treatment with radiation for women with early-stage invasive breast carcinoma or ductal carcinoma in situ. J Clin Oncol 2008;26(3):386–91.

97. Schnall MD, Blume J, Bluemke DA, et al. MRI detection of distinct incidental cancer in women with primary breast cancer studied in IBMC 6883. J Surg Oncol 2005;92(1):32–8.

98. Deurloo EE, Peterse JL, Rutgers EJ, et al. Additional breast lesions in patients eligible for breast-conserving therapy by MRI: impact on preoperative management and potential benefit of computerised analysis. Eur J Cancer 2005;41(10):1393–401.

99. Schelfout K, Van Goethem M, Kersschot E, et al. Contrast-enhanced MR imaging of breast lesions and effect on treatment. Eur J Surg Oncol 2004; 30(5):501–7.

100. Berg WA, Gutierrez L, NessAiver MS, et al. Diagnostic accuracy of mammography, clinical examination, US, and MR imaging in preoperative assessment of breast cancer. Radiology 2004; 233(3):830–49.

101. Hata T, Takahashi H, Watanabe K, et al. Magnetic resonance imaging for preoperative evaluation of breast cancer: a comparative study with mammography and ultrasonography. J Am Coll Surg 2004; 198(2):190–7.

102. Sardanelli F, Giuseppetti GM, Panizza P, et al. Sensitivity of MRI versus mammography for detecting foci of multifocal, multicentric breast cancer in fatty and dense breasts using the whole-breast pathologic examination as a gold standard. AJR Am J Roentgenol 2004;183(4):1149–57.

103. Orel SG, Schnall MD, Powell CM, et al. Staging of suspected breast cancer: effect of MR imaging and MR-guided biopsy. Radiology 1995;196(1): 115–22.

104. Boetes C, Mus RD, Holland R, et al. Breast tumors: comparative accuracy of MR imaging relative to mammography and US for demonstrating extent. Radiology 1995;197(3):743–7.

105. Mumtaz H, Hall-Craggs MA, Davidson T, et al. Staging of symptomatic primary breast cancer with MR imaging. AJR Am J Roentgenol 1997; 169(2):417–24.

106. Kramer S, Schulz-Wendtland R, Hagedorn K, et al. Magnetic resonance imaging and its role in the diagnosis of multicentric breast cancer. Anticancer Res 1998;18(3C):2163–4.

107. Bedrosian I, Mick R, Orel SG, et al. Changes in the surgical management of patients with breast carcinoma based on preoperative magnetic resonance imaging. Cancer 2003;98(3):468–73.

108. Schnall M. MR imaging evaluation of cancer extent: is there clinical relevance? Magn Reson Imaging Clin N Am 2006;14(3):379–81, vii.

109. Morris EA, Schwartz LH, Drotman MB, et al. Evaluation of pectoralis major muscle in patients with posterior breast tumors on breast MR images: early experience. Radiology 2000;214(1):67–72.

110. Kazama T, Nakamura S, Doi O, et al. Prospective evaluation of pectoralis muscle invasion of breast cancer by MR imaging. Breast Cancer 2005; 12(4):312–6.

111. Egan RL. Bilateral breast carcinomas: role of mammography. Cancer 1976;38(2):931–8.

112. Hungness ES, Safa M, Shaughnessy EA, et al. Bilateral synchronous breast cancer: mode of detection and comparison of histologic features between the 2 breasts. Surgery 2000;128(4):702–7.

113. Slanetz PJ, Edmister WB, Yeh ED, et al. Occult contralateral breast carcinoma incidentally

detected by breast magnetic resonance imaging. Breast J 2002;8(3):145–8.

114. Pediconi F, Catalano C, Roselli A, et al. Contrast-enhanced MR mammography for evaluation of the contralateral breast in patients with diagnosed unilateral breast cancer or high-risk lesions. Radiology 2007;243(3):670–80.

115. Liberman L, Morris EA, Kim CM, et al. MR imaging findings in the contralateral breast of women with recently diagnosed breast cancer. AJR Am J Roentgenol 2003;180(2):333–41.

116. Lee SG, Orel SG, Woo IJ, et al. MR imaging screening of the contralateral breast in patients with newly diagnosed breast cancer: preliminary results. Radiology 2003;226(3):773–8.

117. Lehman CD, Blume JD, Thickman D, et al. Added cancer yield of MRI in screening the contralateral breast of women recently diagnosed with breast cancer: results from the International Breast Magnetic Resonance Consortium (IBMC) Trial. J Surg Oncol 2005;92(1):9–15 [discussion: 15–6].

118. Lehman CD, Gatsonis C, Kuhl CK, et al. MRI evaluation of the contralateral breast in women with recently diagnosed breast cancer. N Engl J Med 2007;356(13):1295–303.

119. Morris EA, Schwartz LH, Dershaw DD, et al. MR imaging of the breast in patients with occult primary breast carcinoma. Radiology 1997;205(2):437–40.

120. Tilanus-Linthorst MM, Obdeijn AI, Bontenbal M, et al. MRI in patients with axillary metastases of occult breast carcinoma. Breast Cancer Res Treat 1997;44(2):179–82.

121. Orel SG, Weinstein SP, Schnall MD, et al. Breast MR imaging in patients with axillary node metastases and unknown primary malignancy. Radiology 1999;212(2):543–9.

122. Stomper PC, Waddell BE, Edge SB, et al. Breast MRI in the evaluation of patients with occult primary breast carcinoma. Breast J 1999;5(4):230–4.

123. Henry-Tillman RS, Harms SE, Westbrook KC, et al. Role of breast magnetic resonance imaging in determining breast as a source of unknown metastatic lymphadenopathy. Am J Surg 1999;178(6):496–500.

124. Buchanan CL, Morris EA, Dorn PL, et al. Utility of breast magnetic resonance imaging in patients with occult primary breast cancer. Ann Surg Oncol 2005;12(12):1045–53.

125. Tozaki M, Yamashiro N, Suzuki T, et al. MR-guided vacuum-assisted breast biopsy: is it an essential technique? Breast Cancer 2009;16(2):121–5.

126. Malhaire C, El Khoury C, Thibault F, et al. Vacuum-assisted biopsies under MR guidance: results of 72 procedures. Eur Radiol 2010;20:1554–62.

127. Masood S, Khalbuss WE. Nipple fluid cytology. Clin Lab Med 2005;25(4):787–94, vii–viii.

128. Rovno HD, Siegelman ES, Reynolds C, et al. Solitary intraductal papilloma: findings at MR imaging and MR galactography. AJR Am J Roentgenol 1999;172(1):151–5.

129. Orel SG, Dougherty CS, Reynolds C, et al. MR imaging in patients with nipple discharge: initial experience. Radiology 2000;216(1):248–54.

130. Nakahara H, Namba K, Watanabe R, et al. A comparison of MR imaging, galactography and ultrasonography in patients with nipple discharge. Breast Cancer 2003;10(4):320–9.

131. Morrogh M, Morris EA, Liberman L, et al. The predictive value of ductography and magnetic resonance imaging in the management of nipple discharge. Ann Surg Oncol 2007;14(12):3369–77.

132. Yoshimoto M, Kasumi F, Iwase T, et al. Magnetic resonance galactography for a patient with nipple discharge. Breast Cancer Res Treat 1997;42(1):87–90.

133. Moy L, Elias K, Patel V, et al. Is breast MRI helpful in the evaluation of inconclusive mammographic findings? AJR Am J Roentgenol 2009;193(4):986–93.

134. Fisher B, Brown A, Mamounas E, et al. Effect of preoperative chemotherapy on local-regional disease in women with operable breast cancer: findings from National Surgical Adjuvant Breast and Bowel Project B-18. J Clin Oncol 1997;15(7):2483–93.

135. Fisher B, Bryant J, Wolmark N, et al. Effect of preoperative chemotherapy on the outcome of women with operable breast cancer. J Clin Oncol 1998;16(8):2672–85.

136. Chang YC, Huang CS, Liu YJ, et al. Angiogenic response of locally advanced breast cancer to neoadjuvant chemotherapy evaluated with parametric histogram from dynamic contrast-enhanced MRI. Phys Med Biol 2004;49(16):3593–602.

137. Martincich L, Montemurro F, De Rosa G, et al. Monitoring response to primary chemotherapy in breast cancer using dynamic contrast-enhanced magnetic resonance imaging. Breast Cancer Res Treat 2004;83(1):67–76.

138. Padhani AR, Hayes C, Assersohn L, et al. Prediction of clinicopathologic response of breast cancer to primary chemotherapy at contrast-enhanced MR imaging: initial clinical results. Radiology 2006;239(2):361–74.

139. Pickles MD, Lowry M, Manton DJ, et al. Role of dynamic contrast enhanced MRI in monitoring early response of locally advanced breast cancer to neoadjuvant chemotherapy. Breast Cancer Res Treat 2005;91(1):1–10.

140. Esserman L, Hylton N, Yassa L, et al. Utility of magnetic resonance imaging in the management of breast cancer: evidence for improved preoperative staging. J Clin Oncol 1999;17(1):110–9.

141. Drew PJ, Kerin MJ, Mahapatra T, et al. Evaluation of response to neoadjuvant chemoradiotherapy for locally advanced breast cancer with dynamic contrast-enhanced MRI of the breast. Eur J Surg Oncol 2001;27(7):617–20.

142. Balu-Maestro C, Chapellier C, Bleuse A, et al. Imaging in evaluation of response to neoadjuvant breast cancer treatment benefits of MRI. Breast Cancer Res Treat 2002;72(2):145–52.

143. Partridge SC, Gibbs JE, Lu Y, et al. Accuracy of MR imaging for revealing residual breast cancer in patients who have undergone neoadjuvant chemotherapy. AJR Am J Roentgenol 2002;179(5):1193–9.

144. Partridge SC, Gibbs JE, Lu Y, et al. MRI measurements of breast tumor volume predict response to neoadjuvant chemotherapy and recurrence-free survival. AJR Am J Roentgenol 2005;184(6):1774–81.

145. Jagannathan NR, Kumar M, Seenu V, et al. Evaluation of total choline from in-vivo volume localized proton MR spectroscopy and its response to neoadjuvant chemotherapy in locally advanced breast cancer. Br J Cancer 2001;84(8):1016–22.

146. Meisamy S, Bolan PJ, Baker EH, et al. Neoadjuvant chemotherapy of locally advanced breast cancer: predicting response with in vivo (1)H MR spectroscopy—a pilot study at 4 T. Radiology 2004;233(2): 424–31.

147. Baek HM, Chen JH, Nie K, et al. Predicting pathologic response to neoadjuvant chemotherapy in breast cancer by using MR imaging and quantitative 1H MR spectroscopy. Radiology 2009;251(3): 653–62.

148. Ford D, Easton DF, Bishop DT, et al. Risks of cancer in BRCA1-mutation carriers. Breast Cancer Linkage Consortium. Lancet 1994;343(8899):692–5.

149. Antoniou A, Pharoah PD, Narod S, et al. Average risks of breast and ovarian cancer associated with BRCA1 or BRCA2 mutations detected in case series unselected for family history: a combined analysis of 22 studies. Am J Hum Genet 2003;72(5):1117–30.

150. Kuhl CK, Schrading S, Leutner CC, et al. Mammography, breast ultrasound, and magnetic resonance imaging for surveillance of women at high familial risk for breast cancer. J Clin Oncol 2005;23(33): 8469–76.

151. Weinstein SP, Localio AR, Conant EF, et al. Multimodality screening of high-risk women: a prospective cohort study. J Clin Oncol 2009;27:6124–8.

152. Warren RM, Pointon L, Thompson D, et al. Reading protocol for dynamic contrast-enhanced MR images of the breast: sensitivity and specificity analysis. Radiology 2005;236(3):779–88.

153. Ikeda DM, Hylton NM, Kinkel K, et al. Development, standardization, and testing of a lexicon for reporting contrast-enhanced breast magnetic resonance imaging studies. J Magn Reson Imaging 2001; 13(6):889–95.

154. Berg WA, Campassi C, Langenberg P, et al. Breast Imaging Reporting and Data System: inter- and intraobserver variability in feature analysis and final assessment. AJR Am J Roentgenol 2000;174(6): 1769–77.

155. Warner E, Causer PA. MRI surveillance for hereditary breast-cancer risk. Lancet 2005;365(9473): 1747–9.

156. American College of Radiology. ACR BI-RADS: ACR breast imaging reporting and data system, breast imaging atlas. Reston (VA): American College of Radiology; 2003.

157. Qualheim RE, Gall EA. Breast carcinoma with multiple sites of origin. Cancer 1957;10(3):460–8.

158. Smitt MC, Nowels KW, Zdeblick MJ, et al. The importance of the lumpectomy surgical margin status in long-term results of breast conservation. Cancer 1995;76(2):259–67.

159. Katipamula R, Degnim AC, Hoskin T, et al. Trends in mastectomy rates at the Mayo Clinic Rochester: effect of surgical year and preoperative magnetic resonance imaging. J Clin Oncol 2009;27(25): 4082–8.

160. Alderman AK, Hawley ST, Waljee J, et al. Understanding the impact of breast reconstruction on the surgical decision-making process for breast cancer. Cancer 2008;112(3):489–94.

161. Turnbull L, Brown S, Harvey I, et al. Comparative effectiveness of MRI in breast cancer (COMICE) trial: a randomised controlled trial. Lancet 2010; 375(9714):563–71.

162. Fischer U, Zachariae O, Baum F, et al. The influence of preoperative MRI of the breasts on recurrence rate in patients with breast cancer. Eur Radiol 2004;14(10):1725–31.

Dedicated Breast Computed Tomography: The Optimal Cross-Sectional Imaging Solution?

Karen K. Lindfors, MD, MPH[a],*, John M. Boone, PhD[a],
Mary S. Newell, MD[b], Carl J. D'Orsi, MD[b]

KEYWORDS

- Digital breast tomosynthesis • Full-field digital mammography
- Stereoscopic digital mammography
- Dedicated breast computed tomography

Mammography has widespread acceptance as a screening modality for breast cancer, with mortality reduction of 30% to 40% in screened populations.[1] However, mammography has limitations. Its sensitivity for cancer detection when used for screening is in the 80% range, ranging from 70.8% in the 40- to 44-year-old age group to 84.5% for patients aged 75 to 89 years.[2] In addition, there is an accepted recall rate of 10% (with 90% of the recalled findings proving to be nonactionable) and an expected negative biopsy rate in the range of 60% to 75% for mammographically identified suspicious lesions, both of which result in added cost, anxiety, and potential morbidity.

One inherent limitation of planar mammography is that a three-dimensional, volumetric structure (the breast) is imaged, but the resultant data are displayed in a two-dimensional manner. This leads to superimposition of tissue and limits effectiveness, especially in women with dense breasts. Carney and colleagues[3] showed a decrease in mammographic sensitivity as a function of increasing breast density (87.0% sensitivity in women with fatty density (87.0% sensitivity in women with fatty breasts vs 62.9% in women with extremely dense breasts). Berg and colleagues[4] demonstrated an even lower sensitivity rate of 45% among women with extremely dense breasts. Yankaskas and colleagues[5] showed that as breast density increases, so does the recall rate from 2.4% in almost entirely fat breasts to 6.9% in extremely dense breasts. This makes intuitive sense, as most noncalcified cancers and normal fibroglandular tissue share similar x-ray attenuation values; as a result, the presence of a significant amount of background noise (heterogeneously or extremely dense parenchymal pattern) can lead to misrepresentation of normal tissue as a potential abnormality requiring recall (false-positive) or, more ominously, nondetection of a cancer obscured by adjacent or overlapping tissue (false-negative). Obtaining 2 near-orthogonal mammographic views (rather than a single view) serves as an attempt at three-dimensionality, helping to sort out real from spurious findings, and aiding in localization of potential abnormalities. However, even when additional views (eg, 90° lateral, step-oblique, rolled views)

This was supported, in part, by Grant No. R01 EB002138 from the National Institutes of Health.
[a] Department of Radiology, University of California, Davis School of Medicine, 4860 Y Street, Suite 3100, Sacramento, CA 95817, USA
[b] Section of Breast Imaging, Winship Cancer Institute, Emory University, Atlanta, GA 30322, USA
* Corresponding author.
E-mail address: kklindfors@ucdavis.edu

Radiol Clin N Am 48 (2010) 1043–1054
doi:10.1016/j.rcl.2010.06.001

are obtained, it remains the mammographer's burden to construct a mental three-dimensional virtual image of the breast, and superimposition of tissue in women with any significant degree of density persists as a limiting constraint.

Full-field digital mammography (FFDM), with its improved dynamic range, tissue contrast, and ability to postprocess digital images, was expected to improve cancer detection, particularly in dense-breasted women. This was confirmed in the Digital Mammographic Imaging Screening Trial, which showed statistically significant improved sensitivity for cancer detection with FFDM compared with screen-film mammography, but only in women less than 50 years of age, pre- or perimenopausal, and with dense breasts, the last factor appearing to be the key.[6,7] However, the issue of tissue superimposition lingers, because while the digital images can be manipulated in many ways, they remain planar.

Imaging the breast with ultrasound (US) more closely approximates a three-dimensional examination, with 2 planes (depth and the chosen transducer orientation plane) visualized at any single moment with the third dimension added by the operator's real-time sweep of the transducer. In most cases, all tissue from skin to chest wall can be interrogated in a single frame, such that superimposition of tissue is not a factor. The effectiveness of US as an adjunctive breast cancer screening tool has been demonstrated recently, with American College of Radiology Imaging Network protocol 6666 showing a supplemental detection yield (over and above cancers found by mammography alone) of 4.2 cancers per 1000 high-risk women undergoing screening.[8] However, the real-time nature of breast US introduces operator-dependence to a far greater degree than is found in mammography and US is most effectively used when the imaging physician performs or is present during scanning. This can be time consuming, and therefore physician labor-intensive and cost-ineffective. Another limitation of breast US, as demonstrated by Berg and colleagues,[8] is a low positive predictive value (PPV) for biopsy at 8.9% versus 22.6% for mammography, in the screening setting. Evolving technological enhancements, including elastography and three-/four-dimensional breast US, may improve its performance in the near future.

An additional exciting bonus to the advent of FFDM is its ability to allow novel computer-based technologies. Digital breast tomosynthesis (DBT) is one example that partially addresses the two-dimensional limitations of planar mammography. DBT is performed using a mammographic x-ray tube but differs significantly from standard digital mammography in that it obtains multiple low-dose images at angled increments along an arc centered around the compressed breast. This information is computer-compiled and subsequently displayed on a workstation that allows the breast to be examined on a slice-by-slice basis, at various slice thicknesses, chosen by the interpreter. Each individual slice has the appearance of a planar mammographic view (either craniocaudal or mediolateral oblique, depending on how the breast was positioned at acquisition), albeit displaying information from only one tomographic plane at a time. The third dimension is added as the examiner scrolls through the breast from skin to skin. Using this imaging technique reduces the element of tissue superimposition, theoretically improving lesion detection capability and mass-margin characterization. Smith and colleagues[9] showed that DBT combined with FFDM resulted in improved clinical performance (as measured by area under the receiver operator curve (ROC) and recall rate reduction) compared with the use of FFDM alone, independent of radiologist experience. However, despite its theoretical promise, DBT has not yet found its niche in routine clinical practice, in part perhaps because of a lack of a validated optimal viewing protocol, well-defined indications, dose considerations, and the large number of reconstructed images that must be reviewed.

Stereoscopic digital mammography (SDM) is another spin-off from FFDM the purpose of which is to mitigate the limitations of superimposed breast tissue. The technique is patterned after the concept of binocular vision; having 2 eyes separated by several centimeters allows each eye to receive slightly discrepant views of the world that the brain is able to compile into a three-dimensional construct. In SDM, 2 discrepant images are obtained in both the cranial-caudal (CC) and mediolateral oblique (MLO) projections, each angled $\pm 5°$ relative to standard tube position. These slightly angled images are sent to a specially designed workstation on which each image is projected separately, then filtered through a polarizing screen. The observer, who is wearing cross-polarized viewing glasses, can see only 1 of the 2 angled images with each eye. From this dataset, the observer's brain constructs a virtual three-dimensional image of the breast. While tissue is still superimposed (the way trees viewed in a forest would be), the viewer can perceive the relative depth and location of structures, helping to differentiate significant findings from spurious ones related to simple superimposition. Getty and colleagues[10] reported a PPV of true lesion detection of 32% for SDM and 26% for standard two-dimensional digital mammography. However, these promising results came with a cost. Because each of the 2 stereo views was obtained at a standard dose, each stereo acquisition in the MLO and CC views was twice that of the standard dose. This is untenable in a population-based screening situation and work is underway to duplicate the study with a dose similar to standard digital mammography.

Although strides have been made toward advancing breast imaging beyond planar mammography, each modality described has significant limitations. As a result, the search for other promising technologies continues. Dedicated breast computed tomography (DBCT) represents a new technology that may allow true three-dimensional imaging of the breast using the same fundamental x-ray contrast mechanism with which breast imagers are already familiar.

TECHNICAL ASPECTS OF DBCT
DBCT Basic Geometry

Conventional whole-body CT scanners use detector arrays that are arranged in an arc around the patient (**Fig. 1**A). The detector arrays are composed of individual detector modules, which are small, modular, planar arrays, arranged on an arced support. The arc in conventional whole-body scanners usually spans an angle of about 60°, and the collimated beam width in the z-axis direction typically spans from 20 to 40 mm.

Flat panel detectors for fluoroscopy are the enabling technology behind many cone beam CT systems, including those for DBCT (**Fig. 1**B). Such detectors replace the fluoroscopic imaging detector, including the image intensifier, optical coupling, and optical camera. Presently, flat panel detectors are capable of real-time readout (30 frames per second) in reduced resolution modes.

Prone patient positioning, with the breast imaged as it projects through a hole in the table top, is used for DBCT (**Fig. 2**A). The x-ray tube and flat panel detector rotate around the breast in the horizontal plane and acquire the image data. Prototype breast CT systems[11,12] make use of flat panel detectors, which give rise to the half cone beam geometry (**Fig. 2**B) because the x-ray tube and detector need to rotate below the plane of the table. This geometry is required to obtain x-ray projections far enough posterior into the breast to capture CT images of the chest wall.

System Hardware

All of the currently fabricated DBCT systems use the PAXSCAN flat panel detector (Varian Imaging Systems, Salt Lake City, UT, USA), which has a 40 cm × 30 cm field of view at the detector plane,

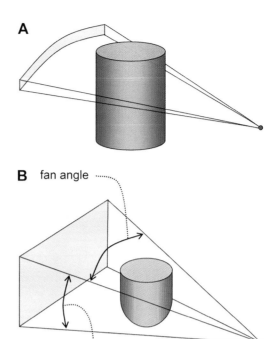

A

B   fan angle

cone angle

Fig. 1. (A) Traditional multiple detector array CT makes use of a fan beam of radiation with very little divergence in the z-dimension. The cone angle of typical whole-body CT scanners is on the order of 2°. (B) Breast CT systems generally use a flat panel detector which covers not only the fan beam of the scanner but also the full extent in the z-dimension. The wider cone beam that results is capable of creating a complete CT dataset of the breast in one rotation of the scanner around the breast.

and represents a 2048 × 1536 array of 194 μm × 194 μm detector elements. To achieve readout of the panel at 30 frames per second, the individual detector elements must be binned into 2 × 2 elements, creating an effective detector element that is 388 μm on a side. The readout array in this mode becomes 1024 × 768.

Scanning Protocols

The scanner developed at the University of Rochester[12] uses a pulsed x-ray source and a 10-second acquisition. A total of 300 views are acquired at 30 frames per second, using the PAXSCAN 4030CB detector. This scanner operates at a maximum of 49 kVp, and uses a digital mammography x-ray tube designed with a tungsten anode. There is a benefit of the pulsed x-ray tube design, in which the short duration (~8 ms) of each x-ray pulse essentially freezes the rotational motion of the gantry, improving spatial resolution. The 10-second scan time should also be accepted well by women who undergo this breath-hold examination.

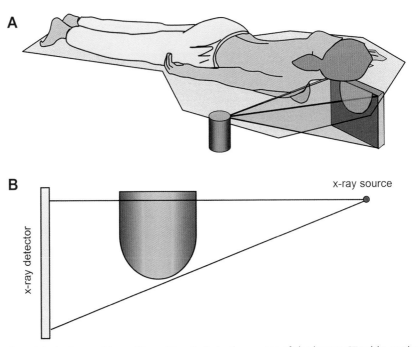

Fig. 2. (*A*) The breast to be imaged is positioned in a hole in the center of the breast CT table, as the women lies prone with her breast in the pendant position. This allows the CT scanner hardware to rotate in the horizontal plane and acquire the projection data necessary for cone beam CT reconstruction. (*B*) The cone angle in breast CT is large compared with whole-body scanners, with cone angles up to about 15°. In whole-body imaging, such a large cone angle would be prone to artifacts, but the breast has no highly attenuating anatomy (ie, bones) and tapers in diameter anteriorly, and this reduces the propensity for cone beam artifacts.

The University of California Davis scanners[11,13–15] use the PAXSCAN 4030CB detector system but also use a continuous (nonpulsed) x-ray source operating typically at 80 kVp. At 30 frames per second, this results in a 33-millisecond acquisition time per frame with a total of 500 frames or projection images acquired over a 16.6-second acquisition sequence. This slightly longer acquisition time has also been well tolerated by patients with a single breath hold.

Data Processing

The reconstruction algorithm uses the entire dataset of projection images acquired during the 360° rotation of the gantry around the breast. For the 500 projection images and the 786,000 pixels in each image, a total of 393 million data points are used to reconstruct the breast CT images. The reconstruction algorithm uses a cone beam reconstruction procedure to produce an isotropic three-dimensional CT volume dataset, consisting of a series of 512 × 512 images.

Radiation Dose from DBCT

The radiation dose from CT in body imaging is substantially more than that required for digital radiography, and thus, for many years it was

thought that CT would be dose prohibitive for breast imaging. However, the smaller dimensions of the breast of 140 mm average diameter (range from 100 to 180 mm) in the pendant position combined with the lower tissue density of adipose (density ∼0.93 g/cm^3) and a higher x-ray beam energy (49–80 kVp) than mammography, suggest that breast CT can be performed at low radiation dose levels.

Monte Carlo techniques, which involve computer simulations of the x-ray beam passing through a mathematically defined breast phantom, x-ray photon by x-ray photon, were used for dose calculation in DBCT.[16] Using these dose coefficients and the measured doses of 2-view mammography, the technique factors for DBCT are adjusted at UC Davis such that the average glandular dose is equal to that of 2-view mammography.

CLINICAL EXPERIENCE WITH DBCT
DBCT Without Contrast

The first prospective comparison of noncontrast DBCT with screen-film mammography was reported in 2008.[15] A prototype scanner was used to image the breasts of 10 healthy volunteers and 69 women with Breast Imaging Reporting and Data System (BIRADS) 4 or 5 (suspicious) lesions. The uncompressed breasts were scanned individually in the pendant position at 80 kVp with the milliamps chosen to deliver the same mean glandular dose as a 2-view mammogram. Scans were viewed in stack mode in coronal, sagittal, and axial planes on dedicated software (**Fig. 3**).

In women with lesions, the DBCT images were compared with mediolateral oblique and craniocaudal mammograms in a nonblinded study. Conspicuity of the lesion in both modalities was subjectively ranked by a single experienced dedicated breast imager. This initial study showed that overall conspicuity of breast lesions on DBCT was equal to that on mammography. There were no significant differences between DBCT and mammography for benign versus malignant lesions or as stratified by breast density; however, masses were significantly more conspicuous on DBCT (P = .002), and calcifications were better seen on mammography (P = .006).

Updated results from the same trial using dedicated noncontrast DBCT amplifies these findings on 180 lesions (**Table 1**). Masses were more conspicuous on DBCT (P<.001), and calcifications were significantly better visualized on mammography (P<.001).

The poor visualization of microcalcifications on unenhanced DBCT poses a significant barrier to the use of this modality for breast cancer screening because many cases of ductal carcinoma in situ (DCIS) might not be visualized. For this reason the utility of contrast enhancement is now being studied.

Contrast-enhanced DBCT

The use of intravenous contrast in other breast imaging modalities, particularly in magnetic resonance (MR) imaging, has been successful in improving lesion conspicuity. Similar improvements would be expected in contrast-enhanced DBCT (CE-DBCT). In addition, in CT the Hounsfield unit (HU) is directly proportional to attenuation and serves as a tool for quantification of differential capillary permeability between normal and malignant tissues.[17–19]

In a pilot study, 46 women with 54 BIRADS 4 or 5 lesions underwent both noncontrast DBCT and CE-DBCT before image-guided biopsy.[20] Lesion conspicuity on CE-DBCT was compared with mediolateral oblique and craniocaudal mammograms. The conspicuity of each lesion was subjectively and independently scored by 2 radiologists on a continuous scale from −5 to 5, where zero corresponded to equivalence between the 2 modalities, negative values corresponded to better conspicuity on CE-DBCT and positive values corresponded to better conspicuity on mammography.

All 29 malignant lesions were significantly more conspicuous on CE-DBCT than on mammography (mean conspicuity = −1.45, P<.001). When divided

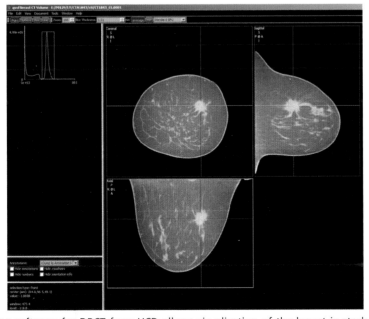

Fig. 3. The viewing software for DBCT from UCD allows visualization of the breast in stack mode in coronal, sagittal, and axial planes. Lesions can be automatically localized in the 3 planes.

Table 1
Conspicuity of lesions on noncontrast dedicated breast CT compared with mammography[a]

Category	No. of Breasts	Score Mean ± SD	Score Median[b]	P value
All	180	5.7 ± 2.1	5.5 (5.4, 5.6)	.20
Lesion Type				
Masses	124	4.9 ± 1.5	5.0 (4.7, 5.3)	<.001[c]
Calcification	56	7.6 ± 1.9	8.0 (7.2, 8.8)	<.001[c]
Lesion Diagnosis				
Malignant	97	5.5 ± 1.9	5.5 (5.3, 5.7)	.90
Benign	83	6.1 ± 2.2	5.5 (5.0, 6.0)	.10

[a] Conspicuity was ranked from 1 to 10. A score of 5.5 indicates equal visualization with DBCT and mammography; a score of less than 5.5 indicates superior visualization with DBCT and a score greater than 5.5 indicates superior visualization with mammography.
[b] Numbers in parentheses are 95% confidence intervals.
[c] Significant.

by lesion type, malignant masses were significantly more conspicuous on CE-DBCT than on mammography (mean conspicuity = −1.84, P<.001) (Fig. 4). The conspicuity of the 7 malignant calcification lesions was slightly better on CE-DBCT than on mammography (mean conspicuity = −0.29, P = .64), but the difference was not statistically significant. Five of the 7 calcification lesions were pure DCIS (Fig. 5).

On CE-DBCT the conspicuity of the 25 benign lesions was similar to that on mammography (mean conspicuity = 0.34, P = .46); however benign calcifications were significantly better seen on mammography (mean conspicuity = 2.33, P<.01), and benign masses were significantly better visualized on CE-DBCT (mean conspicuity = −1.07, P<.01). The poor conspicuity of benign calcifications on CE-DBCT suggests the possibility that specificity in diagnosis of indeterminate calcifications may be improved by the use of CE-DBCT, although the numbers in this study are small and further clinical investigation is necessary.

For 52 of the 54 lesions in this pilot study, mean lesion voxel intensity (in HU) was measured on pre- and postcontrast DBCT scans to provide a quantified measurement of enhancement. Malignant lesions enhanced by a mean of 55.9 HU, and benign lesions enhanced by 17.6 HU (P<.001). The 5 pure DCIS lesions enhanced by a mean of 59.6 HU; benign calcifications enhanced by 24.9 HU.

ROC analysis of the quantitative enhancement of benign and malignant lesions yielded an area under the curve (AUC) of 0.876, suggesting that quantitative enhancement should be useful in predicting malignancy. A large study of the performance of clinical mammography reported an AUC of approximately 0.92,[21] and AUCs of 0.88 have been shown for MR imaging using both kinetic and morphologic information.[22,23] It seems likely that CE-DBCT could equal or surpass these AUCs if morphologic data are combined with quantitative enhancement metrics.

The use of intravenous contrast in DBCT clearly improves visualization of malignant lesions, including DCIS. Current scanner designs allow imaging of one breast at a time, which is a limitation; however the importance of the delay between contrast injection and imaging in tumor detection and diagnosis remains a research topic. In the pilot study of CE-DBCT described, the delay between injection of contrast and imaging varied from 52 to 247 seconds (mean = 96 seconds), however the delay did not significantly affect lesion enhancement. It is plausible that serial imaging of both breasts with CE-DBCT will be diagnostically useful.

PATIENT PERCEPTIONS OF DBCT

From the patient perspective, DBCT offers an advantage over mammography because breast compression is not currently required. Following DBCT and CE-DBCT, 209 women were asked to complete a questionnaire regarding their comfort during the procedure rating from 1 to 10: (1) comfort of their position on the DBCT table, (2) how difficult it was for them to maintain the breath hold of 16.6 seconds, (3) their overall comfort during DBCT, and (4) to compare their comfort during DBCT to their comfort during mammography. Additional comments about DBCT were also solicited at the end of the questionnaire.

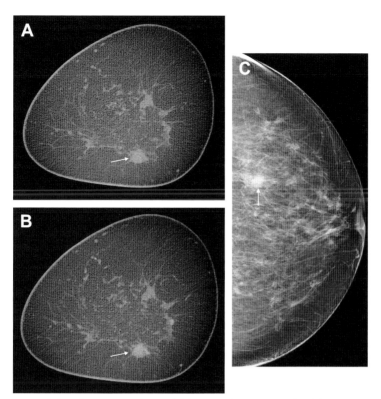

Fig. 4. (A–C) Noncontrast (A) and contrast-enhanced (B) coronal University of California Davis DBCT scans of an enhancing infiltrating ductal carcinoma (arrows) at 6 o'clock in the left breast, which is partially obscured by superimposed tissue on the corresponding craniocaudal screening mammogram (C). The cancer enhanced by 43.7 HU on DBCT, while the normal glandular tissue at 12 o'clock did not enhance.

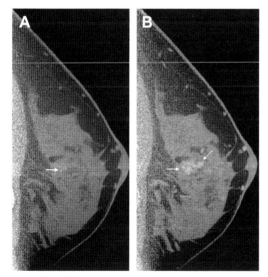

Fig. 5. (A, B) Sagittal DBCT scans of DCIS showing a faint group of microcalcifications (arrow) on the University of California Davis noncontrast scan (A) with enhancement of the tumor (arrows) after contrast administration (B). The DCIS enhanced by 60.9 HU.

Results (Table 2) showed that many women found the position on the DBCT table somewhat uncomfortable. It was difficult for many to arch their backs so as to push their breasts forward into the scanner for maximum coverage. Many women complained that their neck was uncomfortable during scanning. However, when asked to rate the comfort of DBCT compared with mammography most preferred DBCT. Ergonomic refinements in the table top may be possible, but it is unlikely that these will be able to significantly decrease the discomfort of positioning. It is also possible for CE-DBCT, if subtraction imaging or kinetics is desired, that some gentle breast compression will eventually be required to limit patient motion.

THE FUTURE

The development of DBCT is in its infancy. The scanners currently in use for clinical research studies are prototypes. Reductions in noise and increases in spatial resolution are required to improve visualization of calcifications and to improve overall image quality. Changes in acquisition strategies including a pulsed, rather than

Table 2
Breast CT comfort survey results in 209 patients

	Score	
Question	Mean ± SD	Median[a]
Position[b]	6.6 ± 2.5	7 (6.3, 7.7)
Breath hold[c]	7.3 ± 2.3	8 (7.3, 8.7)
Comfort[d]	8.1 ± 5.0	8 (7.1, 8.9)
Breast CT vs mammography[e]	8.8 ± 2.0	10 (10, 10)

[a] Numbers in parentheses are the 95% confidence intervals.
[b] Position refers to comfort of the position on the breast CT table (1 = poor, 10 = excellent).
[c] Breath hold refers to ease of 16.6 second breath hold (1 = very difficult, 10 = not at all difficult).
[d] Comfort refers to the overall comfort of breast CT (1 = very uncomfortable, 10 = extremely comfortable).
[e] Breast CT versus mammography refers to the comfort during breast CT compared with comfort during screen-film mammography (1 = comfort was much worse than that of screen-film mammography, 5.5 = comfort was equal to that of screen-film mammography, 10 = breast CT was much more comfortable than screen-film mammography).

a continuous x-ray source, and new detectors with reduced electronic noise and increased frame rates are being considered for the redesign and upgrading of the UC Davis scanners. Even with the above improvements and/or with reduced kilovolt peak used by some systems,[24] it will be challenging for noncontrast DBCT to equal mammography in the depiction and characterization of microcalcifications.

An additional challenge for DBCT is coverage of the breast including the axillary tail extending to the chest wall. Refinements in table design have increased such coverage from the previous report in which chest wall musculature was visualized in only 17% of scanned patients,[15] but further improvements are still required. X-ray tubes with a more compact housing design and detectors with smaller bezels (the frame surrounding the detector) are in development and will allow greater coverage of the posterior breast.

DBCT may not become a stand-alone replacement for screening mammography in the general population, however DBCT may play an important role in breast cancer imaging. If DBCT is used as a screening modality in conjunction with mammography, as is proposed for DBT, it is likely that the three-dimensional and multiplanar capabilities of DBCT would lead to a reduction in the number of patient recalls for summation artifacts and could increase sensitivity for masses (**Figs. 6** and **7**). Alternatively, DBCT could be used to analyze and validate findings suspected from a screening mammogram because a single scan will create an isotropic image dataset of the breast and produce individual scans in the x, y, and z directions. Regions of interest can be placed on any slice and be located on the full image and the corresponding slices in the other 2 orthogonal planes.

Initial work has shown that malignant lesions are significantly more conspicuous on CE-DBCT compared with mammography and DBCT. DCIS, manifested by microcalcifications alone, clearly enhances on CE-DBCT, although patient numbers are small and further study is necessary to determine whether enhancement is related to the nuclear grade of DCIS, as is now being postulated for DCIS enhancement in breast MR imaging.[25] Quantification of lesion enhancement will likely be helpful in improving both sensitivity and specificity of CE-DBCT, which could conceivably then replace breast MR imaging both in screening of high-risk women and in the assessment of recently diagnosed cancers (**Fig. 8**). The improved spatial resolution of CE-DBCT over MR imaging and similar vascular information with contrast, may lead to greater accuracy of CE-DBCT over breast MR imaging. There are also no metal precautions or issues with claustrophobia. It is likely that both equipment and examination costs for CE-DBCT will be lower than for MR imaging and, theoretically, these units can be easily sited in breast imaging centers. Patient throughput will be faster with CE-DBCT because of the short scan time of 10 to 16 seconds.

The DBCT platform is ideal for integration with other modalities useful in breast cancer detection, diagnosis, and treatment. An integrated robotic biopsy device is under development and there is potential for incorporation of new therapeutic interventions, such as radiofrequency ablation, cryoablation, or high-intensity focused US. DBCT is likely to be useful in external-beam radiation therapy of the breast, because the pendant position will allow more reproducible positioning of the breast. Preliminary work has already shown that a low-energy x-ray source (such as 320 kVp), rather than

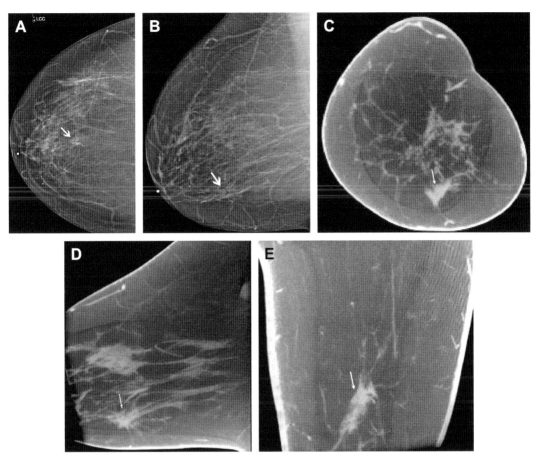

Fig. 6. (*A–E*) Craniocaudal (*A*) and mediolateral oblique (*B*) mammograms showing a spiculated mass (*arrows*), ultimately diagnosed as infiltrating ductal carcinoma at the 6 o'clock position in the right breast. Coronal (*C*), sagittal (*D*), and axial (*E*) DBCT scans from the Koning CBCT System performed on the same patient show the mass (*arrows*) without superimposed tissue.

the typical 6 MVp linear accelerator, can be used to deliver highly conformal dose distributions for partial breast irradiation, and the homogeneous dose distributions of whole breast irradiation. In addition, a small kilovolt peak–based radiation therapy system can be placed above ground in a leaded x-ray room, which would be a very cost-effective solution for breast radiation therapy.

Molecular breast imaging offers significant potential for diagnosis and therapeutic evaluation of breast tumors by providing physiologic information. Today such techniques are based on adionuclides and include single photon emission-computed tomography (SPECT) and positron emission tomography (PET). Dedicated breast SPECT and PET systems have each been integrated with DBCT systems[26,27] to provide high-resolution coregistered anatomic and physiologic information.

In the only clinical study reported to date, 4 patients with mammographic findings that were highly suspicious for breast cancer, underwent dedicated breast PET/CT on a prototype unit.[28]

Among the 4 patients, 3 had invasive cancers, ranging from 9 mm to 25 mm in diameter and one had a 10 mm pure DCIS. All of the invasive cancers were positive on PET, but on DBCT the invasive cancers were seen in only 2 patients (Fig. 9). In the third patient the cancer was close to the chest wall and was not seen as it was out of the DBCT field of view. One patient with an invasive cancer also had an extensive intraductal component, which was well visualized on dedicated breast PET/CT; detailed histologic correlation of the mastectomy specimen with the breast PET/CT in that patient demonstrated excellent comparability. The one case of pure DCIS, seen as microcalcifications on mammography, was seen on the DBCT, but not on the PET images, likely because of patient motion. These are preliminary results, and although technical challenges remain, they seem promising.

The improved spatial resolution of dedicated breast PET/CT compared with whole-body PET/CT (3.7 mm vs 6.4 mm average full width at half

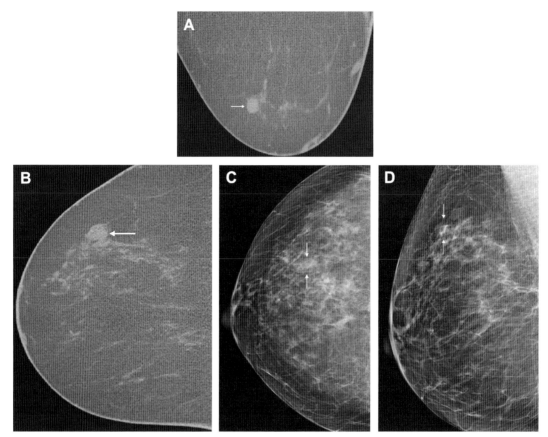

Fig. 7. (A–D) Axial (A) and sagittal (B) DBCT scans done without contrast demonstrate a fibroadenoma (arrows), which is not obscured by the overlying glandular tissue as it is on the corresponding craniocaudal (C) and mediolateral oblique (D) mammograms.

maximum) has the potential to allow detection, diagnosis, and evaluation of smaller lesions and more accurate local staging of cancers.[28] It is also anticipated that quantitative high-resolution PET may play an important enabling role in monitoring response to neoadjuvant therapy. If CE-BCT is performed in conjunction with dedicated breast PET/CT, sensitivity and specificity of the system should improve further. DBCT integrated with PET should find increased utility as new breast cancer specific molecular imaging agents are discovered.

Further clinical comparison of DBCT with other established modalities such as MR imaging and

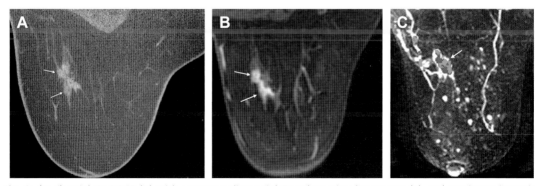

Fig. 8. (A–C) Axial CE-DBCT (A) with corresponding axial T1 subtraction breast MR (B) and maximum-intensity projection MR with angiogenesis color overlay (C) of an infiltrating ductal carcinoma (arrows) of the left breast. The DBCT is comparable with the MR.

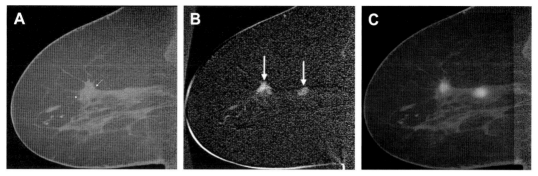

Fig. 9. (*A–C*) Noncontrast sagittal DBCT (*A*) showing a spiculated mass (*arrows*) partially obscured by surrounding dense tissue. Contrast subtraction sagittal scan (*B*) and fused PET/DBCT (*C*) of the same patient showing 2 areas of focal uptake on the PET/DBCT and 2 enhancing lesions (*arrows*), measuring 13 mm and 9 mm, on the subtraction image. Both were infiltrating ductal carcinoma; the second more posterior cancer was not appreciated initially on the corresponding screening mammogram (not shown). (*From* Bowen SL, Wu Y, Chaudhari AJ, et al. Initial characterization of a dedicated breast PET/CT scanner during human imaging. J Nucl Med 2009;50(9):1401–8; with permission.)

with emerging technologies including DBT, SDM, three- and four-dimensional ultrasonography, US elastography, and radionuclide imaging will be required to determine the optimal, most cost-effective strategies for the use of DBCT. In the next decade it is likely that we will move from a standardized approach to breast cancer screening into a more individualized approach based on such factors as risk and breast density. DBCT is likely to play a significant role in breast imaging as this paradigm shift occurs.

SUMMARY

DBCT is a burgeoning technology that has many advantages over current breast imaging systems. Three-dimensional visualization of the breast mitigates the limiting effects of superimposition noted with mammography. Postprocessing capabilities will allow application of advanced technologies, such as creation of maximum-intensity projection and subtraction images, and the use of both computer-aided detection and possible computer-aided diagnosis algorithms. Excellent morphologic detail and soft tissue contrast can be achieved, due in part to the isotropic image data that DBCT produces. The expected cost should be more reasonable than MR imaging. At present, because the breast is not compressed, patients find it more comfortable than mammography. Physiologic information can be obtained when intravenous contrast material is used and/or when DBCT is combined with SPECT or PET. DBCT provides an excellent platform for multimodality systems including integration with interventional and therapeutic procedures. With a slightly altered design, the DBCT platform may also be useful for external-beam radiation with image guidance.

REFERENCES

1. Smith RA, Duffy SW, Gabe R, et al. The randomized trials of breast cancer screening: what have we learned? Radiol Clin North Am 2004;42(5):793–806.
2. NCI-funded breast cancer surveillance consortium co-operative agreement. Performance measures for 3,603,832 screening mammography studies from 1996 to 2006 by age. Rockville (MD): National Cancer Institute; 2008. Available at: http://breastscreening.cancer.gov/data/performance/perf_age.html. Accessed June 1, 2010.
3. Carney PA, Miglioretti DL, Yankaskas BC, et al. Individual and combined effects of age, breast density, and hormone replacement therapy use on the accuracy of screening mammography. Ann Intern Med 2003;138(3):168–75.
4. Berg WA, Gutierrez L, NessAiver MS, et al. Diagnostic accuracy of mammography, clinical examination, US and MR imaging in pre-operative assessment of breast cancer. Radiology 2004;233:830–49.
5. Yankaskas BC, Cleveland RJ, Schell MJ, et al. Association of recall rates with sensitivity and positive predictive values of screening mammography. AJR Am J Roentgenol 2001;177(3):543–9.
6. Pisano ED, Gatsonis C, Hendrick E, et al. Diagnostic performance of digital versus film mammography in breast-cancer screening. N Engl J Med 2005;353(17):1773–83.
7. Pisano ED, Hendrick RE, Yaffe MJ, et al. Diagnostic accuracy of digital versus film mammography: exploratory analysis of selected population subgroups in DMIST. Radiology 2008;246(2):376–83.
8. Berg WA, Blume JD, Cormack JB, et al. Combined screening with ultrasound and mammography vs mammography alone in women at elevated risk of breast cancer. JAMA 2008;299(18):2151–63.

9. Smith AP, Rafferty EA, Niklason L. Clinical performance of breast tomosynthesis as a function of radiologist experience level. LNCS 2008;5116:61–6.

10. Getty DJ, D'Orsi CJ, Newell MS, et al. Improved accuracy of lesion detection in breast cancer screening with stereoscopic digital mammography [abstract]. RSNA Scientific Assembly and Annual Meeting Program. Chicago (IL), November 27, 2007. p. 381–2.

11. Boone JM, Nelson TR, Lindfors KK, et al. Dedicated breast CT: radiation dose and image quality evaluation. Radiology 2001;221(3):657–67.

12. Chen Z, Ning R. Why should breast tumour detection go three dimensional? Phys Med Biol 2003; 48(14):2217–28.

13. Boone JM. Breast CT: its prospect for breast cancer screening and diagnosis. In: Karellas A, Giger ML, editors. 2004 syllabus: advances in breast imaging physics, technology, and clinical applications. Oak Park (IL): Radiological Society of North America; 2004. p. 165–77.

14. Glick SJ. Breast CT. Annu Rev Biomed Eng 2007;9: 501–26.

15. Lindfors KK, Boone JM, Nelson TR, et al. Dedicated breast CT: initial clinical experience. Radiology 2008;246(3):725–33.

16. Boone JM, Shah N, Nelson TR. A comprehensive analysis of DgN (CT) coefficients for pendant-geometry cone-beam breast computed tomography. Med Phys 2004;31(2):226–35.

17. Dawson P. Functional imaging in CT. Eur J Radiol 2006;60(3):331–40.

18. Miles KA. Tumour angiogenesis and its relation to contrast enhancement on computed tomography: a review. Eur J Radiol 1999;30(3):198–205.

19. Cuenod CA, Fournier L, Balvay D, et al. Tumor angiogenesis: pathophysiology and implications for contrast-enhanced MRI and CT assessment. Abdom Imaging 2006;31(2):188–93.

20. Prionas ND, Lindfors KK, Ray S, et al. Contrast-enhanced dedicated breast computed tomography: initial clinical experience. Radiology, in press.

21. Jensen A, Vejborg I, Severinsen N, et al. Performance of clinical mammography: a nationwide study from Denmark. Int J Cancer 2006;119(1):183–91.

22. Warren RM, Thompson D, Pointon LJ, et al. Evaluation of a prospective scoring system designed for a multicenter breast MR imaging screening study. Radiology 2006;239(3):677–85.

23. Schnall MD, Blume J, Bluemke DA, et al. Diagnostic architectural and dynamic features at breast MR imaging: multicenter study. Radiology 2006;238(1): 42–53.

24. Chen B, Ning R. Cone-beam volume CT breast imaging: feasibility study. Med Phys 2002;29(5): 755–70.

25. Kuhl CK. Why do purely intraductal cancers enhance on breast MR images? Radiology 2009; 253(2):281–7.

26. Wu Y, Bowen SL, Yang K, et al. PET characteristics of a dedicated breast PET/CT scanner prototype. Phys Med Biol 2009;54(13):4273–87.

27. McKinley RL, Tornai MP, Brzymialkiewicz C, et al. Analysis of a novel offset cone-beam computed mammotomography system geometry for accommodating various breast sizes. Phys Med 2006; 21(Suppl 1):48–55.

28. Bowen SL, Wu Y, Chaudhari AJ, et al. Initial characterization of a dedicated breast PET/CT scanner during human imaging. J Nucl Med 2009;50(9):1401–8.

Nuclear Medicine Imaging of the Breast: A Novel, Physiologic Approach to Breast Cancer Detection and Diagnosis

Rachel F. Brem, MD*, Lauren R. Rechtman, MA

KEYWORDS

- Breast cancer • Breast-specific gamma imaging
- Molecular breast imaging
- Nuclear medicine imaging of the breast

Mammography has been an effective modality for mortality reduction from breast cancer.[1] From 1975 to 1990, the death rate from breast cancer increased annually by 0.4%. However, from 1990 to 2002 the rate decreased by 2.3% annually,[2] with a 3.3% decrease in women younger than 50 years of age and 2% in women older than 50 years. A recent study by Berry and colleagues[3] utilized 7 screening mammography trials published between 1975 and 2000 with mathematical modeling to estimate the impact of screening as compared with improved therapy in mortality reduction using screening studies published between 1975 and 2000 and found that increased screening accounted for at least 40% and possibly as much as 55% of the mortality reduction. Others have reported mortality reduction of up to 44%.[4]

Mammography, the mainstay for breast cancer screening, is an anatomic approach to breast cancer detection and diagnosis with the goal of identifying the mammographic signs of breast cancer as compared with the normal surrounding breast parenchyma. Similarly, ultrasound, the most common adjuvant imaging modality in breast imaging, also uses an anatomic approach in breast cancer detection. Although effective, mammography is imperfect. Fifteen percent of breast cancers are not mammographically visible. In women with dense breasts, women with implants, or those who have undergone prior breast surgery, the sensitivity of mammography is even lower.[5] Others have reported yet lower sensitivity for mammography.[6] Therefore adjunct imaging modalities to improve the ability to detect breast cancer are needed to improve the sensitivity of breast cancer detection.

The second limitation of mammography and ultrasound is the ability to differentiate detected lesions as benign or malignant. Only 15% to 30% of breast biopsies result in a diagnosis of cancer[7] with the vast majority performed because of the limitation of anatomic imaging to differentiate benign from malignant tissue. Therefore, there is also a need to improve the specificity of breast lesion detection and thereby decrease the number of biopsies performed for benign findings.

The mainstays of breast imaging rely on anatomic approaches to breast cancer diagnosis. However, if physiologic or metabolic approaches to breast imaging were used, the potential to

Disclosure: Dr Brem is a consultant for and is on the Board of Managers of Dilon Technologies.
Department of Radiology, Breast Imaging and Interventional Center, The George Washington University, 2150 Pennsylvania Avenue, NW Washington, DC 20037, USA
* Corresponding author.
E-mail address: rbrem@mfa.gwu.edu

Radiol Clin N Am 48 (2010) 1055–1074
doi:10.1016/j.rcl.2010.06.008

both improve sensitivity and specificity of breast cancer diagnosis exists. It is this challenge that led to the development of nuclear medicine imaging of the breast.

NUCLEAR MEDICINE IMAGING OF THE BREAST

Nuclear medicine imaging of the breast uses functional approaches to image malignant breast tumors, which requires the administration of a radiotracer via an injection and a camera for imaging the radiotracer activity. Radiotracers are designed to preferentially accumulate in malignant tissues and the differential uptake is what is imaged. The ideal radiopharmaceuticals would show high tumor uptake, minimal activity within the normal breast tissue, and minimal or no activity in benign breast lesions. Currently, the most widely used tracer is Tc-99m sestamibi, a small cationic complex of technetium originally introduced for myocardial perfusion imaging that was subsequently proposed as a tumor-seeking agent.[8] Tc-99m sestamibi uptake and retention in cancer cells is dependent on regional blood flow, plasma and mitochondrial membrane potential, angiogenesis, and tissue metabolism, with about 90% of tracer activity concentrated in the mitochondria.[9] Other radiopharmaceuticals that have been used to image the breast include Tc-99m tetrofosmin and fluorodeoxyglucose.

The use of a traditional gamma camera and a radiopharmaceutical to image the breast is termed *scintimammography*, where patients lie prone with the breast dependent with imaging performed in the lateral and anteroposterior positions. This approach was limited in that the gamma camera could not be positioned sufficiently close to the breast and that the breast could not be imaged in positions comparable to mammography. Furthermore, the intrinsic design of the gamma camera did not reliably allow for imaging of subcentimeter cancers. A review by Taillefer[10] in more than 2000 women from 20 studies found the sensitivity, specificity, negative predictive value (NPV), and positive predictive value to be 85%, 89%, 84%, and 89%, respectively. Similar results were reported in a meta-analysis of more than 5000 subjects imaged with a traditional gamma camera[11] as well as a multi-institutional study in the United States[12] where the aggregate findings demonstrated a sensitivity of 85.2%, specificity of 86.6%, negative predictive value of 81.8%, positive predictive value of 88.2%, and accuracy of 85.9%. The majority (80%) of the studies reported sensitivity and specificity values of more than 80%, with nearly half of them yielding values more than 90%. As a result of the findings of these studies, the US Food and Drug Administration (FDA) approved 99m Tc Sestamibi as an adjunct imaging modality for the diagnosis of breast cancer in 1997, which is identical to Technetium Tc99m Sestamibi, the most commonly used radiopharmaceutical for cardiac imaging.

However, it is crucial to interpret these finding in the context of the size of the cancers detected. A multicenter study of 420 subjects with 449 breast lesions reported sensitivity of 26%, 56%, 95%, and 97% for T1a, T1b, T1c, and T2 breast cancers, respectively.[13] Similarly in the report of his multi-institutional trial performed in the United States, Khalkhali showed a sensitivity of 74.2% for cancers greater than 1 cm and 48.2% for cancers less than 1 cm.[12] The ability to detect breast cancer was also dependent on whether the cancer was palpable, with sensitivities of palpable versus nonpalpable cancers reported as 87% versus 61%, respectively. The detection of small, nonpalpable breast cancer is critical for the clinical development and meaningful integration of nuclear medicine imaging of the breast in clinical practice. Although the studies reported that using a traditional gamma camera could not reliably detect small, nonpalpable breast cancers, the results were exciting because there was proof of principle that nuclear medicine imaging of the breast might be a useful adjunct imaging modality. This finding was particularly true because the detection of breast cancer with scintimammography was not impacted by breast density. That is, the sensitivity was the same whether women had dense or fatty breasts.[14] However, until gamma cameras were developed that could reliably image subcentimeter cancers and could image in positions comparable to mammography so that correlative, multimodality imaging was possible, nuclear medicine imaging of the breast could not meaningfully be integrated into clinical practice. The need for a high-resolution, small field of view, breast-specific gamma camera (HRBSG) led to the development of this type of gamma camera (**Fig. 1**).[15] This type of camera allows for greater flexibility in patient positioning, imaging in positions comparable to mammography, and nearly eliminates the dead space of the detector such that the entire detector can be used for imaging. Furthermore, the use of minimal compression allows for the lesion to be closer to the detector by reducing the thickness of the breast resulting in improving resolution. This latter principle is

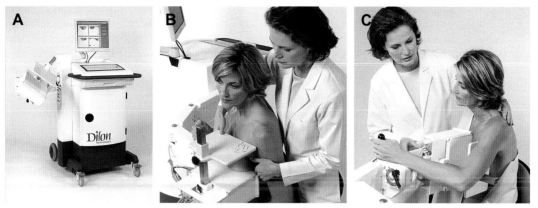

Fig. 1. A high-resolution, breast-specific gamma camera. (*Courtesy of* Dilon Technologies, Newport News, VA; with permission.) (*A*) A mobile high-resolution breast-specific gamma camera imaging unit. (*B*) Patient positioned in the craniocaudal view in the imaging unit. (*C*) Patient positioned in the lateral view in the imaging unit. The detector is on an articulating arm and can be positioned at any angle.

based on always trying to position the lesion as close to the detector as possible to optimize resolution. The HRBSG camera also allows for better spatial resolution with improved contrast of small lesions. The imaging of the breast with a high-resolution gamma camera and a gamma emitting radiopharmaceutical is referred to as either breast-specific gamma imaging (BSGI) or molecular breast imaging (MBI). Various configurations of this type of camera exist that include free standing and mobile units (see **Fig.** 1A) and a camera mounted on a modified mammography system (see **Fig.** 1B).

THE BREAST-SPECIFIC GAMMA IMAGING/ MOLECULAR BREAST IMAGING PROCEDURE

Patients require no preparation prior to the BSGI/ MBI examination. Imaging begins immediately after injection of 15 to 25 mCi of technetium sesta-mibi in the ante cubital vein of the opposite arm to a known breast abnormality to avoid artifactual axillary lymph node uptake from extravasated radiotracer via lymphatic drainage, or in either arm when the examination is performed for surveil-lance in high-risk women. Early reports described injection in the pedal vein to avoid any axillary lymph node uptake. However, this is no longer done because of the discomfort from a pedal injection and the increased awareness of extrava-sated versus metastatic lymph nodes.[16]

The breast is lightly compressed by a plate. Images are obtained to 100,000 counts per image,

which is about 6 minutes. However, in the future it is likely that shorter scans will result in equal infor-mation. Currently the entire examination takes approximately 45 minutes during which time patients can read, watch television, or simply sit comfortably.

The examination should be performed by a mammography technologist because the posi-tioning is similar to that used in breast imaging. The initial craniocaudal and mediolateral oblique images are obtained and reviewed by the radiolo-gist, who can obtain additional images (exagger-ated craniocaudal, true lateral, and others) as needed. Any other position or obliquity that is possible with mammography is easily obtained with BSGI as the detector is on an articulating arm or mounted on a mammography unit.

In women who are premenopausal and obtaining BSGI/MBI for surveillance, the optimal time for the procedure is day 7 to 14 of the menstrual cycle. However, if there is a clinical issue, imaging during any time of the menstrual cycle can be done. In the authors' experience, BSGI/MBI can be done following percutaneous biopsy and there will be essentially no activity, whether the procedure was an fine needle aspiration, core biopsy, or vacuum-assisted biopsy. Imaging can also be per-formed even days following surgery. The postoper-ative seroma should have a thin rim of radiotracer uptake. Any nodular or irregular uptake at the sero-ma site is suggestive of residual disease.

When a focal area of radiotracer uptake is iden-tified, particularly if there was no concern on the mammogram, directed ultrasound can be performed to determine if there is a suspicious finding warranting biopsy. Additionally, the mammogram can be reevaluated to determine if there is a subtle mammographic finding that can be used as a target for biopsy (**Fig. 2**).

The initial recommendations were for the use of 25 mCi of technetium sestamibi. However, although doses as low as 15 mCi allow for optimal image acquisition, even lower doses would be optimal, particularly if BSGI is to be considered for repetitive imaging, such as screening of high-risk women. There are ongoing studies focused on modifying the detectors to allow for doses as low as 4 to 10 mCi and it is highly likely that in the future, BSGI will use far lower doses of radio-tracer than is even currently used.

Positron emission mammography (PEM), a procedure using a dedicated breast positron emission tomography (PET) imager, uses a different approach to nuclear medicine imaging of the breast. PEM uses 2 moving detector heads opposite each other mounted on compression paddles with a 23 cm × 17 cm field of view to obtain tomographic images. A PEM study requires that patients fast for a minimum of 4 hours prior to the study and have an appropriate blood glucose level before the study can be initiated. Ten to 15 mCi of 2-deoxy2-[18F] fluoro-D-glucose (FDG) is injected and, similar to MBI/BSGI studies, injection is preferentially done in the arm contralateral to the side of the known abnormality. Patients must rest quietly for some

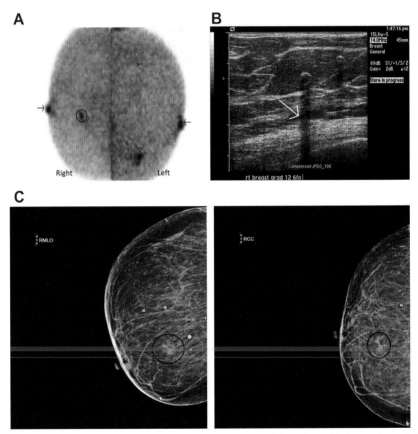

Fig. 2. A 41-year-old patient with biopsy-proven (*left*) breast cancer. (*A*) Right and left craniocaudal BSGI images with normal physiological bilateral nipple uptake (*arrows*). The BSGI demonstrates focal radiotracer uptake (*arrowhead*) in the left breast corresponding to the biopsy-proven DCIS. In the right breast, a focus of suspicious uptake (*circle*) was identified for which directed ultrasound was recommended. (*B*). Ultrasound directed to the inferomedial right breast was unremarkable with a focal area of shadowing (*arrow*) caused by a benign coarse calcification. (*C*) Mediolateral oblique and craniocaudal right mammograms demonstrate a vague asymmetry (*circle*) corresponding to the area of uptake on the BSGI that was initially interpreted as normal. Stereotactic biopsy of this area demonstrated atypical ductal hyperplasia. At surgical excision DCIS was identified.

time prior to initiating imaging, usually 1 to 3 hours, and are asked to void prior to beginning the study.

Equipment cost, radiotracer cost, reimbursement, ease of installation, and space requirements are important when considering new equipment. The different equipment used in nuclear medicine imaging of the breast can range from $300,000 to nearly $1,000,000. The cost of a dose of sestamibi is usually about $75 and the cost of a dose of FDG is usually about $600 and can be as high as $950. With BSGI/MBI, the equipment can easily be situated in a breast-imaging center and although requirements vary by state, generally needs no additional shielding. The requirements for siting a PEM device are similar to that needed for PET imaging. With regard to space requirements, BSGI/MBI is mounted on a modified mammography system and does not require a dedicated room. BSGI/MBI is a mobile system and does not require a dedicated room unless the injection is performed in the same location as the imaging device. In that case, a dedicated room is needed to comply with the requirement for injection of the radiotracer. In some institutions, the injection is done in nuclear medicine and the imaging in breast imaging. In that case, no additional space is needed because the BSGI/MBI device is about the size of an ultrasound unit. Finally with regard to reimbursement, BSGI/MBI uses recognized *Current Procedural Terminology* (CPT) codes and is generally reimbursed. Reimbursement for any PET examination requires a diagnosis of cancer and therefore the use of PEM for screening high-risk populations, or for evaluating equivocal mammographic or clinical findings, is limited at this time.

THE EVOLUTION OF HIGH-RESOLUTION, SMALL FIELD-OF-VIEW GAMMA IMAGING FOR THE DETECTION OF BREAST CANCER

The initial published study evaluating a breast-specific gamma camera evaluated women who initially had scintimammography for various clinical indications and only after completion of that study were images with a prototype HRBSG camera and the results compared.[17] A total of 50 subjects with 28 cancers were studied. Unlike prior scintimammography studies in which the majority of cancers were palpable and larger than 1 cm, in this study 71% of the cancers were not palpable and the cancers ranged in size from 3 to 60 mm (mean 11 mm). The study showed improved sensitivity for the detection of small and nonpalpable breast cancers and that it was feasible to detect and image subcentimeter cancers, image in positions comparable to mammography and thereby optimize breast imaging, and functionally integrate this approach into clinical practice.[17] These encouraging findings further supported the development of a commercial HRBSG camera with the first of these cameras approved by the FDA in 1999.

Two studies addressing the use of functional breast imaging to screen high-risk women, particularly those with dense breasts, for occult disease have been published.[18,19] In one study, 94 high-risk women with normal mammograms and physical examination underwent BSGI to evaluate its role as an adjunct imaging modality for the detection of breast cancer.[18] Of the 94 women, there were 16 positive BSGI examinations all of which had directed ultrasound to the region with focal radiotracer uptake and 11 had sonographically detected abnormalities. All 11 underwent ultrasound-guided biopsy of which 2 were found to have invasive infiltrating ductal cancers measuring 9 and 10 mm. Both of these subjects had a prior history of breast cancer, one with a contralateral cancer and the other with a recurrence in the lumpectomy bed. Nine of the ultrasound-guided biopsies were benign with pathology demonstrating fibrocystic breast tissue in 7 and fat necrosis and fibroadenoma in 1 subject each. In the 5 subjects with no focal finding on directed ultrasound, 6-month and 1-year follow-up did not demonstrate any abnormality. In this small series the sensitivity was 100%, the specificity 84%, and the NPV was 100%. Similarly, Coover reported that of 37 women with dense breasts and a family history of breast cancer imaged with a HRBSG camera, there were 5 positive studies and cancer was diagnosed in 3 subjects.[19] Multi-institutional studies are needed to better define the sensitivity and specificity of BSGI in the detection of occult cancers in women at increased risk for breast cancer. In the authors' practice, they extensively use BSGI to evaluate high-risk women with normal mammograms and physical examinations. The authors have found this to be helpful in many women because the examination is more cost effective, more comfortable for patients, and requires far less time to interpret. In women in whom MRI is not possible or in patients with claustrophobia the use of BSGI is particularly helpful.

The question as to the sensitivity and specificity of BSGI remains germane to its potential role in breast imaging. In a study evaluating 146 consecutive women with BSGI and subsequent biopsy,

167 suspicious lesions were identified.[20] In this study with 83 malignant lesions, BSGI correctly identified 80 as malignant for a sensitivity of 96.4%. BSGI identified 65 of 67 invasive cancers (mean size of 20 mm; sensitivity 97.0%) and 15 of 16 ductal carcinoma in situ (DCIS) (mean size of 18 mm; sensitivity 93.8%). The smallest invasive cancer and DCIS each measured 1 mm at pathologic evaluation. Evaluation of the 1 cm and smaller cancers demonstrated sensitivity of 88.9% and of the 5 lesions that measured less than or equal to 5 mm, 100% were detected by BSGI. These findings are somewhat similar to another study that demonstrated an overall sensitivity of 90% and a sensitivity of 82% for lesions less than 1 cm.[19] However, in this study no cancers smaller than 5 mm were detected. There were differences in these 2 studies, including camera design and subject selection.

Recently, a study evaluating a dual-headed MBI camera in 88 women with 128 cancers reported a sensitivity of 90% for the dual-headed camera as compared with 80% for their single-headed camera. In cancers less than 10 mm the sensitivity of the dual-headed camera was 82% as compared with 68% for the single-headed camera.[21] The sensitivity of the dual-headed camera approaches the sensitivity detected for small cancers with some single-headed detectors.[20] Further detector design is ongoing to allow for decreased radiotracer dose with equal sensitivity.

When imaging women at increased risk for breast cancer, the negative predictive value is important, particularly in women with challenging mammograms. If a woman at high risk is seen with a normal mammogram, but the interpretation is limited because of breast density or multiple findings, then an adjunct imaging modality that demonstrates a normal BSGI can be helpful in reassuring that disease may indeed not be present, but it is important to note that BSGI/MBI does not have a 100% NPV (reported range 94%–98%).[20] (J Weigert, MD, personal communication, 2009).

ADDITIONAL FOCI OF OCCULT CANCER IN WOMEN WITH NEWLY DIAGNOSED BREAST CANCER

When breast cancer is confined to one quadrant of the breast, a woman can be offered lumpectomy and radiation therapy. However, if there is cancer in more than one quadrant the optimal surgical approach is mastectomy. Additionally, with the increasing use of partial breast radiation, it is likely prudent to identify all foci of malignancy at the initial time of diagnosis. When considering options for postmastectomy reconstruction, a trans rectus

musculocutaneous flap (TRAM) can be performed unilaterally or bilaterally at the time of initial surgery. However, if patients are found to have contralateral disease following a TRAM reconstruction, the option of bilateral TRAM is no longer possible because the fibrosis makes dissection of the rectus impossible to harvest at a subsequent surgical procedure. The use of BSGI/MBI to diagnose additional occult foci of breast cancer in women with newly diagnosed breast cancer is helpful in identifying additional occult foci of breast cancer (**Figs. 3–5**). In one study,[20] 7.2% of subjects with breast cancer had an additional occult focus of breast cancer identified with BSGI. Similarly, Zhou and colleagues[22] reported their findings in 138 women with breast cancer where an additional 11 (7%) foci of breast cancer were detected. A recently reported larger series describes detection of additional occult foci of breast cancer in 9% of women with breast cancer.[23] These findings are similar to those reported for contrast-enhanced breast MRI (CE-MRI) for detecting additional occult foci of breast cancer where contralateral occult disease in women with newly diagnosed breast cancer is 3%[24,25] and the multicentricity is 7.7%.[25] Again, additional, multi-institutional studies directly comparing the detection of additional foci with BSGI/MBI and MRI are needed.

With regard to reimbursement, BSGI/MBI is an FDA-approved modality that utilizes existing CPT codes. Although reimbursement is dependent on the individual insurance situation and can be regionally variable, in most locations and in the authors' clinical experience, BSGI is an imaging procedure with an established CPT code and is reimbursed.

DUCTAL CARCINOMA IN SITU AND INVASIVE LOBULAR CARCINOMA AND BREAST-SPECIFIC GAMMA IMAGING

Invasive lobular carcinoma (ILC), the second most common invasive breast cancer, arises from the lobular epithelium and often has an insidious presentation both clinically and with imaging. The malignant cells insinuate themselves between the normal breast parenchyma and do not incite a desmoplastic reaction. Mammographically, ILC can present as a vague asymmetry and difficult to detect both with mammogram and sonography[26,27] and may often present as large node positive cancers.[28] MRI has been shown to be less sensitive in detecting ILC than other cancers.[29] Twenty-eight women from 4 institutions with pure ILC were evaluated, all with mammography and BSGI and some with ultrasound and

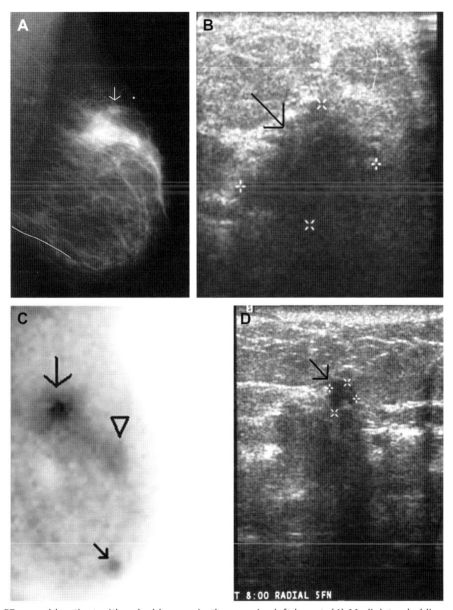

Fig. 3. A 57-year-old patient with palpable mass in the superior left breast. (*A*) Mediolateral oblique mammogram with metallic marker on the palpable mass. A 4-cm ill-defined mass (*arrow*) is seen. (*B*) Ultrasound of the palpable mass demonstrates a microlobulated, suspicious mass (*arrow*). (*C*) BSGI demonstrates the palpable mass corresponding to the pathologic proven invasive duct carcinoma (*arrow*) with segmental extension of path-proven DCIS (*arrowhead*) towards the nipple. A second suspicious area of increased radiotracer uptake (*small arrow*) is seen in the retroareolar portion of the breast. (*D*) Ultrasound directed toward the retroareolar area demonstrates a 6 mm, microlobulated, irregular mass (*arrow*), which on ultrasound-guided core biopsy was a 6-mm invasive ductal carcinoma. This mass was an occult cancer unsuspected prior to the BSGI.

MRI. The sensitivity of mammography, ultrasound, and MRI for ILC was 79%, 68%, and 83%, respectively. The sensitivity of BSGI for the detection of ILC was 93%. It is likely that the physiologic basis of BSGI accounts for its higher sensitivity in the detection of ILC (**Fig. 6**).

Similar to ILC, the sensitivity of MRI for the detection of ductal carcinoma in situ (77%–96%) is lower than that reported for invasive cancers (95%–99%).[30] It is for this reason that the authors chose to investigate the sensitivity of DCIS with BSGI that is 91% to 94%.[20,31,32]

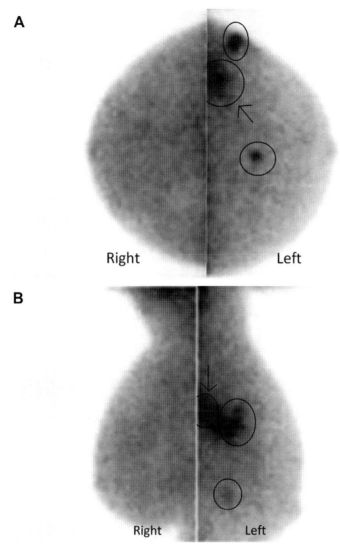

Fig. 4. Patient with known cancer (*circle with arrow*) in the left breast had BSGI that demonstrates 2 additional foci (*circles*) of uptake. These additional areas were identified with directed ultrasound and confirmed to be 2 additional foci of malignancy. (*A*) Right and left craniocaudal BSGI images. (*B*) Right and left mediolateral BSGI images.

POSITRON EMISSION MAMMOGRAPHY

Similar to the situation with conventional gamma cameras, PET scans using FDG lack the resolution for the imaging of small lesions and, although use a metabolic approach to imaging, are not optimally designed for breast imaging. Therefore, PEM has been developed to utilize PET imaging with high resolution as an adjunct imaging modality for breast cancer diagnosis.

In a study by Berg and colleagues,[33] 94 women with known breast cancer or suspicious lesions were studied with PEM. Seventeen women were excluded because of no pathology, incorrect data entry, prior surgery, protocol limitations, and equipment malfunction. Additionally the 2 cases of breast lymphoma and 1 case of breast cancer where the blinded reader panel determined that the cancer was not in the field of view of the PEM device were also excluded. Of the remaining 77 subjects, the sensitivity of PEM was 89% for invasive cancers and 91% for DCIS.[33] Furthermore, the study reported

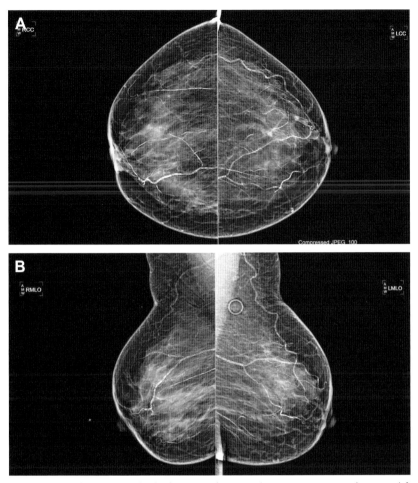

Fig. 5. Patient presented with right nipple discharge and a negative mammogram. Ultrasound found an intraductal mass in the right breast and directed the core biopsy with the finding of DCIS. BSGI-detected contralateral cancer that was identified and biopsied with ultrasound. (A) Right and left craniocaudal mammograms. (B) Right and left mediolateral oblique mammograms. (C) Right and left craniocaudal BSGI images demonstrate bilateral, linear clumped areas of enhancement (arrows) corresponding to bilateral biopsy-proven DCIS. (D) Right and left mediolateral oblique BSGI images again demonstrate the bilateral, linear clumped areas of enhancement (arrows) corresponding to bilateral biopsy-proven DCIS.

that PEM depicted 50% of T1a cancers and 67% of T1b lesions. Tafra and colleagues[34] reported 94 women imaged with PEM with suspected or proven breast cancer. A total of 44 subjects were evaluated for this study because subjects were excluded if they were to undergo a sentinel lymph node biopsy within 6 hours, did not have pathologic correlation, were not deemed suitable surgical candidates, or had studies that could not be evaluated by the reader. In the final 44 subjects, the sensitivity of the index lesion was 89%. The 4 lesions not detected were 3, 6, and 10 mm cancers,

and a 1 mm breast lymphoma. Investigators have suggested integrating anatomical imaging with mammography and ultrasound with results of PEM studies to improve the specificity of breast imaging.[33]

There are some challenges for integrating PEM in clinical practice. There is the requisite wait following injection prior to imaging, certain patients cannot be imaged because of glucose levels, and currently reimbursement is available for any PET study only in subjects who already have a diagnosis of cancer. As such, cost constraints may make PEM limited in its use for

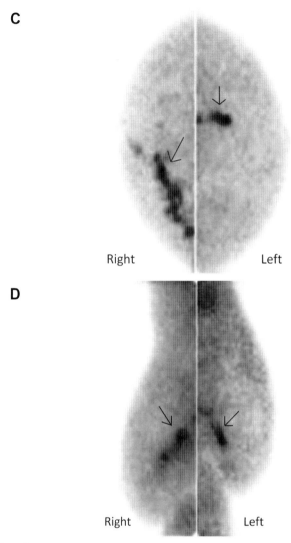

C

Right   Left

D

Right   Left

Fig. 5. (*continued*)

screening high-risk patients or in evaluating equivocal mammographic or clinical findings. Furthermore, in the 2 largest clinical trials[33,34] 18% and 53% of the subjects studied were not included in the analysis, with a significant number excluded because the studies were not interpretable. Additional development will allow for more consistent ability to interpret PEM examinations.

Using the currently available published data comparing PEM and BSGI/MRI, the sensitivity and specificity appear similar. However, the smallest cancers detected with BSGI/MBI are smaller than those reported with PEM. The cost of the equipment also differs with a BSGI unit approximately $300,000 and a PEM unit approximately

$800,000. Additional differences include the ability to image patients with BSGI/MBI immediately after injection, as compared with the requisite time required after injection for any PEM study and the difference in the need for shielding and installation of the 2 types of nuclear medicine imaging of the breast.

MRI AND BREAST-SPECIFIC GAMMA IMAGING/MOLECULAR BREAST IMAGING

Both BSGI/MBI and MRI of the breast are used for surveillance in high-risk women, to help identify additional, occult foci of breast cancer in women with newly diagnosed breast cancer, and as

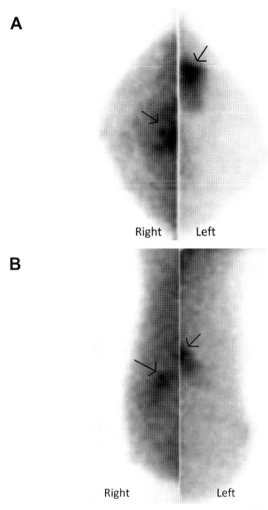

Fig. 6. Images from a patient with known bilateral cancer demonstrate bilateral focal radiotracer uptake (*arrows*) correlating with the biopsy-proven bilateral invasive lobular carcinomas. (*A*) Right and left craniocaudal BSGI images. (*B*) Right and left mediolateral oblique BSGI images.

problem solving tools. Both of these imaging modalities are based on physiologic imaging. Therefore, it is important to compare the sensitivity and specificity of MRI and BSGI. In a study evaluating 122 biopsy-proven lesions in 201 women, the sensitivity of BSGI and MRI were 91.6% and 90.6%, respectively. There were 6 lesions with MRI and 3 lesions with BSGI that were indeterminate (i.e., unclear if they were positive or negative.)[35] Bertrand[36] reported equal sensitivity and high specificity when BSGI is compared with MRI. Furthermore, in this study, all women were able to comply with BSGI examinations, whereas 4 (5.3%) could not undergo MRI examination.

Others have reported that in comparing MRI and BSGI, BSGI can reduce the number of false positive biopsies, corroborate a benign directed ultrasound, mitigate the need for continued short-interval follow-up of MRI studies or confirm the need for biospy.[37]

In a study evaluating the cost effectiveness of BSGI and MRI, based on 75 subjects imaged, using the national Medicare reimbursement average where a BSGI examination is $219.43 and an MRI is $994.43, the use of BSGI alone would have saved $58,107.[36]

The increased specificity of BSGI could be a significant improvement particularly in screening women at increased risk for breast cancer. Certainly, well-designed studies are needed, and several are underway to prospectively compare BSGI and MRI and the authors await those findings. However, until then, the authors' clinical experience has been that BSGI does in fact have equal sensitivity with better specificity than MRI, which is particularly true in premenopausal women with dense breasts (**Fig. 7**).

In comparing the procedures, BSGI has several benefits over MRI. Any patient in whom venous access is possible can have BSGI/MBI, there are no contraindications and all patients can be comfortably imaged. This statement is in contradistinction to MRI, where there are several clinical situations that render performing the examination impossible: implanted cardiac or central nervous system devices, such as pacemakers, automatic

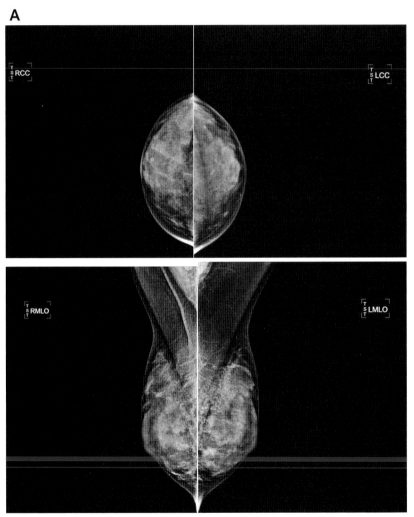

Fig. 7. A 37-year-old with strong family history of breast cancer. (*A*) Right and left craniocaudal and right and left mediolateral oblique mammograms demonstrate extremely dense tissue without suspicious findings. (*B*) MRI demonstrated multiple enhancing masses, with the most concerning in the inferior right breast (*arrow*). This lesion underwent MRI-guided biopsy with pathology demonstrating a fibroadenoma. A different postcontrast T1 fat saturation, postcontrast axial image shows scattered foci of enhancement in both breasts without a suspicious finding in the left. The sagittal left-breast image demonstrates no focal mass in the superior left breast. (*C*) BSGI demonstrates a focal area of uptake in the superior left breast (*arrows*) for which directed ultrasound was performed. The right breast demonstrates the focal area of uptake (*arrowheads*) corresponding to the biopsy-proven fibroadenoma. (*D*) Directed ultrasound to the superior left breast shows a highly suspicious mass (*arrow*) proven at biopsy to be a 1.4-cm invasive ductal carcinoma.

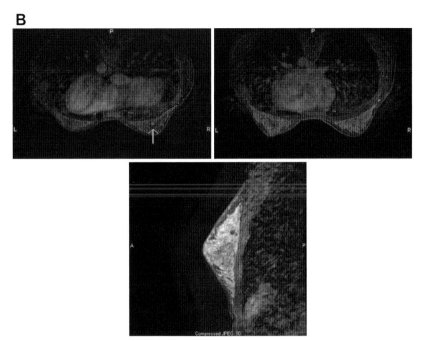

B

Fig. 7. (*continued*)

implantable cardioverter-defibrillators, and many aneurysm clips; larger patients who do not fit in the magnet; patients with claustrophobia; and patients with decreased glomerular filtration rate caused by the potential of nephrogenic systemic fibrosis. The equipment cost of a single-headed, high-resolution, breast-specific gamma camera is lower than an MRI. With a portable BSGI unit, the space requirements for the equipment are minimal and a dedicated space is not required. The possible benefit of improved specificity is much needed. Finally, the BSGI/MBI study generates 4 to 10 images, as compared with hundreds of images generated by a breast MRI. This marked reduction in image number translates into a concomitant decrease in the amount of radiologist time to interpret the examination as well as the ease of the surgeon incorporating this information in surgical planning. However, MRI provides greater anatomic information and may be advantageous in discerning pectoralis muscle involvement and other anatomic features.

It is important to appreciate that BSGI/MBI is not a replacement for CE-MRI, but rather another tool in the armamentarium we have to optimally image breast cancer. In fact, there are clinical situations where both studies are performed. In women who have numerous enhancing foci on MRI

examination, a BSGI can be performed to determine if one of the foci is suspicious and warrants biopsy. This is particularly important in women who are either at increased risk for breast cancer, such as those with BrCA genetic mutations, or in women with newly diagnosed breast cancer. Additionally, there are situations, such as when a targeted ultrasound does not identify a lesion that correlates with the focus of increase radiotracer uptake, where an MRI can be done to target the biopsy of the suspicious lesion. This latter indication is decreasing, as there is now an FDA-approved direct gamma-guided localization device that can be used to target lesions seen only with BSGI.

CLINICAL INDICATIONS FOR BREAST-SPECIFIC GAMMA IMAGING/MOLECULAR BREAST IMAGING

The ability to image the breast metabolically/physiologically can be extremely helpful This statement is particularly true because the sensitivity of nuclear medicine imaging of the breast is equally sensitive in women with dense and fatty breasts.[14] In the authors' institution, every woman with a newly diagnosed breast cancer undergoes either BSGI or MRI to definitive surgery to determine

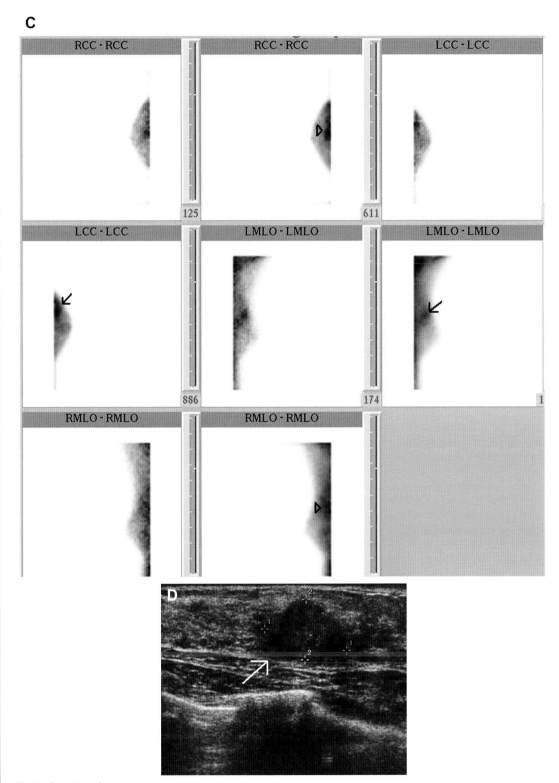

Fig. 7. (*continued*)

extent of disease and for surgical planning. The decision to use either BSGI or MRI is a complicated one. However, in the authors' practice high-risk women who have been followed with BSGI or MRI continue to do so in order to facilitate comparison. Women who have had prior MRI that have demonstrated multiple enhancing areas are directed to BSGI in future evaluation because BSGI has higher specificity.[36,38–41] Although additional data is needed to define the use of BSGI and MRI in women who are BrCA 1 or 2 positive, in the authors' practice they recommend mammography and BSGI alternating at 6 months with MRI. Other indications for BSGI include imaging high-risk women with normal mammograms; women with implants, particularly if they are at increased risk (Fig. 8); patients who have had direct silicone injection (Fig. 9); and as a problem-solving tool in situations of equivocal imaging or clinical findings. Recently, the authors have begun to use BSGI to evaluate women undergoing neoadjuvant chemotherapy and the preliminary results show excellent correlation between tumor size determined by ultrasound at initial diagnosis and at surgical excision and size determined by BSGI. In 11 subjects with prechemotherapy ultrasound measurements, BSGI measurements were within 5 millimeters in 7 and within 1 centimeter in 10 subjects (Fig. 10). Studies to further evaluate the role of BSGI in subjects during neoadjuvant chemotherapy are ongoing.

BIOPSY OF LESIONS IDENTIFIED WITH BREAST-SPECIFIC GAMMA IMAGING

Once a suspicious lesion is identified with BSGI it must be localized for tissue sampling. There is an FDA-approved, gamma-guided, stereotactic localization device (GammaLoc, Dilon Technologies, Newport News, VA, USA) (Fig. 11) allowing direct targeting and biopsy of lesions identified only with BSGI. However, until this was available, the use of multimodality imaging allowed for the biopsy of suspicious lesions identified with BSGI. Initially, ultrasound directed to the location of the abnormality often revealed the finding allowing for ultrasound-guided core needle biopsy (see Fig. 3B). Additionally, reevaluation of the mammogram to identify a subtle, previously unappreciated area can identify the abnormality (see Fig. 2), which allows for the use of stereotactic, vacuum-assisted biopsy to target and sample the lesion. If an area corresponding to the abnormality on BSGI is not identified with directed ultrasound or reevaluation of the mammogram, patients can undergo MRI to target and biopsy the finding with MRI-guided biopsy. In the authors' practice, they have used all of these approaches. However, with the introduction of the direct gamma-guided biopsy device, the use of MRI-guided biopsy to sample lesions identified with BSGI will likely decrease or not be necessary.

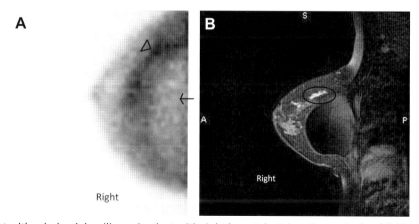

Fig. 8. Patient with subglandular silicone implant with right breast ductal carcinoma in situ. (A) Right breast BSGI demonstrates the subglandular silicone implant (*arrow*) with focal radiotracer uptake (*arrowhead*) in the superior right breast. (B) MRI demonstrates corresponding area of enhancement (*circle*) in the superior right breast. The area seen on both the BSGI and MRI corresponds to biopsy-proven DCIS.

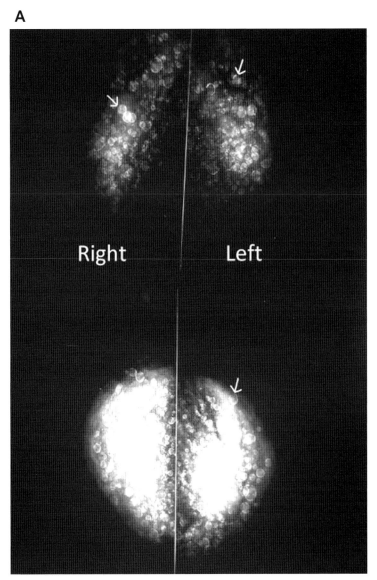

Fig. 9. Patient with direct silicone injection and BSGI. (*A*) Mammogram demonstrates extensive foreign body granulomas (*arrows*) making interpretation challenging. (*B*) BSGI demonstrates no abnormalities. BSGI is not impacted by direct silicone injection based on its physiologic approach to imaging.

Physiologic/metabolic imaging of the breast is an exciting approach for adjuvant imaging of the breast. BSGI/MBI has high sensitivity and specificity and has been shown to be an effective adjunct imaging modality in multiple clinical situations, including screening of high-risk women, especially those with dense breasts; identifying the extent of disease and additional foci of cancer in women with newly diagnosed breast cancer; evaluation of women with implants and who had direct silicone injections; and for problem solving. PEM has demonstrated high sensitivity for detecting breast cancer although its use in screening high-risk populations is currently limited because it is only indicated in women who have a diagnosis of cancer. However, the approach of using metabolic imaging expands the armamentarium of

B

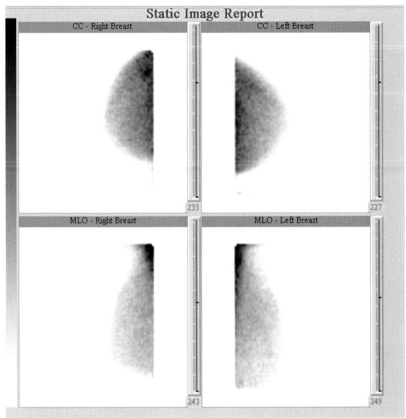

Fig. 9. (*continued*)

approaches to optimal diagnosis of breast cancer. It is best used in conjunction with currently available breast imaging modalities and the integration of all of the available approaches will allow for more versatile breast imaging. Early comparison with MRI suggests that nuclear medicine imaging is equally sensitive with some advantages, including equipment cost and the ability to image all women regardless of body habitus, the presence of implanted devices, or those patients with renal insufficiency. Furthermore, nuclear medicine imaging of the breast results in approximately 4 to 10 images as compared with the numerous images obtained in a breast MRI examination.

Nuclear medicine imaging of the breast is an FDA-approved imaging modality that is being integrated into clinical practice to increase the armamentarium of tools available to diagnose breast cancer. The authors' practice, as well as others that have integrated nuclear medicine imaging of the breast into their clinical protocols, has found it to be a critical tool in optimally evaluating women for breast cancer. Additional studies are needed to further define the addition of breast imaging to the nuclear medicine studies and to compare them to currently available breast imaging modalities. However, the physiologic/metabolic approach of the nuclear medicine breast imaging studies, as well as their utility in clinical situations where other imaging modalities are limited, make them an important part of the entire spectrum of modalities for optimal breast cancer diagnosis.

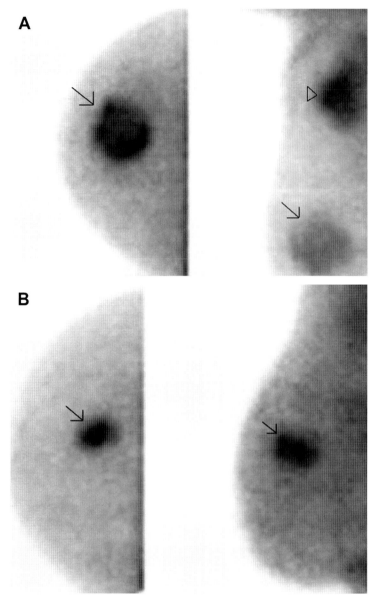

Fig. 10. A 52-year-old patient undergoing neoadjuvant chemotherapy for right-breast invasive ductal carcinoma. (A) Right craniocaudal and right mediolateral oblique BSGI images preneoadjuvant chemotherapy. The right craniocaudal view demonstrates a large mass (*arrow*) with decreased central activity caused by necrosis. The right mediolateral oblique view demonstrates the mass (*arrow*) and extensive bulky adenopathy (*arrowhead*). The cause for the apparent lower activity in the mass is the marked uptake in the nodes. The image can be modified by altering the contrast to make the mass more apparent. (B) Right craniocaudal and right mediolateral oblique BSGI images following neoadjuvant chemotherapy demonstrate complete resolution of uptake in the axillary nodes and marked reduction of activity in the mass (*arrows*) within the breast.

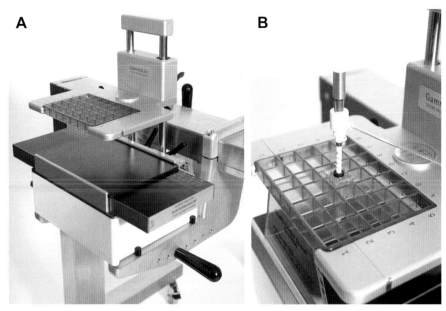

Fig. 11. FDA-approved stereotactic gamma-guided localization device, which allows for direct localization of focal areas of increased radiotracer uptake on BSGI. (*Courtesy of* Dilon Technologies, Newport News, VA; with permission.) (*A*) Gamma Loc utilizes stereotactic gamma images at 20° to determine the precise location of the lesion. (*B*) Gamma Loc localizing obturator in a grid used with vacuum-assisted biopsy devices.

REFERENCES

1. Reddy M, Given-Wilson R. Screening for breast cancer. Women's Health Medicine 2006;3(1):22–7.
2. American Cancer Society. Breast Cancer Facts and Figures 2005–2006. [Online].
3. Berry Donald A, Cronin Dathleen A, Plevritis Sylvia K, et al. Effect of screening and adjuvant therapy on mortality from breast cancer. N Engl J Med 2005;353:1784–92.
4. Tabar L, Fagerberg G, Chen H, et al. Efficacy of breast cancer screening by age. Cancer 2006;75(10):2507–17.
5. Miglioretti DL, Rutter CM, Geller BM. Effect of breast augmentation on the accuracy of mammography and cancer characteristics. JAMA 2004;291(4):442–50.
6. Pisano ED, Gatsonis C, Endrick E, et al. Diagnostic performance of digital versus film mammography for breast cancer screening. N Engl J Med 2005;353:1773.
7. Kopans D, Moore R, McCarthy K, et al. Positive predictive value of breast biopsy performed as a result of mammography: there is no abrupt change at age 50 years. Radiology 1996;200:357–60.
8. Schomacker K, Schicha H. Use of myocardial imaging agents for tumour diagnosis–a success story? Eur J Nucl Med 2000;27:1845–63.
9. Maublant J, Zhang Z, Rapp M, et al. In vitro uptake of technetium-99m-teboroxime in carcinoma cell lines and normal cells: comparison with technetium-99m-sestamibi and thallium-201. J Nucl Med 1993;34:1949–52.
10. Taillefer R. The role of Tc-99m and other conventional radiopharmaceuticals in breast cancer diagnosis. Semin Nucl Med 1999;29:16–40.
11. Liberman M, Sampalis F, Mulder DS, et al. Breast cancer diagnosis by scintimammography: a meta-analysis and review of the literature. Breast Cancer Res Treat 2003;80:115–26.
12. Khalkhali I, Villanueva-Meyer J, Edell SL, et al. Diagnostic accuracy of 99m Tc-sestamibi breast imaging: multicenter trial results. J Nucl Med 2000;41(12):1972–9.
13. Scopinar F, Schillaci O, Ussof W, et al. A three center study on the diagnostic accuracy of Tc-99m MIBI scintimammography. Anticancer Res 1997;17:1631–4.
14. Khalkhali I, Baum JK, Villanueva-Meyer J, et al. (99m) Tc sestamibi breast imaging for the examination of patients with dense and fatty breasts: multicenter study. Radiology 2002;222(1):149–55.
15. Williams MB, Williams B, Goode AR, et al. Performance of a PSPMT based detector for scintimammography. Phys Med Biol 2000;45(3):781–800.
16. Werner J, Rapelyea JA, Yost KG. Quantification of radio-tracer uptake in axillary lymph nodes using breast specific gamma imaging (BSGI): benign radio-tracer extravasation versus uptake secondary to breast cancer. Breast J 2009;15(6):579–82.

17. Brem RF, Schoonjans JM, Kieper DA, et al. Evaluation of a high-resolution, breast-specific gamma camera: a pilot study. J Nucl Med 2002;43:909–15.

18. Brem RF, Rapelyea JA, Zisman G, et al. Occult breast cancer: scintimammography with high-resolution breast-specific gamma camera in women at high risk for breast cancer. Radiology 2005; 237(1):274–80.

19. Coover LR, Caravaglia DO, Kuhn P. Scintimammography with dedicated breast camera detects and localizes occult carcinoma. J Nucl Med 2004;45(4):553–8.

20. Brem RF, Floerke AC, Rapelyea JA, et al. Breast specific gamma imaging as an adjunct imaging modality for the diagnosis of breast cancer. Radiology 2008;247:651–7.

21. Druska CB, Phillips SW, Whaley DH, et al. Molecular breast imaging: use of a dual-head dedicated gamma camera to detect small breast tumors. AJR Am J Roentgenol 2008;191(6):1805–15.

22. Zhou M, Johson N, Gruner S, et al. Clinical utility of breast specific gamma imaging for evaluating disease extent in the newly diagnosed breast cancer patient. Am J Surg 2009;197(2):159–63.

23. Brem RF, Shahan C, Rapelyea JA, et al. Detection of occult foci of breast cancer using breast-specific gamma imaging in women with one mammographic or clinically suspicious breast lesion. Acad Radiol 2010;17(6):735–43.

24. Lehman CD, Gatsonis C, Kuhl CK, et al. MRI evaluation of the contralateral breast in women with recently diagnosed breast cancer. N Engl J Med 2007;356(13):1295–303.

25. Hollingsworth AB, Stough RG, O'Dell CA, et al. Breast magnetic resonance imaging for preoperative locoregional staging. Am J Surg 2009;197(5):691–3.

26. Sickles EA. The subtle and atypical mammographic features of invasive lobular carcinoma. Radiology 1991;153:25–6.

27. Krecke KN, Gisvold JJ. Invasive lobular carcinoma of the breast: mammographic findings and extent of disease at diagnosis in 184 patients. AJR Am J Roentgenol 1993;161:957–60.

28. Selinko VL, Middleton LP, Dempsey PJ. Role of sonography in diagnosing and staging invasive lobular carcinoma. J Clin Ultrasound 2004;32:323–33.

29. Mann RM, Hoogeveen YL, Blickman JG, et al. The role of MRI in invasive lobular carcinoma. Breast Cancer Res Treat 2004;86:31–7.

30. Raza S, Vallejo M, Chikarmane SA, et al. Pure ductal carcinoma in situ: a range of MRI features. AJR Am J Roentgenol 2008;191:689–99.

31. Brem RF, Fishman M, Rapelyea JA. Detection of ductal carcinoma in situ with mammography, breast specific gamma imaging, and magnetic resonance imaging: a comparative study. Acad Radiol 2007; 14:945–50.

32. O'Connor M, Rhodes D, Hruska C. Molecular breast imaging. Expert Rev Anticancer Ther 2009;9(8): 1073–80.

33. Berg WA, Weinberg IN, Naraanan D, et al. High-resolution fluorodeoxyglucose positron emission tomography with compression ("Positron Emission Mammography") is highly accurate in depicting primary breast cancer. Breast J 2006;12(4):309–23.

34. Tafra L, Cheng Z, Uddo J, et al. Pilot clinical trial of 18F-fluorodeoxyglucose positron-emission mammography in the surgical management of breast cancer. Am J Surg 2005;190:628–32.

35. Lanzkowsky L, Zaparinuk B. The use of gamma imaging compared to MRI in breast patients needing additional diagnostic imaging. National Consortium of Breast Centers Annual Conference. Las Vegas (NV), March 15–18, 2009.

36. Bertrand M. First year's experience using breast-specific gamma imaging: a comparative analysis with mammography, ultrasound and MRI in the detection of breast cancer. Miami Breast Cancer Conference. Orlando (FL), February 20–23, 2008.

37. Lanzkowsky L, Rubin D, Fu K, et al. Breast specific gamma imaging in the management of indeterminate lesions detected on breast MRI. National Consortium of Breast Centers Annual Conference. Las Vegas (NV), March 2–5, 2008.

38. Bertrand M, Dambro T. Breast-specific gamma imaging compared to breast MRI in the presurgical planning of patients with known cancer diagnosis. Radiological Society of North America Annual Meeting. Chicago (IL), November 30 to December 5, 2008.

39. Brill K, Rosenberg AL, Stern L, et al. Breast-specific gamma imaging compared to breast MRI in Patients requiring diagnostic imaging after screening mammography. Breast Cancer Symposium. Washington, DC, September 5–7, 2008.

40. Brem RF, Petrovich I, Rapelyea JA, et al. Breast Specific gamma imaging with 99m technetium sestamibi and magnetic resonance imaging in the diagnosis of breast cancer: a comparative study. Breast J 2007;13:465–9.

41. Weinmann AL, Hruska CB, O'Connor MK. Design of optimal collimation for dedicated molecular breast imaging systems. Med Phys 2009;36(3):845–56.

Molecular Imaging of the Breast

Robyn L. Birdwell, MD[a,*], Carolyn E. Mountford, DPhil[b],
J. Dirk Iglehart, MD[c,d]

KEYWORDS

- Breast cancer • Breast cancer screening
- Molecular imaging • Magnetic resonance spectroscopy
- Nuclear medicine

Contrast-enhanced magnetic resonance imaging (MRI), MR spectroscopy (MRS), and nuclear medicine sestamibi imaging using technetium-99m methoxyisobutyl isonitrile (MIBI) or positron emission tomography (PET) techniques provide information beyond that of structural imaging by displaying tumor neoangiogenesis (MRI), tumor metabolites (MRS), increased numbers of tumor cellular mitochondria (sestamibi imaging), and hypermetabolic tumor cells (FDG PET). Much needs to be learned at the molecular level of normal cellular pathways either suppressed or enhanced by tumor-specific molecular changes. These discoveries will allow realization of true individualized patient tumor detection, treatment, and surveillance.

Molecular imaging is defined by Wagenaar and colleagues[1] as

> "the in vivo characterization and measurement of biologic processes at the cellular and molecular levels." This "growing research discipline is aimed at developing and testing novel tools, reagents, and methods to image specific molecular pathways in vivo—particularly those that are key targets in disease processes."

Such methods of imaging at the molecular level have been hailed as the next great advance for imaging.[2] How do these imaging advances provide tumor-specific details that can lead to early assessment of treatment response, the individualization of treatment options, and detection even before there is disease as it now is recognized? To begin looking at these questions, one needs a basic understanding of the molecular basis of breast cancer.

MOLECULAR SUBTYPES OF BREAST CANCER

Technologies allowing the simultaneous determination of expression from several thousand genes in tumor tissue have profoundly changed breast cancer treatment and research. These technologies are based on arrays of oligonucleotides to which tissue RNA or DNA is hybridized.[3–6] Expression arrays are designed to determine the amount of tumor RNA for any gene on the array that is expressed in the tumor. Expression arrays are available commercially from several vendors. Because these arrays measure the functional expression of chromosomal genes, their use is referred to as functional genomics. Arrays of oligonucleotides complementary to genomic DNA determine the presence and amount (copy number) of chromosomal genes. Single nucleotide polymorphisms (SNPs, called snips) are single nucleotide sequence variations among individuals and human populations. SNP arrays, also called genotyping

This article is republished from Birdwell RL, Mountford CE, Iglehart JD. Molecular imaging of the breast. Am J Roentgenol 2009;193:367–76; with permission.

[a] Division of Breast Imaging, Department of Radiology, Brigham and Women's Hospital and Harvard Medical School, 75 Francis Street, Boston, MA 02129, USA

[b] Department of Radiology, Center for Clinical Spectroscopy, Brigham and Women's Hospital and Harvard Medical School, Boston, MA, USA

[c] Department of Surgery, Brigham and Women's Hospital, Boston, MA, USA

[d] Department of Cancer Biology, Dana-Farber Cancer Institute, Boston, MA, USA

* Corresponding author.
E-mail address: rbirdwell@partners.org

arrays, are capable of measuring the presence and amount of the individual polymorphic allele. This article illustrates these technologies and how they have altered thinking about breast cancer and how to approach patients.

The simple diagram shown in **Fig. 1** illustrates how a gene expression array works. RNA isolated from living, frozen, or even fixed-and-paraffin-embedded tissue is labeled with fluorescent dyes and hybridized to the gene array. Complementary sequences stick to the array, and the array is scanned by fluorescent detectors to provide a measure of the amount of tumor RNA bound to the specific gene probe on the array. This experiment can be repeated many times using different tumors, tumors before and after treatment, or tumors from different stages of progression in the same patient. The resulting matrix display provides a striking look at an entire cohort of samples and at the expression of many thousands of genes. Gene arrays, both for RNA and DNA determinations, have several uses in modern cancer research, particularly fundamental investigation of pathogenesis and progression. In gene discovery, the arrays are used to uncover single genes, or chromosomal regions, important for pathogenesis or progression. In breast cancer, recent examples of gene discovery include the work of Chin and colleagues,[7] who used a combination of SNP arrays to measure copy number and expression arrays to relate copy number to gene expression. This team found 66 genes whose expression was dysregulated by copy number increase; nine of these genes were potentially

drugable molecular targets. Gene arrays may be used to study disease progression by measuring important genetic changes that occur during the progression of cancer. These applications are primarily used for the discovery of new genes important for pathogenesis of disease. More relevant to clinical research are two applications: class prediction and class discovery.

Class Prediction

Class prediction attempts to find gene expression signatures that together can foretell the state of a particular sample or population of tumors. A group of genes whose expression (up and down) combines to form a numeric predictor of future behavior and outcome is called a gene signature. Class prediction might be identifying a group of breast cancer patients whose tumors are likely to metastasize or recur at an early time point after treatment. In this sense, class prediction is like prognosis, and the genes that contribute to the signature of recurrence are prognosis factors. Although important, what clinicians want most are predictive factors.

Signatures that predict response to treatment (eg, for instance, to a molecularly targeted drug) are the most valuable clinical tools. For instance, in current practice, oncologists depend on the presence of the estrogen receptor (ER) to predict response to endocrine treatment (eg, tamoxifen or aromatase inhibitors).[8] Another single gene predictor is *HER2* (*erbB2/neu*), a cell surface growth factor receptor-like molecule. When the

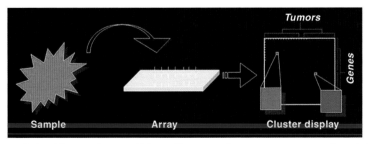

Fig. 1. Gene array analysis of human tumors. Schematic summarizes gene array experiment. DNA or RNA from portion of surgical specimen is extracted and hybridized to commercial array of oligonucleotide probes that may represent every known expressed gene in the human genome. A fluorescent plate reader accumulates intensity of hybridization at each probe on array, and data are captured in a large computerized database. Statistical analysis and data representation are performed by various algorithms, of which the most commonly used is unsupervised clustering. In this analysis, samples are clustered according to similarity of gene expression, in this case, across top and in columns. Genes are clustered according to similarity of their expression in cohort of samples undergoing analysis. Intersection of particular sample and individual gene is point on array and is shown as a box. In this depiction, red means relatively high expression of gene compared with other samples, and blue means relatively low expression compared with other samples. Resulting matrix is snapshot of cohort, showing relatedness of samples on top in evolutionary dendrogram and relatedness of gene expression in dendrogram on side of matrix. (*From* Birdwell RL, Mountford CE, Iglehart JD. Molecular imaging of the breast. Am J Roentgenol 2009;193:367–76; with permission.)

HER2 gene is amplified, it drives high-level overexpression of the cell surface HER2 protein and predicts sensitivity to trastuzumab (marketed as Herceptin) or to small molecule inhibitors of the receptor-linked tyrosine kinase (eg, lapatinib).[9]

Multiple-gene signatures, however, might provide more information, because they integrate information from several genes. For instance, a pressing question in clinical research is whether signatures can be discovered that will accurately tell which patients have tumors sensitive to a particular drug or class of drugs or which patients' tumors will be resistant and suggest prescribing another drug or treatment. A recent example is a signature that predicts sensitivity to tamoxifen in women with primary breast cancer that may benefit from the addition of chemotherapy. This test, marketed as Oncotype Dx, is made up of a panel of 21 genes that are weighted and combined to provide a recurrence score that predicts response to single-agent tamoxifen given as adjuvant treatment after primary surgery.[9]

Class Discovery

Interestingly, information from class discovery has been the most influential on modern clinical research and clinical practice. Class discovery essentially means studying a cohort of tumors, or tissues from any biologic source, and then classifying them according to their genetic relatedness or similarity. Pathologists classify tumors based on their histologic appearance. Their studies have provided definitions of invasive and noninvasive cancer; lobular versus ductal cancers; and, importantly, the histologic grade of tumors. The use of ER, progesterone receptor (PR), and HER2 has been important, because these markers not only predict response to treatment, but also may define important subclasses of breast cancer. Finally, some cancers may go unclassified, because they lack distinguishing features histologically or lack expression of ER, PR, and HER2.

In 2000, a seminal article[4] was published that opened the way to understanding the power of genomics to classify disease. In this study, Perou and colleagues[4] used gene expression arrays to classify a group of 65 breast tumors. These investigators concluded that there were at least five types of human breast cancer broadly defined as luminal, whose histogenesis was putatively from the inner luminal cells lining breast ducts, and basal, coming from cells lining the inner surface of the basement membrane. Basal cells, also called myoepithelial cells, are a specialized epithelium with contractile properties, and they contribute to the formation of the intact basement membrane that confines normal epithelium in the duct. Breast tumors that were basal-like were primarily ER-negative, PR-negative, and HER2-negative, also abbreviated as triple-negative. This early work showed that basal-like or triple-negative breast cancers were remarkably homogeneous and similar to one another; they were not a wastebasket of unclassifiable tumors. Since publication of this article by Perou and colleagues,[4] various groups have profiled hundreds of human breast cancers, providing a unique look at the disease.

Class discovery in breast cancer has uncovered at least four principal subtypes of human breast cancer. Not all classification schemes are the same, and the following example is one way to subdivide the human disease. For instance, the authors profiled 141 human breast cancer specimens before any systemic therapy, taken from the operating room and immediately frozen.[10,11] This group of malignant tumors was compared with 12 semipurified epithelial cells from normal human breast tissue obtained from reduction mammoplasties. RNA was extracted and hybridized to expression arrays. Unsupervised clustering was performed as depicted in **Fig. 1**, and the output is shown in **Fig. 2**. Triple-negative cancers are uniformly high grade and are generally an aggressive group of cancers; these tumors form an unexpectedly homogeneous cluster of very similar tumors and gene expression patterns.[12] In the middle is a large cluster of breast cancers that are nearly uniformly ER-positive. Not shown in this analysis is the division of ER-positive cancers into those that are histologically high grade and those that are lower grade. Although pathologists define low, intermediate, and high grades, the expression analysis produces a more bimodal distribution of grade.[11] High-grade ER-positive tumors may be aggressive and have a poorer outcome on average compared with low-grade ER-positive tumors that pursue a more indolent and less aggressive behavior. Finally, this analysis groups the HER2-positive breast cancers into a single group that includes both ER-positive and ER-negative cancers; these tumors are uniformly intermediate-to-high grade by pathology. HER2-positive cancers all have gene amplification of the HER2 gene on chromosome 17 and may respond to trastuzumab or tyrosine kinase inhibitors.

The resulting amalgamation of these data naturally produces four principal classes of human breast cancer: basal-like, or triple-negative; ER-positive high grade; ER-positive lower grade; and HER2-positive cancers. In fact, clinical oncologists are likely to refer to these subtypes by the names

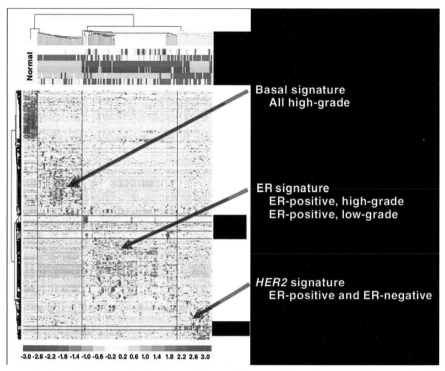

Fig. 2. Unsupervised clustering of cohort of normal breast tissue and breast cancers. Unsupervised clustering of 141 tumors and 12 normal specimens (*yellow box*) is displayed. Gene expression at each intersection of genes and samples is shown in graded shades of red to blue at the bottom of the matrix. At top in colored dendrogram, relatedness of specimens is shown and highlighted by different colors assigned to distinct arms of dendrogram. At top in colored rows above the matrix, the following information (from top to bottom) is depicted: tumor type (*yellow* = ductal, *red* = lobular); histologic grade (*dark gray* = high grade, *light gray* = low grade); estrogen receptor (ER) status (*blue* = positive, *green* = negative); progesterone receptor status (*blue* = positive, *green* = negative); HER2 (*green* = negative, *blue* = positive); and axillary lymph node status (*blue* = positive, *gray* = negative). Principal subtypes of human breast cancer can be seen by viewing whole matrix at low power (at distance). There are at least three obvious breast cancer subtypes: basal-like, or triple-negative; ER-positive; and HER2-positive. (*From* Birdwell RL, Mountford CE, Iglehart DJ. Molecular imaging of the breast. Am J Roentgenol 2009;193:367–76; with permission.)

provided here and may de-emphasize descriptors of tumor stage, such as size and lymph node status. As discussed, this is because treatment is driven by this classification scheme.

IMAGING BREAST CANCER PHENOTYPES

Are there recognizable phenotypic differences between, for example, an ER-positive tumor and a triple-negative tumor that result in unique MR appearances that could in some way predict treatment outcome? Phenotypes are those observable characteristics of an organism caused by the gene expression pattern; phenotype is the result of the genotype and the history and current condition of an organism's developmental environment. Tchou and colleagues[13] found observable differences specific to triple-negative tumors on mammography, ultrasound, and MRI. Triple-negative masses were more likely to be round with smooth margins (no spiculations), show rim enhancement on MRI, and have no calcifications on mammography. Shrading and Kuhl[14] reported phenotypic tumor appearance differences as related to individual breast cancer risk level. In women with either BRCA1 or a family history suggestive of a familial predisposition for breast cancer, 80% of the masses characterized by ultrasound were very similar to fibroadenomas, with an oval shape, relatively smooth margins, and no calcifications; 67% were in a posterior location.

The spectrum of technologies used to image disease encompasses anatomic (or structural) imaging, physiologic imaging, and imaging at the cellular level. Breast MR tumor morphology after injection of gadolinium-based contrast material can be seen in fine detail with high spatial resolution and is based on tumor angiogenesis (ie, changes at a molecular level), with the contrast material literally leaking out of the abnormal tumor vessels, resulting in a brightly enhancing mass.

MR APPLICATIONS
Proton MRS

MRS is perhaps the most established of the molecular imaging techniques, and for this reason, this method is discussed in detail. MRS has been used since the late 1980s to investigate tumor development and progression in cells and biopsies. Proton (1H) MRS can identify pathology in human tissues with a high level of accuracy.[15,16] The MRS method shows the chemical composition of cells and those changes that occur with tumor development and progression.[17] MRS also can identify some abnormalities before disease is morphologically apparent and thus visible by light microscopy.[18–20] In the past 20 years, MRS has been developed for in vivo applications, particularly in the brain,[21] and more recently, the breast.[22] For a recent review,[23] see the special issue on breast in *NMR in Biomedicine*, volume 22, issue 1. The cell studies established what could be expected from the examination of tissue biopsies and assisted in the development of protocols to study the breast in vivo. Of particular importance is the role of choline metabolism in malignant transformation.[24]

A one-dimensional spectrum of a poorly differentiated malignant breast cell line[25] (**Fig. 3**) shows that many of the magnetic resonances are composites and overlap. In a two-dimensional correlated spectroscopy (COSY) spectrum of the same sample (see **Fig. 1**), however, the composite resonances are separated by the use of a second frequency.[26–28] There are approximately 45 cross peaks available for inspection and for comparison with biologically diagnostic and prognostic factors. The cross peaks seen in **Fig. 3** are described and assigned in an article by Lean and colleagues.[29] Of particular interest are the assignments of the methyl-to-methine cross peaks, denoted Fuc I, Fuc II, and Fuc III in **Fig. 4**. Cross peak Fuc II is consistent with the resonance at 1.25 ppm, with a long T2 relaxation rate found in metastatic tumors. Typical 1H MR spectra obtained from breast fine-needle aspiration (FNA) biopsy (**Fig. 5**) show a clear distinction between frankly malignant and benign disease. Research has shown that the choline-to-creatine ratio could provide the distinction from benign and malignant disease with an accuracy of 96%,[30] a finding consistent with the literature on cultured cells. The application to core biopsies

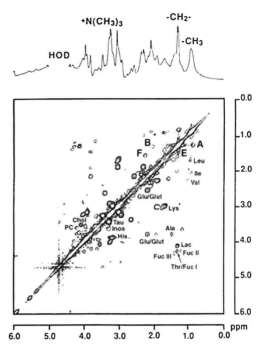

Fig. 3. 8.5-T proton (1H) one-dimensional (1D) magnetic resonance spectrum (number of scans [NS] = 128) and symmetrized COrrelated SpectroscopY (COSY) spectrum (NS = 32, number of increments [INC] = 200) of 108 log phase DU4475, poorly differentiated malignant breast cell line. Cells were suspended in 400 μL phosphate buffered saline and D20. Data were obtained at 37°C with sample spinning. Line broadening of 3 Hz was applied to 1D spectrum and sine bell, and Lorentzian and gaussian (Lb = −30.0, GB = 0.12) window functions were used in t1 and t2 domains, respectively, for COSY spectrum (Lb = −30, GB = 0.2). Expanded methyl–methine coupling regions (F2:1.00–1.70 ppm and F1:3.70–4.50 ppm) of this COSY spectrum are compared in Fig. 4 with those obtained from well-differentiated and moderately differentiated breast cancer cell lines. Fuc I, Fuc II, and Fuc III are methyl and methine cross-peaks. (*Abbreviations:* Ala, alanine; Chol, choline; Glu, glutamine; Glut, glutamate; His, histidine; Ile, isoleucine; Inos, inositol; Lac, lactate; leu, leucine; Lys*, lysine; PC, phosphocreatine; Tau, taurine; Thr, threonine; Val, valine.) (*Reprinted from Roman SA. Proton MRS study of breast cancer [PhD thesis]. Sydney [Australia]: University of Sydney; 1992. p. 184.*)

is compromised by the presence of fat that superimposes over the diagnostic and prognostic spectral features.[15]

One of the most revealing studies into the diagnostic power of 1H MRS applied to breast disease was FNA-analyzed by a pattern recognition method. A multistage statistical classification strategy was developed specifically to address these issues.[31] From the spectra obtained from

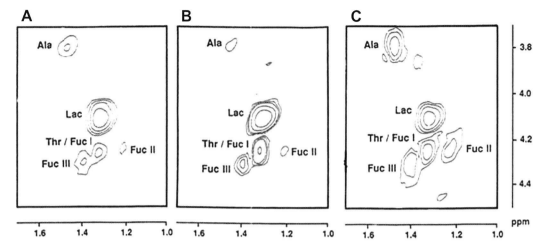

Fig. 4. Expanded methyl—methine coupling regions (F2:1.00—1.70 ppm and F1:3.70—4.50 ppm) of Correlated SpectroscopY (COSY) spectra recorded from breast cancer cell line HBL-100 (*A*), which is transformed and well differentiated; from malignant and moderately differentiated cell line MDA-MB-453 (*B*); and from malignant and poorly differentiated cell line DU4475 (*C*) shown in **Fig. 3.** Data were collected as described in **Fig. 3.** Fuc I, Fuc II, and Fuc III are methyl-to-methine cross peaks. (*Abbreviations:* Ala, alanine; Lac, lactate; Thr, threonine.) (*Reprinted from* Roman SA. Proton MRS study of breast cancer [PhD thesis]. Sydney [Australia]: University of Sydney; 1992. p. 184.)

tissue in the primary tumor alone and using the statistical classification strategy method, prediction of lymph node involvement, vascular invasion, and hormone receptor presence was possible.[32–35]

There is now a series of reports about the application of MRS to breast in vivo at 1.5, 3, and 4 T.

These studies used a range of surface coils and pulse sequences, and the results have been summarized.[36] Investigators initially proposed and continue to propose that the broad-composite resonance from choline and choline-containing compounds at 3.2 ppm alone is a marker for malignant disease.[37–43]

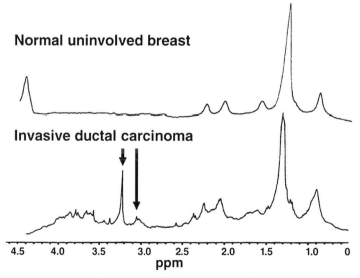

Fig. 5. 1H magnetic resonance spectra (8.5 T, 37°C) of breast fine-needle aspiration biopsies with signal-to-noise ratio greater than 10. Spectra were acquired over sweep width of 3,597 Hz, 8192 data points, 256 accumulations, and relaxation delay of 2 seconds. (*Reprinted from* Mountford CE, Somorjai RL, Malycha P, et al. Diagnosis and prognosis of breast cancer by magnetic resonance spectroscopy of fine-needle aspirates analyzed using statistical classification strategy. Br J Surg 2001;88:1234—40; with permission.)

There are distinct resonances under this composite resonance indicative of disease; however, a degree of technical competence is required to undertake in vivo MRS of the breast and care is required to avoid mistakes in interpretation.[44] Properly used, MRS has the potential to provide preoperative diagnosis, determine the extent of disease, and assess treatment response.

OTHER ADVANCED APPLICATIONS OF MRI

A modification of contrast-enhanced MRI is dynamic contrast-enhanced MRI, so-called DCE, where temporal resolution is emphasized at the expense of spatial resolution. This modified protocol collects information from more than the three or four standard postcontrast injection time points and, using mathematic equations, fits the data to pharmacokinetic models to assess physiologic parameters including tissue perfusion, microvascular vessel wall permeability, extracellular volume fraction, and average intracellular water lifetime. Yankeelov and colleagues[45] found significant changes or trends toward significance in most of these physiologic parameters after neoadjuvant chemotherapy treatment (treatment given before surgery) (**Fig. 6**). These molecular-level changes may provide further insight about the nature of the disease process.

Diffusion-weighted imaging (DWI) is an MRI sequence based on the normal diffusion of water molecules and how this movement is affected by cell swelling or density, the nuclear–cytoplasmic ratio, cell membrane permeability, or surrounding viscosity. The degree of diffusion is estimated by the apparent diffusion coefficient (ADC). A high DWI intensity has a low ADC value, and low ADC values are reported to be seen in breast cancer (**Fig. 7**).[45–47] Recent work from Lo and colleagues[47] on their first experience comparing the sensitivity and specificity of DWI, ADC, and contrast-enhanced MRI at 3 T on 31 mammographic and ultrasound lesions reported sensitivities and specificities of 95% and 91%, respectively, for MRI; 95% and 63.6%, respectively for qualitative DWI; and 90% and 91%, respectively for quantitative ADC.

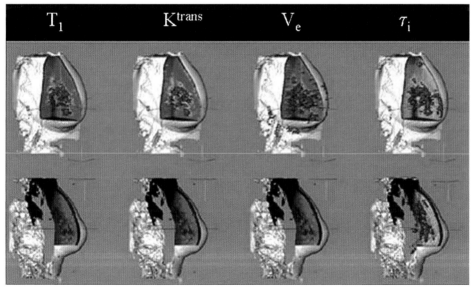

Fig. 6. Pretreatment (*top row*) and post-treatment (*bottom row*) three-dimensional volume renderings of each parameter's assessment of tumor extent of representative patient are presented. Each volume is rendered at 50% of each respective parameter's maximum value obtained from pretreatment study; that is, only those voxels with values greater than 50% of maximum pretreatment value are displayed. Comparing top row with bottom row, quantitative map (T_1), volume transfer constant (K^{trans}), and extravascular extracellular volume fraction (V_e) maps indicate tremendous drop in extent of disease, whereas τi map presents some residual areas of elevated τ_i. It is important to note that T1, Ktrans, and ve maps still have voxel values that are elevated above healthy values, but they are no longer about 50% of maximum value obtained from pretreatment study. Post-treatment apparent diffusion coefficient (ADC) rendering (not shown) revealed increase in overall ADC compared with pretreatment rendering. (*Reprinted from* Yankeelov TE, Lepage M, Chakravarthy A, et al. Integration of quantitative DCE-MRI and ADC mapping to monitor treatment response in human breast cancer: initial results. Magn Reson Imaging 2007;25:1–13, 2007; with permission.)

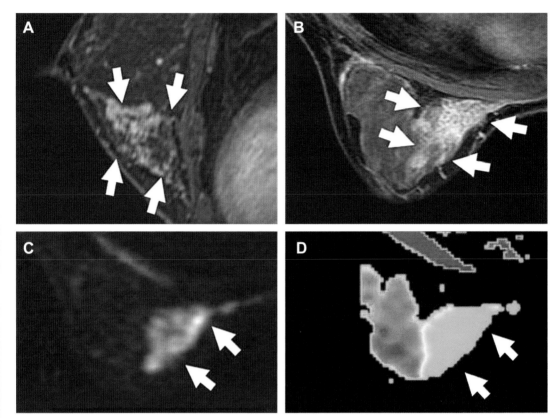

Fig. 7. 51-year-old woman with ductal carcinoma in situ (DCIS). Diffusion-weighted imaging is advanced application of breast magnetic resonance imaging (MRI) and is likely result of cellular and cellular environmental changes that affect normal diffusion of water molecules. (*A*, *B*), Sagittal fat-saturated T1-weighted early phase MR image (*A*) and axial delayed image (*B*) show nonmasslike enhancement in segmental distribution with clumped internal enhancement (*arrows*). These images are highly suspicious for cancer, and MR-guided core biopsy showed DCIS. (*C*) Axial diffusion-weighted MR image shows high signal (*arrows*) within breast segment containing DCIS. (*D*) Accompanying apparent diffusion coefficient (ADC) map shows low ADC values (*green*) within segment of DCIS. In stark contrast to low signal seen within normal tissue on diffusion-weighted image (*C*), high ADC values (*red*) appear within normal breast tissue. (*Courtesy of* Reiko Woodhams, Kitasato University School of Medicine, Japan.)

COMPUTED TOMOGRAPHY

Development and testing of computed tomography (CT) systems for dedicated breast CT offer the advantage of isotropic three-dimensional anatomic detail while limiting the obscuring of abnormalities by overlying tissue.[48] Lindfors and colleagues[49] reported the overall performance of CT to be equal to that of mammography, with differences in the visualization of masses (CT superior) and calcifications (mammography superior) (**Fig. 8**). Only 4 of their 69 patients received iodinated contrast material, and enhancement of the tumors in three patients was likely because of tumor angiogenesis analogous to MR lesion enhancement.

NUCLEAR MEDICINE TECHNIQUES

Sestamibi imaging using 99mTc-MIBI and PET using 18F-FDG identify tumors because of sequestering radionuclide within cells. In the case of the MIBI isotope, there is specific mitochondrial uptake with as much as nine times greater uptake within tumor cells as compared with normal cells. FDG PET is based on normal glucose metabolism, with intracellular phosphorylation trapping the ion within the cell as FDG-6-phosphate. The FDG ion is an example of one of the two molecular imaging probe types, the radiolabeled probes. These probes have continuous signal production and require a time period after injection to allow the removal of the untrapped

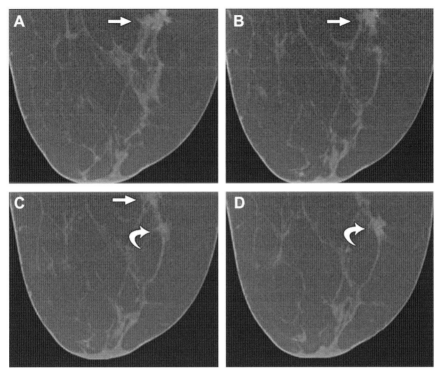

Fig. 8. 59-year-old woman with invasive ductal carcinoma (IDC). (*A–D*), Sequential transverse contrast-enhanced breast computed tomography (CT) scans show two enhancing, speculated masses, both of which are IDC. Only posterior lesion (*straight arrows, A–C*) was seen on screenfilm mammogram (not shown). Second anterior lesion (*curved arrows, C and D*) was not seen at mammography (not shown). (*Reprinted from* Lindfors KK, Boone JM, Nelson TR, et al. Dedicated breast CT: initial clinical experience. Radiology 2008;246:725–33; with permission.)

probe, so the uptake by glucose-consuming tumor cells will be highlighted. Probes capable of activation, such as those used for near-infrared fluorescent optical imaging, produce signal only when they interact with the target of interest (**Fig. 9**).

Breast-specific gamma imaging (**Fig. 10**) and FDG positron emission mammography (PEM) using new high-resolution minicamera detection technology specifically designed for imaging the breast show promise in finding both small invasive cancers and ductal carcinoma in situ (DCIS). Studies of breast-specific gamma imaging report sensitivity with biopsy-proven cancers of 79% to 96%.[50–52] Berg and colleagues[53] found that FDG PEM depicted 90% of the cancers studied: 91% of DCIS and 89% of invasive tumors. Sources of false-positives with both techniques included fibroadenomas, fibrocystic changes, and fat necrosis. Both of these techniques require image-specific biopsy capability, and prototypes are in development.[54]

OPTICAL IMAGING

Optical imaging of the breast combines functional and molecular characteristics of disease using near-infrared light. Research methods include use of intrinsic tissue contrast and exogenous fluorescent probes. These activation-capable probes provide information pertinent to physiologic and molecularly controlled variables related, in particular, to angiogenesis and hypoxia[55,56] and show potential for preclinical imaging and drug discovery (see **Fig. 9**).[57] Conklin and colleagues[58] reported encouraging information regarding the assessment of lifetime imaging of endogenous fluorophores in H and E-stained histologic slides. They were able to differentiate properties of endogenous fluorophores between normal tissue and carcinoma in situ, with the tumor cells producing higher intensity and longer fluorescence lifetimes. These early data are important not only because the information has potential for early detection of in situ cancer, but also because the information was extracted from processed fixed tissue.

A 2008 review on optical imaging of the breast[59] stated the following

Based on the present literature, diagnostic performance of optical breast imaging without contrast agent is expected to be insufficient for clinical application. Development of contrast agents that target specific

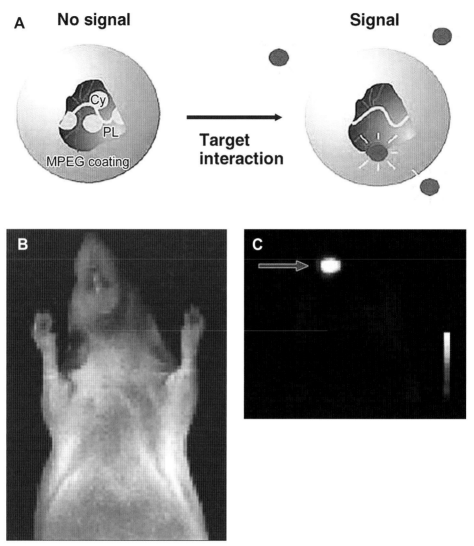

Fig. 9. Activatable fluorescent probe that can be activated. (*A*) Schematic shows near-infrared florescence probe activation. Initial proximity of fluorochrome molecules to each other results in signal quenching. After protease activation, fluorochromes become detectable (light bulb effect). Cy, 5 cyanine fluorochrome; MPEG, 5 methoxy-polyethylene glycol; PL, 5 poly-L-lysine. (*Reprinted from* Weissleder R, Mahmood U. Molecular imaging. Radiology 2001;219:316–33; with permission.) (*B*) Light image of LX1 tumor implanted into mammary fat pad of nude mouse. Tumor is not detectabl. (*Reprinted from* Weissleder R, Tung CH, Mahmood U, et al. In vivo imaging of tumors with protease-activated near-infrared fluorescent probes. Nat Biotechnol 1999;17:375–8, 1999; with permission.) (*C*) False-colored near-infrared fluorescent image superimposed on white light image shows cathepsin B and H enzyme activity, which allows small tumor (*arrow*) in mammary fat pad to be detected. (*Reprinted from* Weissleder R, Tung CH, Mahmood U, et al. In vivo imaging of tumors with protease-activated near-infrared fluorescent probes. Nat Biotechnol 1999;17:375–8; with permission.)

molecular changes associated with breast cancer formation is the opportunity for clinical success of optical breast imaging.

Targeted Imaging and Targeted Therapy

Tumor growth and progression depend in part on the activity of cell surface membrane receptors. These receptors control the intracellular signal transduction pathways that regulate many aspects of cellular activity including proliferation, apoptosis, angiogenesis, cell adhesion, and motility. As the fundamental molecular biologic and biochemical pathways of diseases are better understood, this information can be translated into the clinical setting. In particular, this knowledge can be used to create drugs that are targeted directly to an aspect of the normal biologic

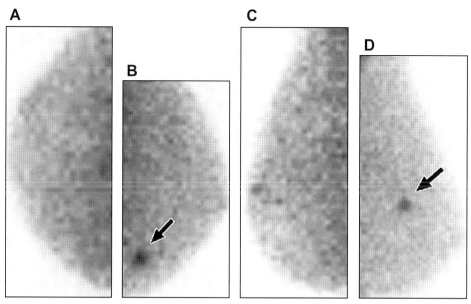

Fig. 10. 57-year-old woman with infiltrating ductal carcinoma. Abnormal scintimammography images in left cra-niocaudal (*A*), right craniocaudal (*B*), left mediolateral oblique (*C*), and right mediolateral oblique (*D*) projections show marked focal radiotracer uptake (*arrow, B* and *D*). Pathologic examination revealed 9 mm infiltrating ductal carcinoma. (*Reprinted from* Brem RF, Rapelyea JA, Zisman G, et al. Occult breast cancer: cintimammography with high-resolution breast-specific gamma camera in women at high risk for breast cancer. Radiology 2005;237:274–80; with permission.)

pathway that has changed or that may change and lead to disease. Novel reagents, new contrast agents, and pathway-specific imaging probes may make it possible to visualize cellular changes from normal to abnormal (**Fig. 11**). Traditional chemotherapeutic drugs target DNA. Extensive basic science research has elucidated many new targets, including mutated or overexpressed oncogene products (*HER2*), vascular endothelial growth factors (VEGFs), tumor suppressor genes (*p53*), cell surface antigens (CD20, CD52), antia-poptotic proteins (bcl-2), and cell cycle regulators (cyclin-dependent kinases).

The goal of modern treatment research is to find predictors of response; it is gratifying that molec-ular subclassification conforms to clinical impres-sions and treatment approaches. Clinical trials, epidemiology, and gene and biomarker discov-eries are all increasingly tailored to specific subtypes of breast cancer. A goal in epidemiology is no longer to find global etiologic factors, but to find factors that predispose to one subtype of breast cancer or another. Treatment is profoundly driven by these subtypes. *HER2*-directed thera-pies with or without endocrine treatment are given to patients with *HER2*-positive cancer; endocrine therapy, with or without chemotherapy, is used for ER-positive cancer. Additionally, clinical inves-tigators are searching for the appropriate treatment strategy for the triple-negative subtype of breast cancer. The goal of modern clinical research in breast cancer is not staging the disease, but finding predictors of response or resistance to available therapies.

THE HORIZON

Recognition of the importance of personal factors, such as the risk for development of breast cancer, is likely to alter the current screening imaging para-digms and many believe that health care providers are

> "Likely to transition from a standardized screening, where all women undergo the same imaging examination (mammography), to selection of a screening modality or modal-ities based on individual risk or other classification"[60]

Hopefully the recognition that one size may indeed not fit all may lead to earlier detection of some of the more aggressive tumors before they have metastasized. These are found, for example, in young women with genetic mutations. For those cancers that are detected, however, limiting unsuc-cessful toxic treatments and maximizing exposure to efficacious drugs may be improved by molecular imaging techniques. Perhaps within hours of

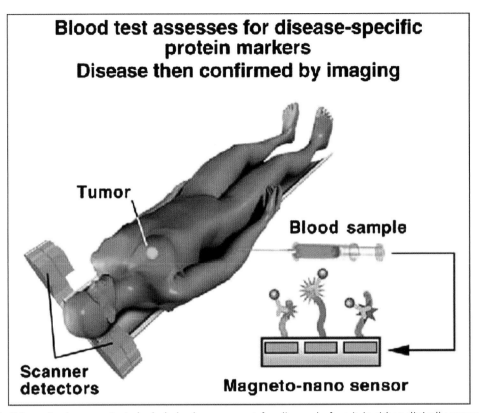

Fig. 11. Schematic shows projected whole-body assessment for disease before it is either clinically apparent or visible using standard imaging techniques. Blood tests would be used to look for protein markers indicative of occult disease, which then would be confirmed by molecular imaging techniques. (*Courtesy of* Sam Gambhir, MD, PhD, Stanford University.)

treatment initiation, changes in tumor metabolism will be shown. In both screening and treatment, the role of the breast imager is expanding, not only encompassing expertise in identifying anatomic imaging changes, but also necessitating the development of new skills focused on the fact that with molecular imaging techniques, the actual molecular signatures of many diseases can be visualized.

REFERENCES

1. Wagenaar DJ, Weissleder R, Hengerer A. Glossary of molecular imaging terminology. Acad Radiol 2001;8:409–20.
2. Hoffman JM, Gambhir SS. Molecular imaging: the vision and opportunity for radiology in the future. Radiology 2007;244:39–47.
3. Golub TR, Slonim DK, Tamayo P, et al. Molecular classification of cancer: class discovery and class prediction by gene expression monitoring. Science 1999;286:531–7.
4. Perou CM, Sorlie T, Elsen MB, et al. Molecular portraits of human breast tumours. Nature 2000; 406:747–53.
5. Lockhart DJ, Winzeler EA. Genomics, gene expression and DNA arrays. Nature 2000;405:827–36.
6. Gresham D, Dunham MJ, Botstein D. Comparing whole genomes using DNA microarrays. Nat Rev Genet 2008;9:291–302.
7. Chin K, DeVries S, Fridlyand J, et al. Genomic and transcriptional aberrations linked to breast cancer pathophysiologies. Cancer Res 2006;10:529–41.
8. Osborne CK. Tamoxifen in the treatment of breast cancer. N Engl J Med 1998;339:1609–18.
9. Dowsett M, Dunbier AK. Emerging biomarkers and new understanding of traditional markers in personalized therapy of breast cancer. Clin Cancer Res 2008;14:8019–26.
10. Wang ZC, Lin M, Wei LJ, et al. Loss of heterozygosity and its correlation with expression profiles in subclasses of invasive breast cancers. Cancer Res 2004;64:64–7.
11. Lu X, Lu X, Wang ZC, et al. Predicting features of breast cancer with gene expression patterns. Breast Cancer Res Treat 2008;108:191–201.
12. Sorlie T, Perou CM, Tibshirani R, et al. Gene expression patterns of breast carcinomas distinguish tumor subclasses with clinical implications. Proc Natl Acad Sci U S A 2001;98:10869–74.

13. Tchou JC, Wang L-P, Sargen M, et al. Do triple-native breast cancers have a distinct imaging phenotype? [abstract]. Breast Cancer Res Treat 2006;100(Suppl 1):S128.

14. Schrading S, Kuhl CK. Mammographic, US, and MR imaging phenotypes of familial breast cancer. Radiology 2008;246:58–70.

15. Mountford CE, Doran S, Lean C, et al. Proton MRS can determine the pathology of human cancers with a high level of accuracy. Chem Rev 2004;104:3677–704.

16. Mountford C, Lean C, Malycha P, et al. Spectroscopy provides accurate pathology on biopsy and in vivo. J Magn Reson Imaging 2006;24:459–77.

17. Mountford CE, Doran S, Lean CL, et al. Cancer pathology in the year 2000. Biophys Chem 1997;68:127–35.

18. Russell P, Lean CL, Delbridge L, et al. Proton magnetic resonance and human thyroid neoplasia. I. Discrimination between benign and malignant neoplasms. Am J Med 1994;96:383–8.

19. Lean CL, Delbridge L, Russell P, et al. Diagnosis of follicular thyroid lesions by proton magnetic resonance on fine needle biopsy. J Clin Endocrinol Metab 1995;80:1306–11.

20. Barry P, Wadstrom C, Falk G, et al. What is the value of 1H MRS in detecting early malignant changes?. In: Giuli R, Galmiche JP, Jamieson GC, et al, editors. The oesophagogastric junction. Montrouge (France): John Libby; 1998. p. 1122–7.

21. Danielsen E, Ross B. Magnetic resonance spectroscopy: diagnosis of neurological diseases. New York: Marcel Dekker; 1999.

22. Stanwell P, Gluch L, Clark D, et al. Specificity of choline metabolites for in vivo diagnosis of breast cancer using 1H MRS at 1.5T. Eur Radiol 2005;15:1037–43.

23. Mountford CE, Stanwell P, Ramadan S, et al. Proton MRS of the breast in the clinical setting. NMR Biomed 2009;22:54–64.

24. Aboagye EO, Bhujwalla ZM. Malignant transformation alters membrane choline phospholipid metabolism of human mammary epithelial cells. Cancer Res 1999;59:80–4.

25. Roman SA. Proton MRS study of breast cancer [PhD thesis]. Sydney (Australia): University of Sidney; 1992.

26. Cross KJ, Holmes KT, Mountford CE, et al. Assignment of acyl chain resonances from membranes of mammalian cells by two-dimensional NMR methods. Biochemistry 1984;23:5895–7.

27. Delikatny E, Hull W, Mountford C. The effect of altering time domains and window functions in two-dimensional proton COSY spectra of biological specimens. J Magn Reson 1991;94:563–73.

28. Ernst R, Bodenhausen G, Wokaun A. Principles of nuclear magnetic resonance in one and two dimensions. Oxford (UK): Clarendon Press; 1987.

29. Lean CL, Mackinnon WB, Delikatny EJ, et al. Cell-surface fucosylation and magnetic resonance spectroscopy characterization of human malignant colorectal cells. Biochemistry 1992;31:11095–105.

30. Mackinnon WB, Barry PA, Malycha PL, et al. Fine-needle biopsy specimens of benign breast lesions distinguished from invasive cancer ex vivo with proton MR spectroscopy. Radiology 1997;204:661–6.

31. Somorjai RL, Alexander M, Baumgartner R, et al. A data-driven, flexible machine learning strategy for the classification of biomedical data. In: Dubitzky W, Azuaje F, editors. Artificial intelligence methods and tools for systems biology. Boston: Springer-Verlag and Kluwer; 2004.

32. Mountford CE, Somorjai RL, Malycha P, et al. Diagnosis and prognosis of breast cancer by magnetic resonance spectroscopy of fine-needle aspirates analysed using a statistical classification strategy. Br J Surg 2001;88:1234–40.

33. Lean C, Doran S, Somorjai RL, et al. Determination of grade and receptor status from the primary breast lesion by magnetic resonance spectroscopy. Technol Cancer Res Treat 2004;3:551–6.

34. Sitter B, Lundgren S, Bathen TF, et al. Comparison of HR MAS MR spectroscopic profiles of breast cancer tissue with clinical parameters. NMR Biomed 2006;19:30–40.

35. Bathen TF, Jensen LR, Sitter B, et al. MR-determined metabolic phenotype of breast cancer in prediction of lymphatic spread, grade, and hormone status. Breast Cancer Res Treat 2007;104:181–9.

36. Sharma U, Jaganathan NR, editors. In vivo magnetic resonance spectroscopy in breast cancer. London: Springer-Verlag; 2007.

37. Katz-Brull R, Lavin P, Lenkinski R. Clinical utility of proton magnetic resonance spectroscopy in characterizing breast lesions. J Natl Cancer Inst 2002;94:1197–203.

38. Gribbestad IS, Singstad TE, Nilsen G, et al. In vivo 1H MRS of normal breast and breast tumors using a dedicated double breast coil. J Magn Reson Imaging 1998;8:1191–7.

39. Cecil KM, Schnall MD, Siegelman ES, et al. The evaluation of human breast lesions with magnetic resonance imaging and proton magnetic resonance spectroscopy. Breast Cancer Res Treat 2001;68:45–54.

40. Jagannathan NR, Kumar M, Seenu V, et al. Evaluation of total choline from in-vivo volume localized proton MR spectroscopy and its response to neoadjuvant chemotherapy in locally advanced breast cancer. Br J Cancer 2001;84:1016–22.

41. Yeung DK, Cheung HS, Tse GM. Human breast lesions: characterization with contrast-enhanced in vivo proton MR spectroscopy—initial results. Radiology 2001;220:40–6.

42. Jacobs MA, Barker PB, Bottomley PA, et al. Proton MR spectroscopic imaging of human breast cancer: a preliminary study. J Magn Reson Imaging 2004;19: 68–75.

43. Bartella L, Morris EA, Dershaw DD, et al. Proton MR spectroscopy with choline peak as malignancy marker improves positive predictive value for breast cancer diagnosis: preliminary study. Radiology 2006;239:686–92.

44. Stanwell P, Mountford C. In vivo proton MR spectroscopy of the breast. Radiographics 2007;27(Suppl 1): S253–66.

45. Yankeelov TE, Lepage M, Chakravarthy A, et al. Integration of quantitative DCE-MRI and ADC mapping to monitor treatment response in human breast cancer: initial results. Magn Reson Imaging 2007; 25:1–13.

46. Kuroki Y, Nasu K. Advances in breast MRI: diffusion-weighted imaging of the breast. Breast Cancer 2008;15:212–7.

47. Lo GG, Ai V, Chan JK, et al. Diffusion-weighted magnetic resonance imaging of the breast lesions: first experiences at 3 T. J Comput Assist Tomogr 2009;33:63–9.

48. Boone JM, Kwan AT, Yang K, et al. Computed tomography for imaging the breast. J Mammary Gland Biol Neoplasia 2006;11:103–11.

49. Lindfors KK, Boone JM, Nelson TR, et al. Dedicated breast CT: initial clinical experience. Radiology 2008;246:725–33.

50. Brem RF, Schoonjans JM, Kieper DA, et al. High-resolution scintimammography: a pilot study. J Nucl Med 2002;43:909–15.

51. Taillefer R. Clinical applications of 99mTc-sestamibi scintimammography. Semin Nucl Med 2005;35: 100–15.

52. Brem RF, Floerke AC, Rapelyea JA, et al. Breast-specific gamma imaging as an adjunct imaging modality for the diagnosis of breast cancer. Radiology 2008;247:651–7.

53. Berg WA, Weinberg I, Narayanan D, et al. High-resolution fluorodeoxyglucose positron emission tomography with compression (positron emission mammography) is highly accurate in depicting primary breast cancer. Breast J 2006;12:309–23.

54. Raylman RR, Majewski S, Smith MF, et al. The positron emission mammography/tomography breast imaging and biopsy system (PEM/PET): design, construction, and phantom-based measurements. Phys Med Biol 2008;53:637–53.

55. Flexman ML, Li Y, Bur AM, et al. The design and characterization of a digital optical breast cancer imaging system. Conf Proc IEEE Eng Med Biol Soc 2008;2008:3735–8.

56. Amoh Y, Katsuoka K, Hoffman RM. Color-coded fluorescent protein imaging of angiogenesis: the Angio-Mouse models. Curr Pharm Des 2008;14:3810–9.

57. Baeten J, Haller J, Shih H, et al. In vivo investigation of breast cancer progression by use of an internal control. Neoplasia 2009;11:220–7.

58. Conklin MW, Provenzano PP, Eliceiri KW, et al. Fluorescence lifetime imaging of endogenous fluorophores in histopathology sections reveals differences between normal and tumor epithelium in carcinoma in situ of the breast. Cell Biochem Biophys 2009;53:145–57.

59. van de Ven SM, Elias SG, van den Bosch MA, et al. Optical imaging of the breast. Cancer Imaging 2008;25:206–15.

60. Karellas A, Vedantham S. Breast cancer imaging: a perspective for the next decade. Med Phys 2008;35:4878–97.

Index

Note: Page numbers of article titles are in **boldface** type.

A

Abscesses
    and breast cysts, 946–947, 949, 952, 965, 976, 978

Accreditation process
    for digital mammography, 903–904

ACP. See *American College of Physicians.*

ACR. See *American College of Radiology.*

ACRIN. See *American College of Radiology Imaging Network.*

ADH. See *Atypical ductal hyperplasia.*

ADU. See *Analog to digital units.*

Age creep
    and mammography screening, 850

Age grouping
    and mammography screening, 854

ALH. See *Atypical lobular hyperplasia.*

ALND. See *Axillary lymph node dissection.*

American College of Physicians
    and recommendations for mammography screening, 851

American College of Radiology
    breast imaging guidelines, 1017

American College of Radiology Imaging Network
    6666 screening protocol
    and breast cysts, 931–985

Analog to digital units
    and digital mammography, 894–895

Apocrine metaplasia
    and breast cysts, 955, 959, 963–964, 967–969, 976, 978

Artifacts
    and digital mammography, 911–913

Atypical ductal hyperplasia
    and high-risk breast lesions, 1000–1008

Atypical lobular hyperplasia
    and high-risk breast lesions, 1000–1002, 1007–1008

Axillary lymph node
    metastasis of, 989–990

Axillary lymph node dissection
    and breast cancer, 990

Axillary ultrasound
    and breast cancer, 991–992

B

The basics and implementation of digital mammography, **893–901**

BCDDP. See *Breast Cancer Detection Demonstration Project.*

Benign papillomas
    and surgical versus imaging follow-up, 1003–1004
    understimation rates for, 1008

BRCA gene mutations
    and breast cancer risk, 860–861, 865–866, 870, 883–885, 1034–1036

Breast cancer
    and axillary lymph node dissection, 990
    and axillary lymph node metastasis, 989–990
    and axillary ultrasound, 991–992
    and class discovery, 1077–1078
    and class prediction, 1076–1077
    and core needle biopsy, 993
    and detection by magnetic resonance imaging, 1013–1037
    imaging of phenotypes, 1078–1079
    individualized therapy for, 852
    and internal mammary lymph nodes, 995
    and lymph node staging, 989–995
    and lymphoscintigraphy, 990
    molecular subtypes of, 1075–1078
    risk factors for, 859–860
    and sentinel lymph node biopsy, 990–991
    and ultrasound-guided fine needle aspiration, 991–995

Breast cancer death rates
    and mammography screening, 843–846, 852, 855

Breast Cancer Detection Demonstration Project
    and mammography screening, 846

Breast cancer risk
    and *BRCA* gene mutations, 860–861, 865–866, 870, 883–885, 1034–1036
    and family history, 860
    and genetic abnormalities, 860–861
    and guidelines for screening, 862–873
    and lobular carcinoma in situ, 860
    and mammographic breast density, 861–862
    and previous breast biopsy malignancies, 859–860
    and previous mediastinal radiation therapy, 860

Breast cancer screening, 843–855

Breast cancer staging
    and magnetic resonance imaging, 1023–1028

Breast compression
    and digital mammography, 905–906

Radiol Clin N Am 48 (2010) 1089–1094
doi:10.1016/S0033-8389(10)00176-4

Moving?

Make sure your subscription moves with you!

To notify us of your new address, find your **Clinics Account Number** (located on your mailing label above your name), and contact customer service at:

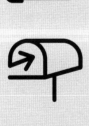

Email: journalscustomerservice-usa@elsevier.com

800-654-2452 (subscribers in the U.S. & Canada)
314-447-8871 (subscribers outside of the U.S. & Canada)

Fax number: 314-447-8029

**Elsevier Health Sciences Division
Subscription Customer Service
3251 Riverport Lane
Maryland Heights, MO 63043**

*To ensure uninterrupted delivery of your subscription, please notify us at least 4 weeks in advance of move.